Frontiers in Biomaterials
The Design, Synthetic Strategies and Biocompatibility of Polymer Scaffolds for Biomedical Application

Volume 1

Editor

Shunsheng Cao
School of Materials Science & Engineering,
Jiangsu University,
Zhenjiang, 212013,
China

Co-Editor

Huijun Zhu
Cranfield Health,
Cranfield University, Cranfield,
Bedfordshire, MK43 0AL,
UK

CONTENTS

CHAPTERS

contd…..

FOREWORD

The area of medical services and products currently contributes to in access of 10% of the gross domestic product for many countries in the world, and implantable biomaterial related devices make up a significant growth area within this sector of the economy. This will continue to represent a phenomenal financial and social impact for any technology focused society over the next couple of decades, as diseases of the aging continue to dominate healthcare and life expectancy increases. Fueling this drive is the need for more efficient and cheaper medical technologies since healthcare provision is reaching an unsustainable level in most jurisdictions. US demand alone for implantable medical devices is anticipated to increase by 8.3 percent annually into 2014, driving an excess of $33 billion US annually into the implantable medical device market alone. Gains will be further driven over the next decade by the development of next generation devices based on new innovative technologies and improved biomaterials. Spinal implants, cardiac stents and orthobiologics will be among the fastest growing product categories, with new biomaterials related to microelectronics, specialty metals, polymers, and elastomers becoming transformational material areas to enable targeted technologies for orthopedic, cardiac, neurological, ophthalmic, breast, drug, urological, cochlear, and dermal applications.

Specifically, the implantable medical device industry is poised to be a significant contributor to these dynamic changes. For example, it anticipated that the world will see the quality of life improve for this aging society with implantable monitoring systems, functional electrical stimulation, and well controlled targeted drug delivery technologies, facilitated by nano-technologies. These approaches provide the capacity to be pro-active in the maintenance of a healthy state rather than only reactive and intervening when illness is at an end-stage. It is anticipated that medical device technologies will become able to better manage biofilm related infections which is still waiting for a technology disruption. The tremendous advances in systems biology (*i.e.* omics technologies), tissue engineering and more broadly regenerative medicine are being integrated within biomedical engineering at a phenomenal pace and will make available replacement tissue for diseased vascular, and both hard and soft tissue loss from cancer surgery or other injuries. What was futuristic in 1995 with vascular graft replacement is now anticipated by 2020. Replacement of coronary and peripheral arteries and veins grown with the patient's own cells are entirely conceivable. There have already been regenerated skin products introduced to the market and we are approaching reproducible technologies in the area of bone tissue engineering products thanks to advances in biomaterials and our understanding of molecular biology.

Given the impact that biomaterials will play in medical device development over the coming decade, the timing of this new eBook " *Frontiers in Biomaterials: The Design, Synthetic Strategies and Biocompatibility of Polymer Scaffolds for Biomedical Application*" is very relevant to the key topics of regenerative medicine and tissue engineering, biodegradable polymers and their processing, nanotechnology advances and related toxicity challenges, combination drug/devices, surface heterogeneity and its chemical function distribution, and biomimetic chemistry. The frontier knowledge on these topics is conveyed by an experienced group of international scholars that describe the fundamental underpinnings of these emerging areas and open the reader's vision towards the possibilities of the future. Chapters 1 and 2 by professors Xiaohua (expertise in the areas of injectable scaffold materials and the manipulation of cell-tissue matrix interactions through drug delivery strategies), and Banerjee (research focused on molecular self-assembly and supra-molecular nanostructures applied to tissue regeneration, drug delivery, tumor cell targeting, bio-imaging, antibacterial materials, and enzyme catalysis) provide an excellent assessment of the current frontiers in scaffold manufacturing for tissue engineering applications, and describe the advances that are on-going with respect to the field's understanding of cellular and biomaterials interactions at the molecular and 3-dimentional tissue construct levels.

The specific areas of tissue engineering applications for biomaterials in Dentistry (Chapter 5 by Dr. Mozafari) and skin (Chapter 8 by Dr. Zhu), and the expansive application of polyesters in the broader field of tissue engineering (Chapter 6 by Dr. Dubruel) are all accentuated and elaborated on in the respective chapters, from the authors' proliferative experience in the areas of polymers and ceramics and their applications with stem cells, and within the emerging sector of biosensors for regenerative medicine and molecular recognition work. The materials processing of biomaterials, into the form of elaborate and organized nanostructures, is proving to be a valuable strategy for enhancing and manipulating the bio-reactivity of materials, and much research activity on this related topic is progressing thanks to the en-roads being made with electro-spinning concepts. The area of electro-spun polymers and related composites is covered in Chapter 7 (by Dr. Baiguera) and Chapter 9 (Dr. Hem Raj Pant) and provides readers with informative and brilliant new perspectives on these nano-fibre constructs. Chapter 10 (Dr. Lino Ferreira, specializes in biomaterials and their influence on stem cell differentiation for tissue engineering applications), Chapter 11 (Dr. Shunsheng Cao, expertise focus is primarily on the design of functional biomaterials with particular attention on silica-based materials), and Chapter 4 (Dr. Sharma, whose work experience covers more than four decades of research in the area of biomaterials and biocompatibility assessment) provide an expansive look at the area of inorganic biomaterials and their contributions to emerging and innovative fields ranging from the regeneration of bone to the assessment of nano-particle toxicology, and from non-fouling surfaces to drug delivery carriers and antimicrobial materials. Chapter 3 (Dr. Pennisi, expertise is concentrated on novel materials for biosensor interfaces and their applications to tissue engineering) is particularly intriguing as it describes novel inorganic material development and their expanding applications into the micro- and nano-electronics areas, a particular topic which is starting to garner much attention for its relevance in bio-sensor design. Here, the exciting possibilities for the area of implantable sensors will be facilitated in the future by both nano-biomaterials and their integration with molecular biology. Accentuating the excitement in the area of the implantable electronic sensor field, is the fact that the world market for microelectronic implants in health care, accessories and supplies, was reported to be worth approximately US$15.4 billion in 2010. That market is projected to grow to US$24.8 billion in 2016. According to BCC Research, an international market research group with activity in the medical devices and biomaterials sectors, the fastest-growing segments of the sensor market are ear implants with a projected compounded annual growth rate (CAGR) of 18.2%, neurostimulators (10.5%) and implantable drug pumps (10.5%).

It is hoped that the readers will be motivated to embrace the exciting vision that the authors of the different chapters have shared with us in this eBook, as they represent some of the most exciting frontiers in the biomaterials field and point to much future work that still needs to be led by innovative scientists and engineers in the biomedical field.

J. Paul Santerre
Faculty of Dentistry
University of Toronto
Edward St, Room 464D
Toronto
Ontario, M5G 1G6
Canada
E-mail: paul.santerre@utoronto.ca

PREFACE

Biomaterials are involved in almost everything that interacts with biological system. They can be either a living structure or a biomedical device that performs, evaluates, treats, augments, or replaces any tissue, organ or function of the body. The need for the development of biomaterials as scaffold for tissue regeneration is driven by the increasing demands for materials that mimic functions of extracellular matrices of body tissues. Significant progress has been made over the past decade in improving the biological and mechanical performance, biocompatibility and degradability of scaffold materials by adopting novel strategies, such as bio-nanotechnology, protein engineering and bionano-fabrication. Despite all the endeavors, it has proved challenging to achieve a simple, predictable and cost-effective design for biocompatible scaffold materials. A large body of knowledge in biomaterials is now available. Unfortunately, apart from sporadic papers, no books have yet been published to assess methodologies involved in biomaterial design, synthesis and their impaction the biocompatibility of biomaterials. With contributions from a group of frontier researchers with their expertise ranged from biomaterial synthesis and functionality, to preclinical and clinical research in tissue regeneration, this eBook is the first of the kind that capitalizes the *state of the art* design strategies for biocompatible scaffold materials. In particular, this eBook discusses some of the latest work that demonstrated challenges on the biocompatibility of scaffold over time after implantation, and addresses the need of new technologies and strategies to develop materials with long-lasting biocompatibility and scaffold function. The eBook is composed of 11 Chapters with 3 distinctive focus areas. It begins with overview on current understanding of the cellular and molecular basis of biomaterial-biological system interaction (Chapter 1, and 2), followed by Chapter 3 to 5 focusing on scaffold design and fabrication. Chapter 6 to 11 presents cases involving application of different biomaterials in tissue regeneration. Without doubt; the publication of such a eBook will potentially draw social and commercial interest in advancement of scaffold materials for improvement of human health.

Shunsheng Cao
School of Materials Science and Engineering
Jiangsu University
Zhenjiang, 212013
P.R. China

Huijun Zhu
Cranfield Health, Cranfield University
Bedfordshire
MK43 0AL
UK

LIST OF CONTRIBUTORS

A.C. Jayalekshmi
Division of Biosurface Technology, Biomedical Technology Wing, Sree Chitra Tirunal Institute for Medical Sciences and Technology, Poojappura, Thiruvananthapuram 695012, Kerala, India

A.M. Urbanska
Division of Digestive and Liver Diseases, Department of Medicine, Irving Cancer Research Center, Columbia University New York, NY 10032, USA

Akhilesh Rai
CNC-Center for Neurosciences and Cell Biology, University of Coimbra, 3004-517 Coimbra, Portugal; Biocant, Biotechnology Innovation Center, 3060-197 Cantanhede, Portugal

Alessandra Bianco
University of Rome "Tor Vergata", Department of Enterprise Engineering, Intrauniversitary Consortium for Material Science and Technology (INSTM), Research Unit Tor Vergata, Rome, Italy

Chandra P. Sharma
Division of Biosurface Technology, Biomedical Technology Wing, Sree Chitra Tirunal Institute for Medical Sciences and Technology, Poojappura, Thiruvananthapuram 695012, Kerala, India

Cheol Sang Kim
Bio-nano System Engineering Department, Chonbuk National University, Jeonju 561-756, Republic of Korea

Claudia Moia
School of Applied Sciences, Cranfield University, Bedfordshire, MK43 0AL, UK

Costantino Del Gaudio
University of Rome "Tor Vergata", Department of Enterprise Engineering, Intrauniversitary Consortium for Material Science and Technology (INSTM), Research Unit Tor Vergata, Rome, Italy

Cristian Pablo Pennisi
Department of Health Science and Technology, Aalborg University, Aalborg, Denmark

Cristiana Paulo
Matera, Biocant, Biotechnology Innovation Center, 3060-197 Cantanhede, Portugal

Diana-Elena Mogosanu
Polymer Chemistry and Biomaterials Research Group, Ghent University, Krijgslaan 281 S4bis, Ghent 9000, Belgium; Center for Microsystems Technology (CMST), Ghent University - IMEC, Technologiepark - Building 914-A, Gent-Zwijnaarde 9052, Belgium

Diana-Maria Dragusin
Polymer Chemistry and Biomaterials Research Group, Ghent University, Krijgslaan 281 S4bis, Ghent 9000, Belgium

Elena-Diana Giol
Polymer Chemistry and Biomaterials Research Group, Ghent University, Krijgslaan 281 S4bis, Ghent 9000, Belgium

H.H. Caicedo
Biologics Research, Biotechnology Center of Excellence, Janssen R&D, LLC, Pharmaceutical Companies of Johnson & Johnson, Spring House, PA 19477, USA; National Biotechnology & Pharmaceutical Association, Chicago, IL 60606, USA

Hem Raj Pant
Department of Engineering Science and Humanities, Pulchowk Campus, Institute of Engineering, Tribhuvan University, Kathmandu, Nepal; Bio-nano System Engineering Department, Chonbuk National University, Jeonju 561-756, Republic of Korea

Huijun Zhu
School of Applied Sciences, Cranfield University, Bedfordshire, MK43 0AL, UK

Huijun Zhu
Cranfield Health, Vincent Building, Cranfield University, Cranfield, Bedfordshire, MK43 0AL, UK

Ipsita A. Banerjee
Department of Chemistry, Fordham University 441 East Fordham Road, Bronx New York, 10458, USA

Juanrong Chen

School of Environment and Safety Engineering, Jiangsu University, Xuefu Road 301, Zhenjiang, 212013, P.R. China; Cranfield Health, Vincent Building, Cranfield University, Cranfield, Bedfordshire, MK43 0AL, UK

Lino Ferreira

CNC-Center for Neurosciences and Cell Biology, University of Coimbra, 3004-517 Coimbra, Portugal; Biocant, Biotechnology Innovation Center, 3060-197 Cantanhede, Portugal

Long Fang

School of Materials Science and Engineering, Jiangsu University, Xuefu Road 301, Zhenjiang, 212013, P.R. China

M. Jafarkhani

School of Chemical Engineering, College of Engineering, University of Tehran, P.O. Box 11155-4563, Tehran, Iran

M. Mozafari

Bioengineering Research Group, Nanotechnology and Advanced Materials Department, Materials and Energy Research Center (MERC), P.O. Box 14155-4777, Tehran, Iran

María Alcaide

Department of Health Science and Technology, Aalborg University, Aalborg, Denmark

Michela Comune

CNC-Center for Neurosciences and Cell Biology, University of Coimbra, 3004-517 Coimbra, Portugal; Biocant, Biotechnology Innovation Center, 3060-197 Cantanhede, Portugal

Mieke Vandenhaute

Polymer Chemistry and Biomaterials Research Group, Ghent University, Krijgslaan 281 S4bis, Ghent 9000, Belgium

Paolo Macchiarini

Advanced Center for Translational Regenerative Medicine (ACTREM), Karolinska Institutet, Stockholm, Sweden

Patrick Vilela

School of Applied Sciences, Cranfield University, Bedfordshire, MK43 0AL, UK

Peter Dubruel

Polymer Chemistry and Biomaterials Research Group, Ghent University, Krijgslaan 281 S4bis, Ghent 9000, Belgium

Princess U. Chukwuneke

Department of Chemistry, Fordham University 441 East Fordham Road, Bronx New York, 10458, USA

S. Shahrabi Farahani

Division of Oral & Maxillofacial Pathology, Department of Diagnostic Sciences and Oral Medicine, College of Dentistry, University of Tennessee Health Science Center, Memphis, TN 38163, USA

Sandra Pinto

CNC-Center for Neurosciences and Cell Biology, University of Coimbra, 3004-517 Coimbra, Portugal; Biocant, Biotechnology Innovation Center, 3060-197 Cantanhede, Portugal

Sangram Keshari Samal

Polymer Chemistry and Biomaterials Research Group, Ghent University, Krijgslaan 281 S4bis, Ghent 9000, Belgium

Shunsheng Cao

School of Materials Science and Engineering, Jiangsu University, Xuefu Road 301, Zhenjiang, 212013, P.R. China; Cranfield Health, Vincent Building, Cranfield University, Cranfield, Bedfordshire, MK43 0AL, UK

Silvia Baiguera

BIOAIRlab, University Hospital Careggi, Florence, Italy

Xiaohua Liu

Plastic and Aesthetic Surgery, Southwest Hospital, Third Military Medical University, Chongqing 400038, P.R. China

Ying Zhang

School of Materials Science and Engineering, Jiangsu University, Xuefu Road 301, Zhenjiang, 212013, P.R. China

Zhe Li

Department of Biomedical Sciences and Center for Craniofacial Research and Diagnosis, Texas A&M University Baylor College of Dentistry, Dallas, TX 75246, USA; Plastic and Aesthetic Surgery, Southwest Hospital, Third Military Medical University, Chongqing 400038, P.R. China

Frontiers in Biomaterials, Vol. 1, 2014, 3-30

CHAPTER 1

Control Over Cell-Scaffold Interactions in Three Dimensions

Zhe Li [1,2] and Xiaohua Liu[*,1]

[1]Department of Biomedical Sciences and Center for Craniofacial Research and Diagnosis, Texas A&M University Baylor College of Dentistry, Dallas, TX 75246, USA; and [2]Plastic and Aesthetic Surgery, Southwest Hospital, Third Military Medical University, Chongqing 400038, P.R. China

Abstract: Understanding cell-matrix interactions is crucial for the development of suitable three-dimensional (3D) scaffolds for tissue regeneration. Cell adhesion, migration, proliferation, differentiation, and signaling on two-dimensional (2D) planar substrates have been extensively studied for over three decades, generating considerable knowledge suggesting that cells can sense multiple features of the extracellular matrix (ECM), integrate that information, and respond to it. However, the cells in the body reside in and interact with a nano-structured 3D ECM network, and increasing evidence has shown that the cellular responses to the 3D environment are significantly different from those of 2D substrates. This chapter describes the current advances in controlling cellular responses to 3D scaffolds. The techniques of tailoring scaffolding chemical composition, architecture, and rigidity are highlighted from the biomaterials aspect, and their applications to regulating cell-scaffold interactions are illustrated.

Keywords: Biomaterials, cell-material interaction, scaffold, three-dimensional, tissue engineering.

INTRODUCTION

In tissue engineering, a scaffold (an artificial extracellular matrix) is one of the key components for critical defects repair. Generally, a scaffold should not only meet basic requirements, including biocompatibility, biodegradability, and suitable mechanical strength, but should also be capable of providing an appropriate microenvironment to guide cell growth and new tissue formation. This microenvironment is modulated by cell-material interactions on the surfaces of the scaffolding material. Therefore, the control of cell-scaffold interactions is

Corresponding Author Xiaohua Liu: Department of Biomedical Sciences and Center for Craniofacial Research and Diagnosis, Texas A&M University Baylor College of Dentistry, Dallas, TX 75246, USA; Tel: 214-370-7007; Fax: 214-874-4538; E-mail: xliu@bcd.tamhsc.edu

pivotal for the success of tissue regeneration. Cell adhesion, migration, proliferation, differentiation, and signaling on two-dimensional (2D) planar substrates have been extensively studied for the past 30 years, and considerable knowledge has been gathered suggesting that cells can sense multiple features of the extracellular matrix (ECM), integrate that information, and respond to it. However, the cells reside in and interact with a nano-structured three-dimensional (3D) ECM network in the body, and increasing evidence has shown that cellular responses to 3D environments are significantly different from those of 2D substrates. In view of this difference, increasing efforts have been made recently to explore how cells respond to biomaterials in 3D architecture. In this chapter, we discuss the control of cell-matrix interactions in three dimensions. We first describe protein adsorption on biomaterials, which is the first step prior to cell attachment to the biomaterial. Both the chemical composition and physical architecture of a scaffold affect the cellular responses; the techniques of tailoring scaffolding chemical composition and architecture are illustrated in section (*Effects of chemical composition on cell-matrix interactions*) and section (*Effects of physical architecture on cell-matrix interactions*). The use of biomaterial rigidity to control cell-scaffold interaction is emphasized in the final section of this chapter.

PROTEIN ADHESION ON BIOMATERIALS

Soon after a biomaterial contacts with body fluid, the proteins in the fluid adhere and accumulate on the surface of the biomaterial. By the time the cells arrive, the surface of the biomaterial is already covered with a thin layer of host proteins [1]. In other words, cell attachment to a biomaterial is not a direct cell-material contact, but happens through the protein coating on the biomaterial surfaces. Because of the bridging characteristic of the proteins during cell attachment to a biomaterial, protein adhesion to the biomaterial surface has a dominant effect on cell-material interactions. This adhesion is a dynamic process influenced by several factors including the physical and chemical properties of both the protein and the biomaterial.

Protein Properties

When a protein interacts with a biomaterial, ionic bonds, hydrophobic interactions, and charge-transfer are the main intramolecular bonds that are influenced by the protein properties, including protein size, charge, hydrophilicity/hydrophobicity, and stability [2]. The movement of a protein toward a biomaterial in body fluid is controlled by a diffusion process. Small-sized proteins have a higher diffusion rate than large ones; therefore, they can more easily reach and adhere to the biomaterial surfaces before the large proteins arrive. However, large proteins may have more binding sites, which make their adsorption on the surface of the biomaterial more stable than that of small proteins. Prior to saturation, a high concentration of a protein leads to a greater accumulation on the biomaterial surface. The protein composition is the main factor affecting protein adhesion to a biomaterial. Each protein is composed of different amino acid sequences, which determine the charges and the hydrophilicity/hydrophobicity of the protein. Secondary and higher order structures of a protein further influence its adhesion to a material surface. A structurally less stable protein that has more binding sites by unfolding the protein tends to adsorb more readily on a material surface. Some binding sites of a protein may be buried when the protein molecule is in a specific conformation, which thus greatly influences the protein adhesion to a material surface.

Surface Properties of Biomaterials

A material's surface properties are another crucial factor in protein adhesion, which affects the type, quantity, and function of the proteins that adhere to it. The surface properties of a biomaterial include hydrophilicity/hydrophobicity, surface topography, and surface functionality. Generally, more proteins adsorb on hydrophobic surfaces than on hydrophilic surfaces. A hydrophilic biomaterial surface can form a hydrogen bond with water, therefore decreasing its interaction with proteins. Topography is another feature that impacts protein adhesion. Rough surfaces, such as grooves and patterns, provide a larger surface area for protein adhesion. The effects of surface architecture on cellular responses will be discussed in Section (Micro/nanopattern). The surface functionality of a material changes the chemical composition and surface hydrophilicity/hydrophobicity and, therefore, the protein adsorption to the material. For example, increasing the fraction of surface hydroxyl groups of a biomaterial through UV irradiation enhanced the hydrophilicity and reduced the affinity of plasma proteins to the biomaterial [3]. The details of surface functionality will be included in Section (Surface modification).

EFFECTS OF CHEMICAL COMPOSITION ON CELL-MATRIX INTERACTIONS

Novel Biomaterials Synthesis

A variety of materials have been utilized in tissue engineering to fabricate 3D biodegradable scaffolds. Among all the materials (metals, ceramics, and polymers), polymers have excellent processing flexibility, and their biodegradability can be imparted through molecular design. Therefore, polymers are the most widely studied scaffolding biomaterials. Naturally derived polymers often have the advantages of positively supporting cell adhesion and function through biological recognition cues in the molecular chain. However, natural polymers are composed of complex structures and have the risks of immunogenicity and pathogen transmission. Compared to natural polymers, synthetic polymers have a higher degree of processing flexibility and no immunological concerns. Poly(α-hydroxy acids), including poly(lactic acid) (PLA), poly(glycolic acid) (PGA), and their copolymer poly[(lactic acid)-co-(glycolic acid)] (PLGA), are the most widely used synthetic polymeric materials. These polymers gained FDA approval for certain human use and have been fabricated into 3D scaffolds *via* a number of techniques. However, there are no functional groups (*e.g.*, hydroxyl and amino groups) available on the poly(α-hydroxy acids) molecular chains, which limits the capacity to incorporate biological moieties onto the scaffolding surface to modulate cell-material interactions.

Considerable efforts have been made to synthesize novel functionalized polymeric biomaterials to control cell-material interactions. The copolymerization of α-hydroxy acids with other monomers containing functional pendant groups is a simple process of incorporating functional groups in the copolymer chains. For example, 3-[N-(carbonylbenzoxy)-L-lysyl]-6-L-methyl-2,5-morpholinedione and L-lactide were copolymerized to form poly(lactic acid-co-lysine) with a functional lysine residue, which was further coupled with Arg-Gly-Asp (RGD) peptide to promote cell adhesion on the materials [4]. In another study, acryloyl carbonate and methacryloyl carbonate were copolymerized with D,L-lactide to incorporate acryloyl groups in the copolymers [5]. The acryloyl groups were amenable to the Michael-type addition reaction with varying thiol-containing molecules such as RGD peptide under mild conditions. A cell culture study showed that RGD-modified copolymer films supported better fibroblast adhesion and growth compared to their unmodified counterparts [5].

While using the copolymerization reaction is an effective strategy to generate functional groups in the random poly(α-hydroxy acids) copolymers, this method often changes the physical properties of the initial homopolymers. To address this problem, a series of block and graft copolymers have been designed and synthesized [6-9]. Poly(ethylene glycol) (PEG) is the most extensively used segment, and block copolymers of PLGA/PEG have been synthesized by the ring-opening polymerization of lactide/glycolide using PEG as an initiator [10-12]. However, the functional groups in PEG-containing block copolymers exist only at the end of each PEG segment, and their content in the block copolymers is often too low for subsequent chemical modification to take place. Several non-PEG block and graft copolymers have been developed [13-18]. We recently designed and synthesized a series of amphiphilic poly(hydroxyalkyl (meth)acrylate)-graft-poly(L-lactic acid) (PHAA-g-PLLA) copolymers [19]. These copolymers contain pendant hydroxyl groups in the molecular chains and have been fabricated into 3D nano-fibrous scaffolds. Compared to poly(L-lactic acid), they can be readily functionalized, are more hydrophilic, and have faster degradation rates; therefore, these copolymers are advantageous for certain tissue engineering applications. In another study, we synthesized star-shaped functional PLLA by using poly(amidoamine) (PAMAM) dendrimers as initiators [20]. The star-shaped polymers were further assembled to create hollow microspheres with nanofibrous architecture and open pores on the surfaces (Fig. **1**). The ECM-mimicking nanofibrous architecture of the microspheres advantageously enhanced the cell material interactions; the channels/pores of multiple scales promoted cell migration, proliferation and mass transport conditions, facilitating tissue regeneration and integration with the host. In addition, the amino groups on the star-shaped polymer can be used to incorporate biological molecules. The nanofibrous hollow microspheres have been demonstrated to be an excellent injectable cell carrier for cartilage regeneration [20].

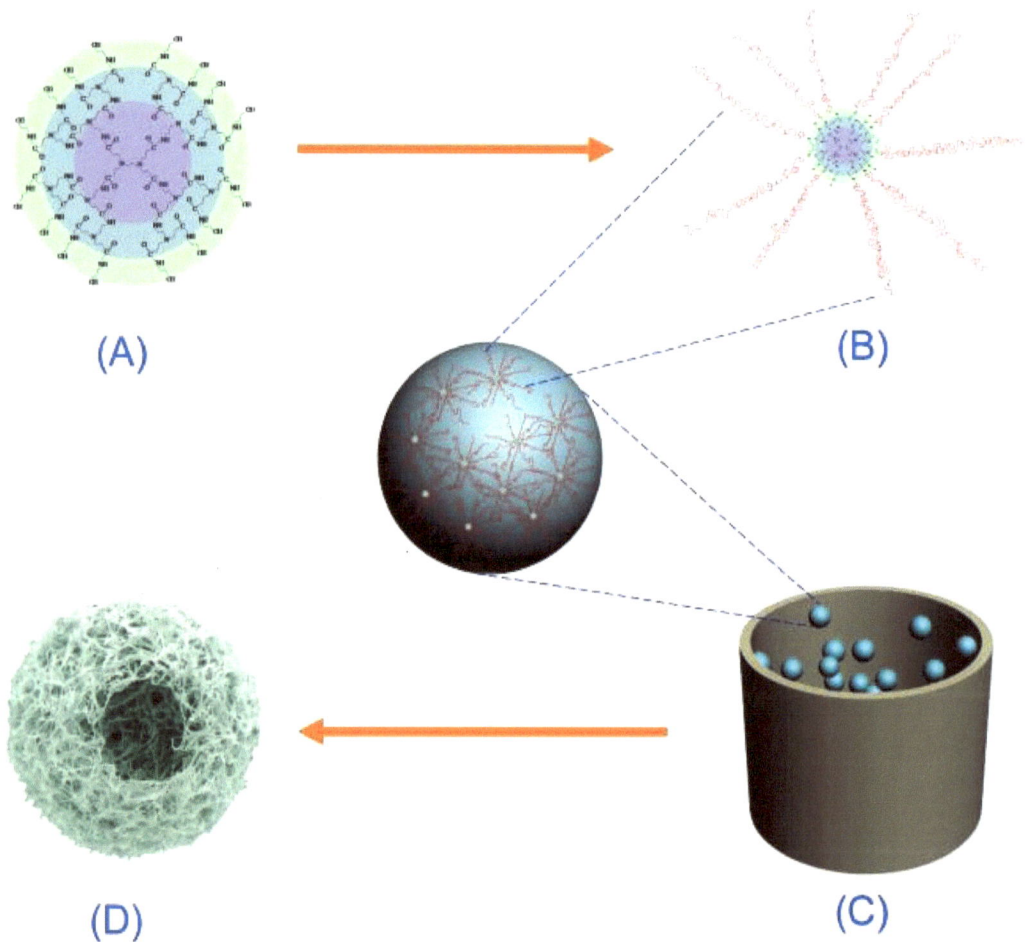

Fig. (1). Synthesis of star-shaped PLLA and fabrication of nanofibrous PLLA hollow microspheres. (a, b) Synthesis of star-shaped PLLA. Poly(amidoamine) dendtrimer was used as an initiator for the synthesis. Red coils represent the PLLA chains. (c) Preparation of star-shaped PLLA microspheres using a surfactant-free emulsification process. (d) Nanofibrous hollow microspheres were obtained after phase separation, solvent extraction and freeze-drying. Reprinted with permission from Ref. [20].

Efforts to functionalize other biodegradable synthetic polymers, such as poly(epsilon-caprolactone) (PCL), poly(3-hydroxybutyrate) (PHB), polyurethanes (PU), and polycarbonate (PC), have also been made to expand their usage as scaffolding materials. However, there are significantly fewer reports on functionalizing these biomaterials compared to the poly(α-hydroxy acids). Some of the reports include the syntheses of functionalized PCL and PC [21-24].

The incorporation of proteinase-sensitive motifs into biomaterials is an exciting approach to prepare cell-responsive functional biomaterials. Recently, cell-responsive PEG-based hydrogels were prepared for tissue regeneration [25, 26]. The hydrogel networks contain pendant oligopeptides (RGDSP) to enhance cell adhesion and matrix metalloproteinase (MMP)-sensitive peptides as crosslinkers for the hydrogel. The MMP-sensitive crosslinker determines the response of the material in the presence of cell-secreted MMPs. Therefore, this PEG-based hydrogel is a cell-responsive functional biomaterial. Primary human fibroblasts were observed to proteolytically invade the hydrogel networks, which depended on MMP substrate activity, adhesion ligand concentration, and network crosslinking density.

Composites

Numerous biomaterials have been investigated for use in tissue engineering over the past three decades. However, no single-component biomaterial has met all the requirements for tissue regeneration. One obvious reason is that natural ECM is a mixture of many organic and inorganic molecules. In order to mimic the architecture and function of natural ECM, composite materials consisting of two or more components have been widely studied in tissue engineering. Generally, these materials exhibit improved characteristics compared with the individual components [27]. In this section, we will limit the discussion to designing and synthesizing biodegradable composites for enhanced bone tissue regeneration.

Bone is a mineralized connective tissue with a hierarchical 3D structure. Chemically, the ECM of bone is mainly composed of collagen fibers and mineral hydroxyapatite (HAP). HAP possesses good mechanical and osteoconductive properties and has been tested for bone tissue regeneration. However, HAP alone is brittle, and its processability is limited. To address these drawbacks, synthetic biodegradable polymers are combined with HAP. For example, PLGA was blended with HAP to prepare a composite scaffold to enhance cell attachment, function, and mineral formation [28, 29]. However, the porosity of the composite scaffold was very low, which might not be ideal for long-term cell proliferation and tissue formation. A gas-forming and particulate-leaching process was reported to increase scaffolding porosity and expose HA nanoparticles on the PLGA surfaces [30]. Enhanced bone formation on the composite scaffolds was attributed to the higher exposure of HA nanoparticles at the scaffold surface, which allowed direct contact with the transplanted cells and stimulated cell proliferation and osteogenic differentiation.

To mimic the chemical composition and physical architecture of natural bone ECM, a biomimetic nanofibrous 3D gelatin/apatite composite scaffold has been developed [31]. A thermally induced phase separation (TIPS) technique was used to prepare a nanofibrous gelatin (NF-gelatin) matrix that mimicked natural collagen fibers and had an average fiber diameter of about 150 nm. By integrating the TIPS method with porogen leaching, three-dimensional NF-gelatin scaffolds with well-defined macropores were fabricated. To further enhance osteoblast cell differentiation and improve mechanical strength, apatite microparticles were incorporated onto the surface of the NF-gelatin scaffolds *via* a simulated body fluid incubation process (Fig. **2**). The composite scaffolds showed significantly higher mechanical strength than the NF-gelatin scaffolds after simulated body fluid treatment. Furthermore, the incorporated apatite in the composite scaffold enhanced osteogenic differentiation. The expression of BSP and OCN (two-bone specific markers) in the osteoblast-composite constructs was about 5 times and 2 times higher, respectively, than in the osteoblast–(NF-gelatin) constructs 4 weeks after cell culture [31]. These results suggest that the strategy of using composite scaffolds with biodegradable polymers and bone mineral-like inorganic components is a viable approach for bone tissue regeneration.

Surface Modification

It is well known that the cell-material interaction in a scaffold takes place on its surfaces. The nature of the scaffolding surface directly affects cellular response, ultimately influencing new tissue formation. The surface chemistry of a biomaterial determines whether protein molecules can adsorb on the material.

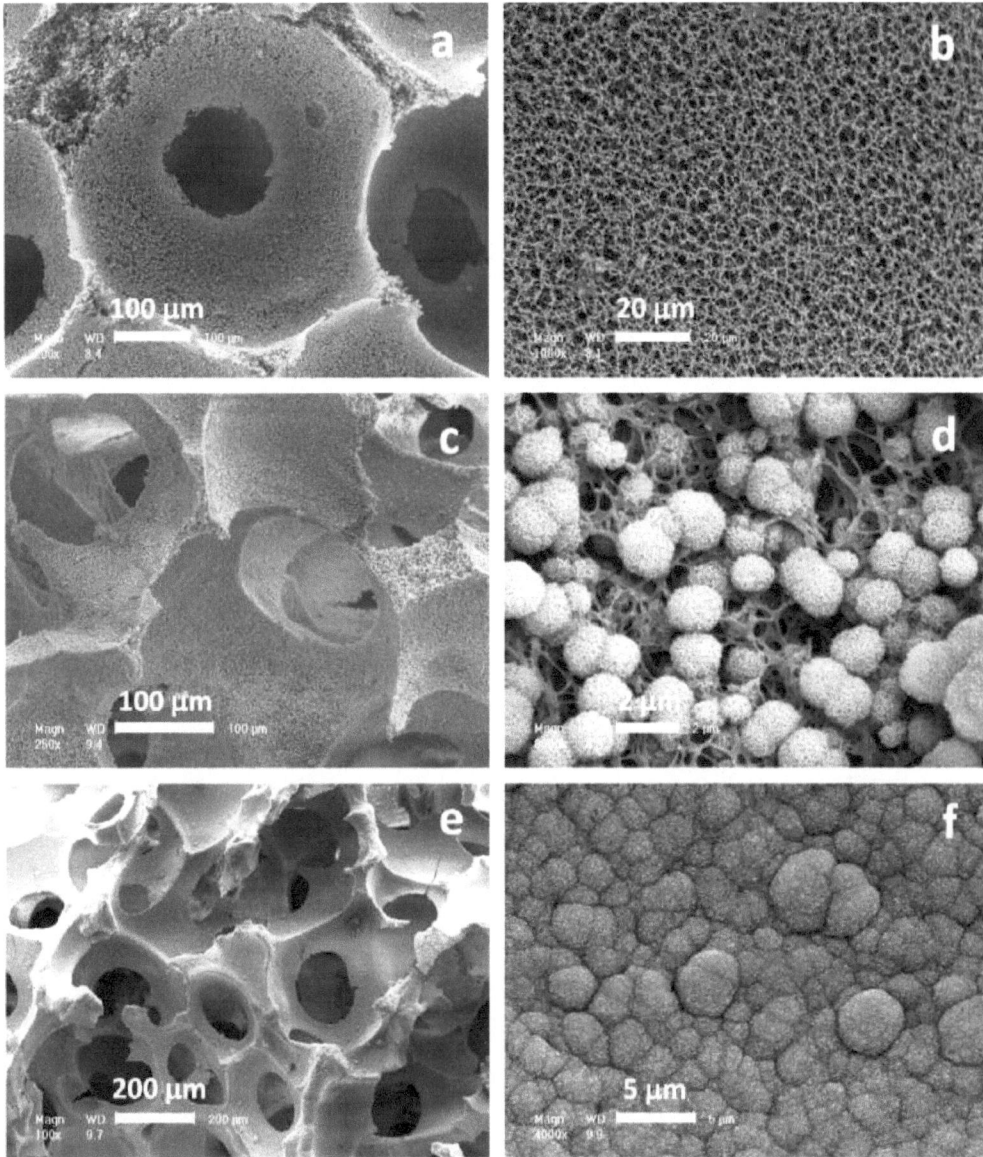

Fig. (2). SEM images of 3D nanofibrous-gelatin/apatite composite scaffolds after incubating simulated body fluid for varying times. (**a**) 1-day overview; (**b**) 1-day pore-wall structure; (**c**) 7-day overview; (**d**) 7-daypore-wall structure; (**e**) 21-day overview; (**f**) 21-day pore-wall structure. Reprinted with permission from Ref. [31].

Proteins (sometimes polysaccharides) on the material surface act as ligands and provide specific binding sites for cell receptors (*e.g.*, integrins). Once the ligand-receptor binding is formed, the receptor is activated to start a cascade of intracellular signaling pathways that regulate various biological processes. Therefore, one important aspect of controlling cellular response to a biomaterial is to couple bioactive molecules onto the scaffold surface by surface modification.

A simple surface-modification approach is to coat the biomaterial surface with natural ECM proteins such as fibronectin (FN), vitronectin (VN), and laminin (LN). These proteins all have specific motifs to bind with the integrins on the cell surfaces. Biomaterials coated with these proteins showed enhanced biocompatibility [32]. However, the binding domains on these long-chain ECM proteins are not always sterically available after their random adsorption to the biomaterial surface. Short peptides fragments, such as Arg-Gly-Asp (RGD), Gly-Arg-Gly-Asp-Ser (GRGDS), Arg-Glu-Asp-Val (REDV), and Gly-Phe-Hyd-Gly-Glu-Arg (GFOGER), were recently examined and found to have the same functions as the long-chain ECM proteins [33, 34]. However, one major limitation of surface coating is that it is not an effective method because the adsorbed proteins/peptides can easily dissolve into the surrounding solutions.

Chemical vapor deposition (CVD) is a chemical reaction process and has been explored to prepare surface-modification layers on scaffold surfaces. In a study incorporating amino groups on scaffolding surfaces, poly(4-amino-p-xylylene-co-p-xylylene) was deposited on PCL surfaces through CVD polymerization [35]. Biotin was conjugated onto the modified PCL surface to immobilize avidin for the binding of biotinylated adenovirus. Besides CVD, plasma treatment is another procedure for surface etching. Oxygen plasma treatment was used to incorporate hydroxyl and peroxyl groups onto poly(α-hydroxy acids) films [36, 37]. However, it has been shown that this plasma etching process alters both surface chemistry and surface morphology, which makes it difficult to predict how cells will respond to this surface-modified material [36]. Furthermore, both CVD and plasma treatment are only effective for 2D films and very thin 3D constructs. To overcome this hurdle, we have developed several techniques to modify true 3D scaffolding surfaces [38-40].

The first method is based on the electrostatic layer-by-layer self-assembly (LBL-SA) technique, which utilizes the alternating adsorption of multiple-charged cationic and anionic species. This technique provides a molecular-level control over the composition and surface functionality of materials; it is thus a novel and promising technique for preparing well-defined surfaces. PLLA scaffolds will be used as an example to illustrate this surface-modification process. Poly(diallyldimethylammonium chloride) (PDAC) and gelatin were selected as the positive- and negative-charged species. The PLLA scaffolds were first pretreated and activated in PDAC solution to obtain stable positively-charged surfaces. After washing the scaffolds with water, they were dipped into gelatin solution and washed again with water. Repeating the same process created PDAC/gelatin multilayers on the scaffolding surfaces. This *in vitro* work confirmed that the surface-modified scaffolds provided a better environment for cell adhesion and proliferation. The advantages of this process include a high degree of molecular control of the surface chemistry, coating thickness, and maintenance of 3D scaffold architecture. Since this process involves an aqueous solution, it is easy to carry out and universally applicable to complex 3D geometry as long as the pores of the scaffolds are interconnected.

Another approach is a surface entrapment method to incorporate bioactive agents onto scaffold surfaces [39] by means of a solvent mixture, which is crucial to the surface entrapment process. In a study of this technique, the introduction of this mixture (H_2O/dioxane) in PLLA solution ensured that certain amounts of gelatin molecules were trapped on the surface of the PLLA scaffolds. Water is a good solvent for gelatin, while 1,4-dixoane is a poor solvent for gelatin. The H_2O/dioxane solvent mixture caused the surface of the PLLA scaffold to swell but not to dissolve. Gelatin molecules in the solvent mixture diffused onto the scaffold surface and were entangled with the PLLA molecules. As the surface-swollen scaffold was removed from the gelatin solution and quickly dipped into cold water, which is a non-solvent for the scaffold, the surface rapidly shrank, and the gelatin molecules on the scaffold surface were trapped and immobilized. The surface entrapment procedure is simple, and no functional groups in polymer chains are needed for this surface modification method. Any scaffold can be modified using this entrapment process as long as a suitable solvent mixture is employed. In contrast to the method of incorporating functional groups by copolymerization, the entrapment method maintains the bulk properties of materials. When osteoblasts were cultured on the surface-modified scaffolds *in vitro*, they had a higher proliferation rate than on the control scaffolds. Furthermore, more ECM was secreted by the cells in the surface-modified scaffolds than in the controls (Fig. **3**).

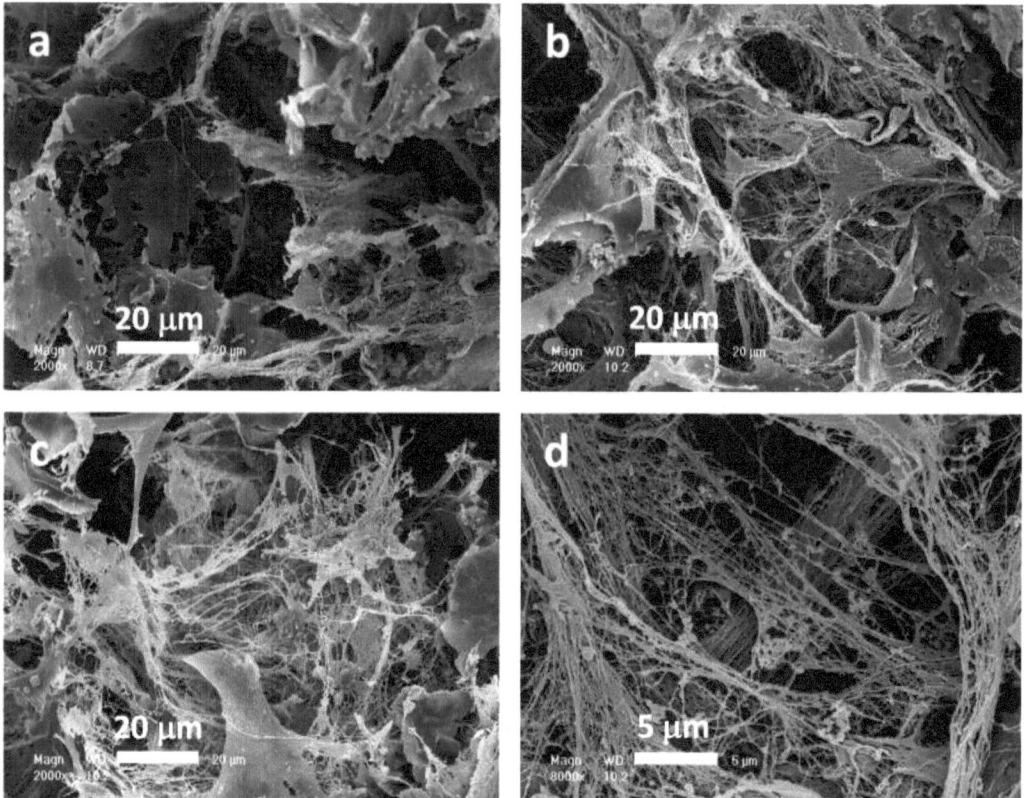

Fig. (3). SEM images of PLLA/osteoblasts constructs after culture for 4 weeks. (**a**) PLLA control; (**b**) physical entrapment in gelatin solution of dioxane/water mixture; (**c**) chemical crosslinking following the physical entrapment; (**d**) high magnification of (c). Reprinted with permission from Ref. [39].

EFFECTS OF PHYSICAL ARCHITECTURE ON CELL-MATRIX INTERACTIONS

Micro/Nanopattern

Considerable efforts have been devoted to regulating cell-material interaction by surface topographical features such as grooves, pits, ridges, and pillars. Because of its relative ease of fabrication, micropatterns were first proposed to control cell fates [41, 42]. Rat bone marrow cells seeded on microgrooved PLLA surfaces for eight days exhibited a distinct orientation along the direction of the surface grooves [43]. In addition, the PLA surfaces having 1 μm deep and 1-2 μm wide grooves exhibited higher calcification levels than other surfaces. Similar results were observed when myoblast cells were seeded on the topographic surfaces with ridges and grooves ranging from 5 to 75 μm [44]. However, the surface micropattern did not affect cell differentiation in this study.

With the rapid advancement of nanotechnology, the surface modification of biomaterials has now been achieved at the nanoscale level. A variety of nanopatterns has been incorporated into biomaterials. Research using the nanopattern scaffolds revealed that nanotopography strongly influences cellular morphology and function [45].

When cells approach a material, they first detect a suitable site for adhesion, and then focal adhesions and mature actin fibers are formed. However, the formation of focal contacts and development of the cell cytoskeleton vary with material types and surface features [46]. In one study, human corneal epithelial cells presented a stellate shape on the nanoscale holes, while they were more expanded on the microscale features [47]. Further study indicated that even small changes in architecture (nanoscale) can profoundly influence cell shape [48]. The adhesion of human corneal epithelial cells was more enhanced on synthetic substrates with nanoscale holes compared to the microscale controls [47]. Similar findings were reported using endothelial cells [49]. This effect may be attributed to the large surface area of nano-structured biomaterials, which can adsorb more proteins compared to other surfaces. However, a nanoscale pattern does not always increase cell adhesion. One example is that significantly fewer platelet cells adhered on titanium with nanoscale features than on a flat group under the same culture conditions [50].

Recent work has indicated that nanotopography can guide stem cells to differentiate in different directions, such as osteogenic, myogenic, and neuronal differentiation [51]. Human mesenchymal stem cells (hMSCs) were seeded on Ti surfaces with pillar-like structures of different heights (15, 55 and 100 nm); the 15 nm height topography feature resulted in the greatest cellular response toward osteogenic lineage [52]. In another study, hMSCs were cultured on poly(dimethylsiloxan) (PDMS) with nano/microgratings of various widths (350 nm, 1 nm and 10 nm); higher neuronal marker expressions were detected on the nano-gratings compared to the unpatterned and micropatterned groups [53]. The combination of nanotopography and biochemical cues further enhanced the expressions of the neuronal markers. However, nanotopography produced a stronger effect than retinoic acid alone on an unpatterned surface. This work demonstrated the significance of nanotopography in directing adult stem cell differentiation.

Nanofibrous Architecture

In the body, the ECM is in the form of a nanoscale 3D network, and collagen (type I) is one of the major ECM components of many tissues. Collagen (type I) exhibits a nanofibrous architecture and has been demonstrated to influence many cellular functions, including adhesion, proliferation, and differentiation [54]. For this reason, nanofibrous biomaterials have received considerable interest regarding mimicking natural collagen fibers and modulating cell behaviors.

Cells often adopt a different morphology on nanofibrous substrates compared with smooth substrates. In many cases, cells have a round shape with a smaller projected area when cultured on nanofibers, compared to flat substrates. Osteoblasts cultured on a nanofibrous PLLA matrix showed a round phenotype with small processes interacting with the substrate nanofibers [55]. In contrast, the cells were spread over large areas on PLLA flat films. Few stress fibers formed in the cells cultured on nanofibrous matrices, while abundant long actin fibers were observed on flat films. Furthermore, there was no typical focal adhesion structure formation on the nanofibrous matrix. Chondrocytes cultured on nanofibrous microspheres exhibited a more rounded morphology, whereas they were flat and spread over significantly larger areas on the smooth microspheres (Fig. **4**) [20]. Almost all of the seeded chondrocytes attached to the nanofibrous microspheres, whereas less than 60% of the seeded chondrocytes attached to the solid-interior microspheres 24 h after cell seeding. The high attachment efficiency of the cells to the nanofibrous microspheres was attributed to their nanofibrous architecture, which has a high surface area and can adsorb cell adhesion proteins (*e.g.*, fibronectin and vitronectin) at significantly higher levels than smooth surfaces.

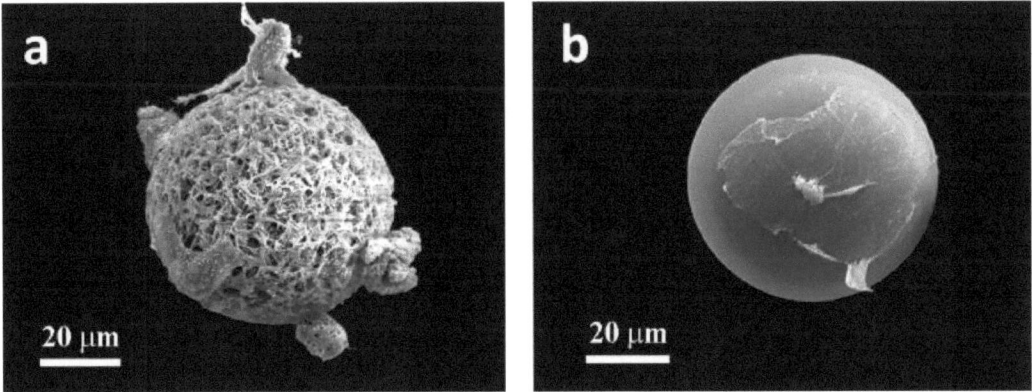

Fig. (4). SEM images of chondrocytes adhesion on (**a**) nanofibrous and (**b**) smooth PLLA microspheres 24 hours after cell seeding. Reprinted with permission from Ref. [31].

Many studies have shown that cells such as smooth muscle cells and neural stem cells aligned in the direction of the nanofibers in the scaffolds [56, 57]. Neural stem cells seeded on PLLA nanofibers migrated parallel to the aligned nanofibers. The interfiber distance was a factor affecting cell migration. At a large interfiber distance (>15 μm), neurites migrated along the fibers and avoided areas of high fiber density, while at interfiber distances less than 15 μm, the neurites traversed between the fibers [58].

Nanofibrous structures also affect cell proliferation and differentiation. Chondrocytes seeded on nanofibrous microspheres had significantly higher proliferation rates and produced higher amounts of glycosaminoglycans than on smooth microspheres [20]. After culturing *in vitro* for three weeks, the cartilage-specific genes (*e.g.*, aggrecan and collagen type II) were down-regulated on the smooth microspheres, whereas the gene expression level of collagen type I was similar for both nanofibrous and smooth microspheres. In contrast, the continuous expression of aggrecan and collagen type II genes at high levels was detected in cells on the nanofibrous microspheres, indicating that the nanofibrous architecture helps retain the chondrocyte phenotype. Under the same culture medium, the

MC3T3-E1 osteoblasts proliferated slower on nanofibrous PLLA matrices than on PLLA flat films [55]. When a differentiation medium was added, the expression levels of bone sialoprotein (BSP) and osteocalcin (OCN) were significantly higher on the nanofibrous PLLA matrix than on the flat ones. Strikingly, the BSP gene expression on a nanofibrous matrix was two orders of magnitude higher than that on the flat films. Even without the addition of ascorbic acid (thus blocking the natural collagen formation), the expression of BSP was still significantly enhanced on the nanofibrous matrix, indicating that there is a direct interaction between the PLLA nanofibers and osteoblasts. Further study indicated that the enhanced BSP gene expression on the nanofibrous matrix was attributed to the down-regulation of the small GTPase RhoA activities. Consistent with higher differential gene expression, the alkaline phosphatase (ALP) content of cells on the nanofibrous matrix was higher than that on flat films after 6 days' culture in a complete induction medium [55].

We recently developed an approach using confocal microscopy as a tool for visualizing, analyzing, and quantifying osteoblast-matrix interactions and bone tissue formation on 3D nanofibrous gelatin (3D-NF-gelatin) matrices [59]. Integrin β1, vinculin, and phosphor-paxillin were utilized to detect osteoblast responses to the nanofibrous architecture of the 3D-NF-gelatin matrix. In contrast to the osteoblasts cultured on 2D substrates, the osteoblasts seeded on 3D-NF-gelatin had fewer focal adhesions for phospho-paxillin and vinculin, and the expression of integrin β1 was weak after being cultured for 5 days (Fig. **5**). The expression of BSP on the 3D-NF-gelatin was present mostly in the cell cytoplasm at 5 days and inside the secretory vesicles at 2 weeks, whereas most of the BSP on the 2D gelatin substrates was concentrated either at the cell interface toward the periphery or at focal adhesion sites. The confocal images further showed that the osteoblasts migrated throughout the entire 3D matrix after 5 days. By 2 weeks, they were organized as nodular aggregations inside the matrix pores, and a considerable amount of collagen and other cell secretions covered and remodeled the 3D-NF-gelatin surfaces. These nodules were mineralized and uniformly distributed inside the entire 3D-NF-gelatin scaffold. These results provide insight into the osteoblast-matrix interactions in biomimetic nanofibrous 3D scaffolds.

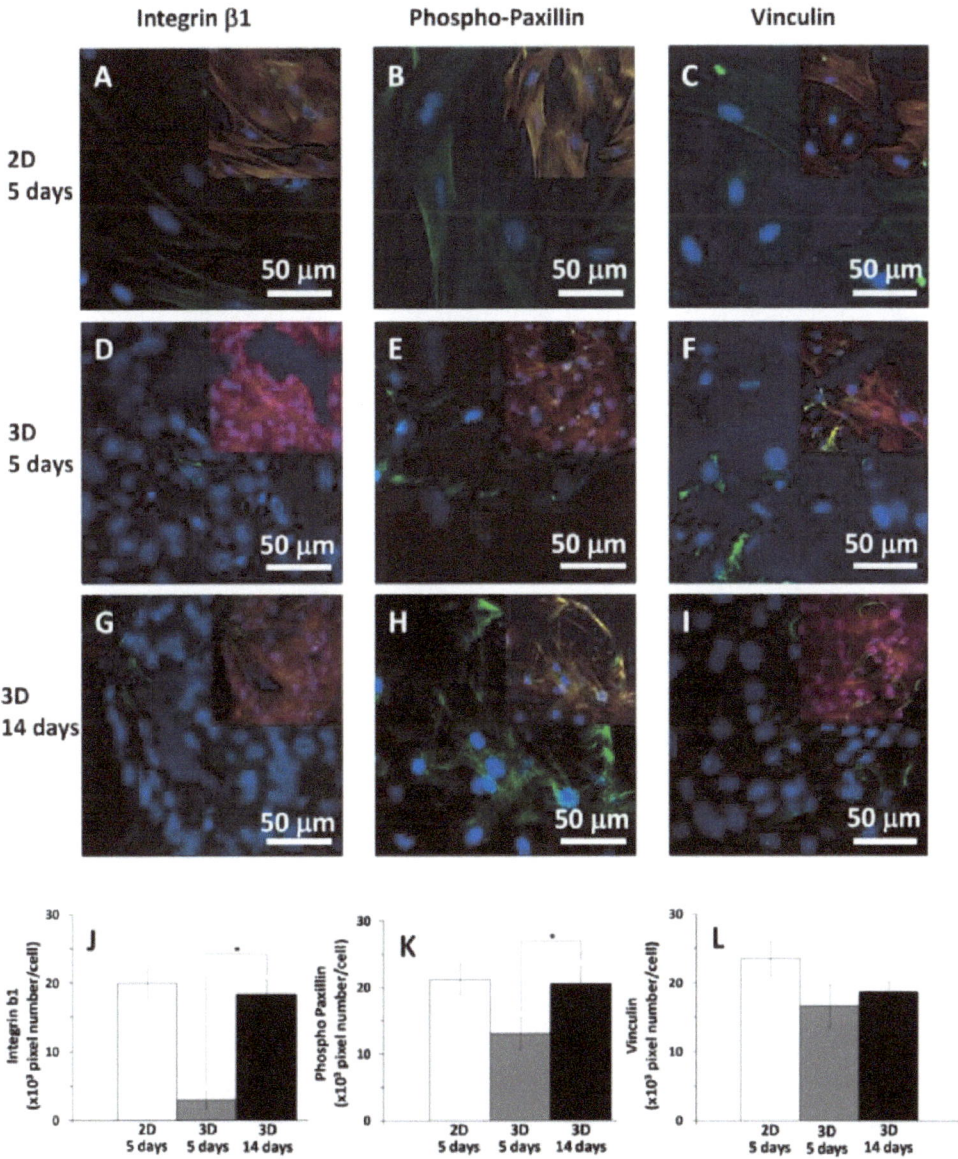

Fig. (5). Focal adhesions of MC3T3-E1 osteoblasts on 3D-NF-gelatin and 2D gelatin substrate after cultured for 5 and 14 days. (**A-C**) Projected z stack confocal images of osteoblasts cultured for 5 days on 2D gelatin surface; (**D-F**) projected z stack confocal images of osteoblasts cultured for 5 days on 3D-NF-gelatin; (**G-I**) projected z stack confocal images of osteoblasts cultured for 14 days on 3D-NF-gelatin. The cell/substrate was stained for focal adhesions using integrin β1 (**A, D, G**), phospho-paxillin (**B, E, H**), and vinculin (**C, F, I**) antibodies (red-actin, blue-nuclei, green-focal adhesions, and yellow-overlap of focal adhesions on actin). Quantification shows significant increase in the adhesions from 5 days to 14 days of culture on the 3D-NF-gelatin. Reprinted with permission from Ref. [59].

EFFECTS OF MATRIX RIGIDITY ON CELL-MATRIX INTERACTIONS

Besides responding to biochemical cues, cells sense and respond to physical signals from the surrounding environment. Matrix rigidity is an important physical signal regulating the fate and activity of a number of cells, such as osteoblasts, neurons, fibroblasts, myoblasts, and endothelial cells. Natural ECM is a complex mixture that includes a large number of proteins, proteoglycans, and inorganic components, which makes it difficult, if not possible, to examine the cellular responses on the ECM with different stiffness. Because of the complexity of the ECM, studying the effects of the matrix stiffness on cellular behavior usually takes place in a synthetic system in which the rigidity of the substrate can be precisely tailored. One widely used synthetic matrix model is the coating of type I collagen on the surface of polyacrylamide [60, 61]. While the chemical composition of the substrates is identical, the rigidity is different and controlled by the crosslinking density of polyacrylamide. The purpose of coating collagen on the substrate surface is to promote cell-material interaction because polyacrylamide is typically inert to cell adhesion. A study has shown that fibroblast cells on soft substrates tend to form little spreading morphology and weak cell adhesion with an irregular shape. With increasing substrate rigidity, the fibroblasts increase their stress fiber formation and cytoskeletal organization [62]. Also, the recruitment of vinculin to the adhesion sites increases and forms transient actin-based adhesive structures called "podosomes" on stiffer substrates [62, 63]. Other types of cells, including smooth muscle cells, myoblasts, and osteoblasts, show similar results and exhibit increased spreading and stronger adhesion with stiffer matrices [64-66]. For example, myocytes cultured on plastic tissue culture dishes had a higher percentage of focal adhesions than on soft polyacrylamide gels [67]. Furthermore, highly aligned sarcomeric striations were visible on stiff polyacrylamide (18kPa and 50kPa), whereas cells on soft polyacrylamide (1 kPa) showed only non-aligned diffused striations [67]. After culturing for 12 days, the human liver hepatocellular carcinoma cell line (C3A) in alginate hydrogels with low stiffness (1kPa) proliferated to form multispheroids with a mean size of 40-50 μm. In contrast, the cell size in the hydrogels with high stiffness (18kPa) was approximately 20-30 μm, which is significantly smaller than that in low-stiffness hydrogels [68]. However, the stiffness of natural ECM in different tissues varies widely. Therefore, different types of cells may show quantitative and qualitative differences in their responses to the matrix stiffness. For instance, myocytes prefer moderately stiff substrates (Young's modulus E ~ 12 kPa), whereas neurons have significantly more branches on softer gels (Young's modulus E ~ 50-300 Pa) compared to stiffer gels (Young's modulus E ~ 300-550 Pa) [66].

The matrix stiffness also influences cell migration. In a 2D substrate model, fibroblasts are capable of sensing the stiffness of the environment and moving toward very rigid substrates, a phenomenon called "durotaxis" [60, 62]. As the leading edge of the fibroblast crosses onto a rigid substrate, the lamella and lamellipodia expand, leading to directed migration onto the rigid substrate. Conversely, as the leading edge of the cell approaches the soft side, local retraction takes place, resulting in a change of direction. However, the rigid guided movement (durotaxis) takes place only when there are no other cells in the vicinity. At high cell density, cells from the soft and the rigid sides of the substrate can move freely across the rigid gradient, most likely as a result of the pulling/pushing forces from neighboring cells [60]. In contrast to migration in 2D, the cells in the body must overcome the biophysical barriers of their surrounding milieu. Correspondingly, cells in a 3D system migrate in two different ways: using either proteolytic or nonproteolytic strategies. In proteteolytic migration, the cells secrete proteases (*e.g.*, MMP) to break down the ECM and thus create macroscopic cavities to allow their movement. Alternatively, many inflammatory cell types (*e.g.*, lymphocytes and dendritic cells) utilize nonproteolytic strategies to overcome matrix resistance by squeezing through the ECM [69]. The three-dimensional migration of fibroblasts in stiff poly(ethylene glycol) (PEG) is strictly dependent on proteolysis [70]. With the low stiffness of the PEG, the fibroblasts can overcome the resistance of the matrix through a nonproteolytic migration mode, suggesting the use of pre-existing or de novo-formed macroscopic gel defects [69].

Human dermal fibroblasts in free-floating collagen matrices (detached from the underlying culture plastic) demonstrated no proliferation. In contrast, fibroblasts cultured in the same matrices, but attached, showed some proliferation [71]. Furthermore, the fibroblasts seeded within collagen matrices with high stiffness had a higher dividing rate. The gene expressions of matrix metalloproteinase 2 (MMP2), TIMP metallopeptidase inhibitor 2 (TIMP2), and collagen type III expression in fibroblasts were significantly up-regulated in constructs of increased stiffness [72]. One possible mechanism is that increasing matrix density results in alterations of the number of binding sites, which would ultimately lead to changes in the gene expressions related to cell division [73]. However, cell proliferation on matrices is cell type-dependent, and different cell types may have different responses to matrix stiffness. For example, when C3A cells were cultured inside alginate, the proliferation rate of the cells decreased with increasing stiffness of the 3D matrix [68]. The cells in stiff alginate exhibited a more prolonged lag phase than those in their soft counterparts. Consequently, the viability of the cells in soft hydrogels was higher than that in stiff alginates. The C3A cells exhibited an dedifferentiated phenotype in stiff alginate, whereas in soft alginate, they remained a differentiated phenotype [68]. Similarly, the MC3T3-E1 osteoblast cells decreased in cell number with increasing compressive modulus of the 3D matrices (from 10 kPa to 300 kPa) [74], in contrast to the results of the MC3T3-E1 osteoblast responses to 2D matrices in which the cell number increased with increasing compressive modulus [75]. Interestingly, the differentiation and mineralization of MC3T3-E1 increased with increasing modulus on both 2D and 3D matrices [74, 75]. Further, the differentiation of osteoblasts in the 3D hydrogel was maximized when the scaffolding modulus matched the modulus of the mineralized bone tissue *in vivo* [74]. Until now, the intracellular signaling transduction pathways that direct osteoblast response to 3D scaffold rigidity have been poorly understood. In contrast, culturing MC3T3-E1 cells on 2D substrates indicates that extracellular signal-regulated kinase/mitogen-activated protein kinase (ERK/MAPK) signaling pathways may play an important role in responding to matrix stiffness [76].

Understanding how to control stem cell fate (*e.g.*, proliferation and differentiation) is critical for tissue regeneration. Recent studies indicated that ECM stiffness could influence stem cell fates. For human embryonic stem cells in the lineage-specification gastrulation phase, the embryo is transformed from a spherical ball of cells to a multi-layered (endoderm, mesoderm, and ectoderm) organism. The differentiation of each germ layer is promoted by the different stiffness threshold of each of the 3D scaffolds, namely, the high, intermediate and low elastic moduli of the scaffold promote mesodermal, endodermal and ectodermal differentiation, respectively [77]. When naive mesenchymal stem cells (MSCs) were cultured at low density, the matrix could specify their destination: toward neurons, myoblasts, and osteoblasts under the same serum conditions. Soft matrices (E ~ 0.1-1 kPa) mimicking the mechanical strength of brain tissue were neurogenic; the matrices of intermediate stiffness (E ~ 8-17 kPa) that mimic muscle were myogenic, and relatively rigid substrates (E ~ 25-40 kPa) mimicking bone matrices were osteogenic [78]. Furthermore, the soluble induction factors were less selective than matrix stiffness in driving their specification and could not reprogram the MSCs that had been pre-committed for several weeks on a given matrix. Similarly, substrate stiffness directed adult neural stem cell differentiation [79]. Soft gels (E ~100-500 Pa) favored neuronal differentiation, whereas stiffer gels (E ~ 10-100 kPa) promoted glial differentiation. In addition, the neurogenic differentiation of human mesenchymal stem cells in gelatin gels with softer stiffness expressed many more neuronal protein markers compared to those cultured in stiffer gelatin gels for the same period of time [80]. For the adipose progenitor cells (APCs), increased matrix rigidity promoted APC self-renewal and angiogenic capacity, whereas it inhibited adipose differentiation [81]. All the results listed here indicate the powerful effect of matrix stiffness on stem cell differentiation. The combination of matrix stiffness with biochemical signals (for example, growth factors) will provide better control of stem cell fate, which is critical for developing differentiated cells from stem cells for therapeutic applications.

PERSPECTIVES

Cells in the body live in a 3D ECM network and have extensive mass exchange and information communication with their surrounding ECMs. Therefore, it is crucial to recapitulate these cell-material interactions using tissue engineering strategy in order to regenerate neo tissues. However, compared to extensive *in vitro* studies of cell-material interactions in 2D, our understanding of cell-material interactions in 3D is very limited, which is partially due to the complexity of the 3D environment as well as the difficulty in designing suitable 3D biomimetic scaffolds. Recent work has shown that the composition, surface morphology, 3D architecture, and rigidity of the scaffolding material all have significant effects on cell adhesion, proliferation, differentiation, and tissue formation. In addition, a few signaling transduction pathways for 3D cell-material interactions have been characterized in recent years. With the advances in material science and nanotechnology, the future is promising with the integration of this knowledge with 3D biomimetic scaffold design, which will lead to the development of the next-generation biomaterials for successful tissue regeneration.

ACKNOWLEDGEMENTS

Declared none.

CONFLICT OF INTEREST

The authors confirm that this chapter contents have no conflict of interest.

ABBREVIATIONS

2D	=	Two-dimensional
3D	=	Three-dimensional
ALP	=	Alkaline phosphatase
APCs	=	Adipose progenitor cells
BSP	=	Bone sialoprotein
CVD	=	Chemical vapor deposition
ECM	=	Extracellular matrix
FN	=	Fibronectin
GFOGER	=	Gly-Phe-Hyd-Gly-Glu-Arg
GRGDS	=	Gly-Arg-Gly-Asp-Ser
HAP	=	Hydroxyapatite
hMSCs	=	Human mesenchymal stem cells

LBL-SA	=	Layer-by-layer self-assembly
LN	=	Laminin
MMP	=	Matrix metalloproteinase
MMP2	=	Matrix metalloproteinase 2
MSCs	=	Mesenchymal stem cells
NF-gelatin	=	Nanofibrous gelatin
OCN	=	Osteocalcin
PAMAM	=	Poly(amidoamine)
PC	=	Polycarbonate
PCL	=	Poly(epsilon-caprolactone)
PDAC	=	Poly(diallyldimethylammonium chloride)
PDMS	=	Poly(dimethylsiloxan)
PEG	=	Poly(ethylene glycol)
PEG	=	Poly(ethylene glycol)
PGA	=	Poly(glycolic acid)
PHAA-g-PLLA	=	Poly(hydroxyalkyl (meth)acrylate)-graft-poly(L-lactic acid)
PHB	=	Poly(3-hydroxybutyrate)
PLA	=	Poly(lactic acid)
PLGA	=	Poly[(lactic acid)-co-(glycolic acid)]
PU	=	Polyurethanes
REDV	=	Arg-Glu-Asp-Val
RGD	=	Arg-Gly-Asp
TIMP2	=	Metallopeptidase inhibitor 2

TIPS   = Thermally induced phase separation

VN   = Vitronectin

REFERENCES

[1]   Wilson, C.J., *et al.*, Mediation of biomaterial-cell interactions by adsorbed proteins: A review. *Tissue Eng.*, 2005, 11, 1-18.

[2]   Schmidt, D., H. Waldeck, and W. Kao, Protein Adsorption to Biomaterials, in Biological Interactions on Materials Surfaces, *Springer*, 2009, 1-18.

[3]   Rupp, F., *et al.*, Multifunctional nature of UV-irradiated nanocrystalline anatase thin films for biomedical applications. *Acta Biomater.*, 2010, 6, 4566-4577.

[4]   Barrera, D.A., *et al.*, Synthesis and RGD peptide modification of a new biodegradable copolymer - poly(lactic acid-co-lysine). *J. Am. Chem. Soc.*, 1993, 115, 11010-11011.

[5]   Chen, W., *et al.*, Versatile synthesis of functional biodegradable polymers by combining ring-opening polymerization and postpolymerization modification *via* michael-type addition reaction. *Macromolecules*, 2010, 43, 201-207.

[6]   Westedt, U., *et al.*, Paclitaxel releasing films consisting of poly(vinyl alcohol)-graft-poly(lactide-co-glycolide) and their potential as biodegradable stent coatings. *J. Control. Release*, 2006, 111, 235-246.

[7]   Huang, Y.R., *et al.*, Application of electrolyzed water in the food industry. *Food Control*, 2008, 19, 329-345.

[8]   Wolf, F.F., N. Friedemann, and H. Frey, Poly(lactide)-block-Poly(HEMA) Block Copolymers: An Orthogonal One-Pot Combination of ROP and ATRP, Using a Bifunctional Initiator. *Macromolecules*, 2009, 42, 5622-5628.

[9]   Wolf, F.K. and H. Frey, Inimer-Promoted Synthesis of Branched and Hyperbranched Polylactide Copolymers. *Macromolecules*, 2009, 42, 9443-9456.

[10] Li, S.M. and M. Vert, Synthesis, characterization, and stereocomplex-induced gelation of block copolymers prepared by ring-opening polymerization of L(D)-lactide in the presence of poly(ethylene glycol). *Macromolecules*, 2003, 36, 8008-8014.

[11] Rashkov, I., *et al.*, Synthesis, characterization, and hydrolytic degradation of PLA/PEO/PLA triblock copolymers with short poly(L-lactic acid) chains. *Macromolecules*, 1996, 29, 50-56.

[12] Wan, Y.Q., *et al.*, Biodegradable poly(L-lactide)-poly(ethylene glycol) multiblock copolymer: synthesis and evaluation of cell affinity. *Biomaterials*, 2003, 24, 2195-2203.

[13] Yang, Y.N., *et al.*, pH-dependent self-assembly of amphiphilic poly(L-glutamic acid)-block-poly(lactic-co-glycolic acid) copolymers. *Polymer*, 2010, 51, 2676-2682.

[14] Li, Y.X., J. Nothnagel, and T. Kissel, Biodegradable brush-like graft polymers from poly(D,L-lactide) or poly(D,L-lactide-co-glycolide) and charge-modified, hydrophilic dextrans as backbone - Synthesis, characterization and *in vitro* degradation properties. *Polymer*, 1997, 38, 6197-6206.

[15] Nouvel, C., *et al.*, Controlled synthesis of amphiphilic biodegradable polylactide-grafted dextran copolymers. *J. Polym. Sci. Part A-Polym. Chem.*, 2004, 42, 2577-2588.

[16] Palumbo, F.S., *et al.*, New graft copolymers of hyaluronic acid and polylactic acid: Synthesis and characterization. *Carbohyd. Polym.*, 2006, 66, 379-385.

[17]   Teramoto, Y. and Y. Nishio, Cellulose diacetate-graft-poly(lactic acid)s: synthesis of wide-ranging compositions and their thermal and mechanical properties. *Polymer*, 2003, 44, 2701-2709.

[18]   Li, Y., *et al.*, Amphiphilic poly(L-lactide)-b-dendritic poly(L-lysine)s synthesized with a metal-free catalyst and new dendron initiators: Chemical preparation and characterization. *Biomacromolecules*, 2006, 7, 224-231.

[19]   Liu, X.H. and P.X. Ma, The nanofibrous architecture of poly(L-lactic acid)-based functional copolymers. *Biomaterials*, 2010, 31, 259-269.

[20]   Liu, X.H., X.B. Jin, and P.X. Ma, Nanofibrous hollow microspheres self-assembled from star-shaped polymers as injectable cell carriers for knee repair. *Nat. Mater.*, 2011, 10, 398-406.

[21]   Tian, D., *et al.*, Ring-opening polymerization of 1,4,8-trioxaspiro 4.6 -9-undecanone: A new route to aliphatic polyesters bearing functional pendent groups. *Macromolecules*, 1997, 30, 406-409.

[22]   Hu, X.L., *et al.*, Biodegradable amphiphilic block copolymers bearing protected hydroxyl groups: Synthesis and characterization. *Biomacromolecules*, 2008, 9, 553-560.

[23]   Wu, R., T.F. Al-Azemi, and K.S. Bisht, Functionalized Polycarbonate Derived from Tartaric Acid: Enzymatic Ring-Opening Polymerization of a Seven-Membered Cyclic Carbonate. *Biomacromolecules*, 2008, 9, 2921-2928.

[24]   Zhou, Y., R.X. Zhuo, and Z.L. Liu, Synthesis and characterization of novel aliphatic poly(carbonate-ester)s with functional pendent groups. *Macromol. Rapid Commun.*, 2005, 26, 1309-1314.

[25]   Lutolf, M.P., *et al.*, Synthetic matrix metalloproteinase-sensitive hydrogels for the conduction of tissue regeneration: Engineering cell-invasion characteristics. *Proc. Natl. Acad. Sci. U. S. A.*, 2003, 100, 5413-5418.

[26]   Lutolf, M.P., *et al.*, Cell-responsive synthetic hydrogels. *Adv. Mater.*, 2003, 15, 888-892.

[27]   Liu, X. and P.X. Ma, Polymeric scaffolds for bone tissue engineering. *Ann. Biomed. Eng.*, 2004, 32, 477-86.

[28]   Devin, J.E., M.A. Attawia, and C.T. Laurencin, Three-dimensional degradable porous polymer-ceramic matrices for use in bone repair. *J. Biomater. Sci.-Polym. Ed.*, 1996, 7, 661-669.

[29]   Laurencin, C.T., *et al.*, Tissue engineered bone-regeneration using degradable polymers: The formation of mineralized matrices. *Bone*, 1996, 19, S93-S99.

[30]   Kim, S.S., *et al.*, Poly(lactide-co-glycolide)/hydroxyapatite composite scaffolds for bone tissue engineering. *Biomaterials*, 2006, 27, 1399-1409.

[31]   Liu, X., *et al.*, Biomimetic nanofibrous gelatin/apatite composite scaffolds for bone tissue engineering. *Biomaterials*, 2009, 30, 2252-2258.

[32]   Shin, H., S. Jo, and A.G. Mikos, Biomimetic materials for tissue engineering. *Biomaterials*, 2003, 24, 4353-4364.

[33]   Stile, R.A. and K.E. Healy, Thermo-responsive peptide-modified hydrogels for tissue regeneration. *Biomacromolecules*, 2001, 2, 185-194.

[34]   Heuts, J., *et al.*, Bio-functionalized star PEG-coated PVDF surfaces for cytocompatibility-improved implant Components. *Journal of Biomedical Materials Research Part A*, 2010, 92A, 1538-1551.

[35]   Hu, W.W., *et al.*, The use of reactive polymer coatings to facilitate gene delivery from poly (epsilon-caprolactone) scaffolds. *Biomaterials*, 2009, 30, 5785-5792.

[36] Wang, Y.Q., *et al.*, Characterization of surface property of poly(lactide-co-glycolide) after oxygen plasma treatment. *Biomaterials*, 2004, 25, 4777-4783.

[37] Yang, J., J.Z. Bei, and S.G. Wang, Enhanced cell affinity of poly (D,L-lactide) by combining plasma treatment with collagen anchorage. *Biomaterials*, 2002, 23, 2607-2614.

[38] Liu, X.H., *et al.*, Surface engineering of nano-fibrous poly(L-Lactic Acid) scaffolds *via* self-assembly technique for bone tissue engineering. *J. Biomed. Nanotech.*, 2005, 1, 54-60.

[39] Liu, X.H., Y.J. Won, and P.X. Ma, Surface modification of interconnected porous scaffolds. *J. Biomed. Mater. Res. Part A*, 2005, 74A, 84-91.

[40] Liu, X.H., Y.J. Won, and P.X. Ma, Porogen-induced surface modification of nano-fibrous poly(L-lactic acid) scaffolds for tissue engineering. *Biomaterials*, 2006, 27, 3980-3987.

[41] Buser, D., *et al.*, Influence of Surface Characteristics on Bone Integration of Titanium Implants - a Histomorphometric Study in Miniature Pigs. *J. Biomed. Mater. Res.*, 1991, 25, 889-902.

[42] Boyan, B.D., *et al.*, Role of material surfaces in regulating bone and cartilage cell response. *Biomaterials*, 1996, 17, 137-46.

[43] Matsuzaka, K., *et al.*, The effect of poly-L-lactic acid with parallel surface micro groove on osteoblast-like cells *in vitro*. *Biomaterials*, 1999, 20, 1293-1301.

[44] Charest, J.L., A.J. Garcia, and W.P. King, Myoblast alignment and differentiation on cell culture substrates with microscale topography and model chemistries. *Biomaterials*, 2007, 28, 2202-2210.

[45] Kim, D.H., *et al.*, Matrix nanotopography as a regulator of cell function. *J. Cell Biol.*, 2012, 197, 351-360.

[46] Dalby, M.J., *et al.*, Fibroblast reaction to island topography: changes in cytoskeleton and morphology with time. *Biomaterials*, 2003, 24, 927-935.

[47] Karuri, N.W., *et al.*, Nano- and microscale holes modulate cell-substrate adhesion, cytoskeletal organization, and -beta 1 integrin localization in SV40 human corneal epithelial cells. *Ieee T. Nanobiosci.*, 2006, 5, 273-280.

[48] Teixeira, A.I., *et al.*, Epithelial contact guidance on well-defined micro- and nanostructured substrates. *J Cell Sci*, 2003, 116, 1881-1892.

[49] Ranjan, A. and T.J. Webster, Increased endothelial cell adhesion and elongation on micron-patterned nano-rough poly(dimethylsiloxane) films. *Nanotechnology*, 2009, 20.

[50] Lu, J., *et al.*, Decreased Platelet Adhesion and Enhanced Endothelial Cell Functions on Nano and Submicron-Rough Titanium Stents. *Tissue Eng Pt A*, 2012, 18, 1389-1398.

[51] Teo, B.K.K., *et al.*, Nanotopography/Mechanical Induction of Stem-Cell Differentiation. *Method. Cell Biol.*, 2010, 98, 241-294.

[52] Sjostrom, T., *et al.*, Fabrication of pillar-like titania nanostructures on titanium and their interactions with human skeletal stem cells. *Acta Biomater.*, 2009, 5, 1433-1441.

[53] Yim, E.K.F., S.W. Pang, and K.W. Leong, Synthetic nanostructures inducing differentiation of human mesenchymal stem cells into neuronal lineage. *Exp Cell Res*, 2007, 313, 1820-1829.

[54] Kleinman, H.K., R.J. Klebe, and G.R. Martin, Role of collagenous matrices in the adhesion and growth of cells. *J. Cell Biol.*, 1981, 88, 473-485.

[55] Hu, J., X.H. Liu, and P.X. Ma, Induction of osteoblast differentiation phenotype on poly(L-lactic acid) nanofibrous matrix. *Biomaterials*, 2008, 29, 3815-3821.

[56] Yang, F., *et al.*, Electrospinning of nano/micro scale poly(L-lactic acid) aligned fibers and their potential in neural tissue engineering. *Biomaterials*, 2005, 26, 2603-2610.

[57]   Xu, C.Y., *et al.*, Aligned biodegradable nanofibrous structure: a potential scaffold for blood vessel engineering. *Biomaterials*, 2004, 25, 877-886.

[58]   Nisbet, D.R., *et al.*, Interaction of embryonic cortical neurons on nanofibrous scaffolds for neural tissue engineering. *J. Neur. Eng.*, 2007, 4, 35-41.

[59]   Sachar, A., *et al.*, Osteoblasts responses to three-dimensional nanofibrous gelatin scaffolds. *J. Biomed. Mater. Res. Part A*, 2012, 100A, 3029-3041.

[60]   Lo, C.M., *et al.*, Cell movement is guided by the rigidity of the substrate. *Biophys. J.*, 2000, 79, 144-152.

[61]   Pelham, R.J. and Y.L. Wang, Cell locomotion and focal adhesions are regulated by substrate flexibility. *Proc. Natl. Acad. Sci. U. S. A.*, 1997, 94, 13661-13665.

[62]   Guo, W.H., *et al.*, Substrate rigidity regulates the formation and maintenance of tissues. *Biophys. J.*, 2006, 90, 2213-2220.

[63]   Paszek, M.J., *et al.*, Tensional homeostasis and the malignant phenotype. *Cancer Cell*, 2005, 8, 241-254.

[64]   Georges, P.C., *et al.*, Matrices with compliance comparable to that of brain tissue select neuronal over glial growth in mixed cortical cultures. *Biophys. J.*, 2006, 90, 3012-3018.

[65]   Califano, J.P. and C.A. Reinhart-King, A Balance of Substrate Mechanics and Matrix Chemistry Regulates Endothelial Cell Network Assembly. *Cell. Mol. Bioeng.*, 2008, 1, 122-132.

[66]   Engler, A.J., *et al.*, Myotubes differentiate optimally on substrates with tissue-like stiffness: pathological implications for soft or stiff microenvironments. *J. Cell Biol.*, 2004, 166, 877-887.

[67]   Bajaj, P., *et al.*, Stiffness of the substrate influences the phenotype of embryonic chicken cardiac myocytes. *J. Biomed. Mater. Res. Part A*, 2010, 95A, 1261-1269.

[68]   Huang, X.B., *et al.*, Matrix Stiffness in Three-Dimensional Systems Effects on the Behavior of C3A Cells. *Artif. Organs*, 2013, 37, 166-174.

[69]   Ehrbar, M., *et al.*, Elucidating the Role of Matrix Stiffness in 3D Cell Migration and Remodeling. *Biophys. J.*, 2011, 100, 284-293.

[70]   Raeber, G.P., M.P. Lutolf, and J.A. Hubbell, Mechanisms of 3-D migration and matrix remodeling of fibroblasts within artificial ECMs. *Acta Biomater.*, 2007, 3, 615-629.

[71]   Hadjipanayi, E., V. Mudera, and R.A. Brown, Close dependence of fibroblast proliferation on collagen scaffold matrix stiffness. *J. Tissue Eng. Regen. Med.*, 2009, 3, 77-84.

[72]   Karamichos, D., R.A. Brown, and V. Mudera, Collagen stiffness regulates cellular contraction and matrix remodeling gene expression. *J. Biomed. Mater. Res. Part A*, 2007, 83A, 887-894.

[73]   Juliano, R.L. and S. Haskill, Signal transduction fromt he extracellular matrix. *J. Cell Biol.*, 1993, 120, 577-585.

[74]   Chatterjee, K., *et al.*, The effect of 3D hydrogel scaffold modulus on osteoblast differentiation and mineralization revealed by combinatorial screening. *Biomaterials*, 2010, 31, 5051-5062.

[75]   Khatiwala, C.B., S.R. Peyton, and A.J. Putnam, Intrinsic mechanical properties of the extracellular matrix affect the behavior of pre-osteoblastic MC3T3-E1 cells. *Am. J. Physiol. - Cell Physiol.*, 2006, 290, C1640-C1650.

[76]   Khatiwala, C.B., *et al.*, ECM Compliance Regulates Osteogenesis by Influencing MAPK Signaling Downstream of RhoA and ROCK. *J. Bone Miner. Res.*, 2009, 24, 886-898.

[77]   Zoldan, J., *et al.*, The influence of scaffold elasticity on germ layer specification of human embryonic stem cells. *Biomaterials*, 2011, 32, 9612-9621.

[78]   Engler, A.J., *et al.*, Matrix elasticity directs stem cell lineage specification. *Cell*, 2006, 126, 677-689.

[79]   Saha, K., *et al.*, Substrate Modulus Directs Neural Stem Cell Behavior. *Biophys. J.*, 2008, 95, 4426-4438.

[80]   Wang, L.S., *et al.*, Injectable biodegradable hydrogels with tunable mechanical properties for the stimulation of neurogenesic differentiation of human mesenchymal stem cells in 3D culture. *Biomaterials*, 2010, 31, 1148-1157.

[81]   Chandler, E.M., *et al.*, Stiffness of Photocrosslinked RGD-Alginate Gels Regulates Adipose Progenitor Cell Behavior. *Biotechnol. Bioeng.*, 2011, 108, 1683-1692.

CHAPTER 2

Biomaterials - From Engineered Scaffolds to Potential Synthetic Organs: A Review

Ipsita A. Banerjee* and **Princess U. Chukwuneke**

Department of Chemistry, Fordham University 441 East Fordham Road, Bronx New York, 10458, USA

Abstract: Biodegradable materials have played a significant role in the construction of numerous types of scaffolds for tissue regeneration applications. Over the years several fabrication techniques have been developed for the preparation of three dimensional scaffolds with high affinities toward specific cell lines. This review chapter provides a succinct overview of some of the key aspects involved in engineering scaffolds that have been applied to three varied types of tissues- namely bone, skin and the myocardium. We have discussed some of the methods involved in the formation of highly fine-tuned biomaterials that can mimic natural tissues and encourage the regeneration of a desired tissue. It is expected that a combination of the appropriate scaffold material with ideal mechanical, electrical, and biological properties, along with biomedical imaging and computer generated datasets, will revolutionize the field of tissue engineering and bring us closer to the development of functional organs.

Keywords: Biomaterials, biomimetic, hydroxyapatite, microfabrication, poly glycerol dendrimers, polymers, scaffolds, self-assembly, tissue engineering.

INTRODUCTION

Repair and restoration of tissues have been the major objectives of scientists and medical professionals in order to reinstate the quality of human life. While surgery and organ transplantation have been the main pathways undertaken toward achieving this goal, researchers have developed several alternative techniques to overcome the tribulations related to surgery. Over the past two decades, research in the field of tissue engineering and development of organ specific tailored biocompatible synthetic materials have gained tremendous importance. Traditionally scientists have resorted to plastics, metals, or ceramics

*****Corresponding Author Ipsita A. Banerjee:** Department of Chemistry, Fordham University 441 East Fordham Road, Bronx New York, 10458, USA; Fax: (718)-817-4432; E-mail: banerjee@fordham.edu

Shunsheng Cao & Huijun Zhu (Eds)

as synthetic materials of choice. However, in many cases those materials have been found to integrate poorly with host tissue, trigger immunological response and wear out over time [1]. For example, common bioceramics including hydroxyapatite (HAp), β-tricalcium phosphate (β-TCP), HAp/β-TCP and bioglass 45S5 are frequently used as bone repair materials [2]. However, some major drawbacks of such materials are their poor mechanical strength and low fracture endurance which significantly restrict their range of applications. Consequently, tissue engineering which involves the use of an appropriate combination of scaffolds, living cells, and growth factors for formation of an engineered construct that can support the growth and regeneration of a specific tissue has been gaining popularity [3]. Ideally, an appropriate scaffold should (a) have surface properties conducive to cell attachment, migration, proliferation; permit vascularization; and (b) allow for the flow of nutrients and metabolic waste. Further, they should display biodegradability, balance mechanical function, and have minimal immune response [4]. Morphological aspects such as size, shape, and porosity of the scaffold also play a vital role in designing an optimal construct [5].

A wide variety of biomaterials have been utilized for multiple tissue engineering applications. These include many biodegradable synthetic polymers such as polyesters like poly(l-lactic acid), poly(glycolic acid) and their copolymers; [6] polycaprolactone; polyorthoester, polyanhydrides, polyhydroxyalkanoate, polypyrroles and poly(ether ester amides) [7]. ABA-type tri-block copolymers composed of poly(L-lactide) (PLA) or poly (lactide-co-glycolide) (PLGA) as A block and poly(ε-caprolactone) (PCL) as B block were also utilized for the preparation of tissue engineering scaffolds with desirable elastic properties [8]. Another class of polymers, namely elastic shape-memory polymers have also emerged as interesting materials for the development of tissue engineering scaffolds [9]. In general, shape memory polymers (SMPs) possess similar shape and elasticity memory effects as shape memory alloys. SMPs can significantly alter their elastic modulus around their glass transition temperatures. Combination of shape and elasticity memory effects make them highly applicable for the development of tissue engineering material systems [10]. In addition to polymers, supramolecular assemblies formed from biomimetic materials have also attracted significant attention. For example, researchers have demonstrated that various biologically derived materials from proteins, oligopeptides, or carbohydrates can be utilized for the preparation of scaffolds. Some examples include collagen, fibrin, gelatin, hyaluronic acid, chitosan, alginate, and chondroitin sulfate (CS) [11-16]. In order to enhance the biocompatiblity and structural characteristics of scaffolds, numerous research groups have blended synthetic biodegradable polymers with some of the aforementioned natural biomaterials. For example Lee and co-workers prepared amphiphilic copolymers by combining CS with PLA which self-assembled into micellar aggregates that could efficiently undergo endocytosis [17]. Fisher and co-workers developed a tissue engineering approach for orbital bone repair by combining 5-ethyl-5-(hydroxymethyl)-β,β-dimethyl-1,3-dioxane-2-ethanol diacrylate (EHD) and poly(ethylene glycol) diacrylate (PEGDA) [18]. EHD and PEGDA were fabricated into macroporous hydrogels by radical polymerization followed by porogen leaching. They then examined the viability and differentiation of human mesenchymal stem cells (hMSCs) as well as the expression of bone morphogenetic protein-2 (BMP-2), BMP receptor type 1A, and BMP receptor type 2 by hMSCs. Their results demonstrated that macroporous EHD-PEGDA hydrogels supported hMSCs and promoted a remarkable increase in BMP-2 expression. Cooper-White and co-workers used the electrostatic layer-by-layer (LbL) method to deposit high molecular weight hyaluronic acid and chitosan onto PLGA surfaces to form a strong, protein-resistant coating [19]. Furthermore, they functionalized the surface by covalent attachment of collagen IV, for developing a template for the self-assembly of basement membrane components from dilute Matrigel. The interactions of NIH-3T3 fibroblasts to these surfaces were then examined.

Several researchers have shown that self assembling peptide nanostructures formed by non-covalent inter and intra-molecular interactions may also play an utilitarian role in the development of tissue engineering scaffolds. For example, Zhang and coworkers developed nanofibrillar gels cross-linked by assembly of self-complementary amphiphilic peptides which were able to support neuronal cell attachment and demonstrated widespread neurite outgrowth [20]. A wide variety of similar scaffolds prepared by using self-assembling peptide moieties have been tailored to deliver growth factors and adhere to cells. For example, RAD gels in which the amino acids arginine and aspartate substitute lysine and glutamine residues form a class of self-assembling peptides that have been used to encapsulate growth factors to speed up dermal and myocardial repair [21-22]. Although such nanofibrous gels biomechanically arrange cells in a three-dimensional manner, they require specificity, for cellular interactions. To promote receptor-mediated specificity, functional groups from the extra-cellular matrix (ECM) have been used to significantly enhance the interactions of supramolecular assemblies with cells and tissues. For example, scaffolds functionalized with laminin-derived peptide sequences could successfully entrap neural progenitor cells and were found to promote neuronal cell growth and proliferation [23]. In another study, self-assembled peptide microtubular assemblies were functionalized with the glycoprotein mucin. Subsequently, *in vitro* cell attachment, cell proliferation, and cytotoxicity analysis in the presence normal rat kidney (NRK) cells revealed that the biomaterials were nontoxic, biocompatible, and showed significant adhesion to the cells [24].

Another class of materials with potential uses in tissue engineering applications include carbon nanotubes (CNT). To alleviate the toxicity issues related to carbon nanotubes, they are often bio-functionalized [25]. For example, multiwalled carbon nanotubes (MWCNT) were functionalized with chitosan, in order to prepare well-defined micro-channel porous structures with biocompatible and biodegradable properties that could support cell growth and proliferation [26]. In another study, porous bio-glass scaffolds were fabricated by replica technique and electrophoretic deposition and utilized for deposition of homogeneous layers of MWCNTs throughout the scaffold pore structure. Results indicated that the incorporation of CNTs induced a nanostructured internal surface of the pores, which is advantageous for osteoblast cell attachment and proliferation [27]. Single walled carbon nanotubes (SWCNTs) have also been utilized for potential tissue engineering applications. For example, Yildirum and co-workers functionalized alginate with SWCNTs in order to prepare composite scaffolds [28]. Those scaffolds were found to show significantly higher cellular attachment and proliferation in comparison to control SWCNTs. Furthermore, incorporation of the SWCNTs showed improvement in the mechanical strength of the scaffolds.

To prepare microstructured scaffolds, several techniques have been utilized. Examples include solvent casting [29], gas foaming [30], particulate leaching [31], emulsion freeze drying [32], phase separation [33], electronspinning [34] and laser sintering [35]. However, traditional scaffold fabrication techniques are unable to precisely control pore size, pore geometry, spatial distribution and construction of internal channels within the scaffolds. To this regard, scaffolds prepared by solvent-casting and particulate-leaching cannot ensure interconnection of pores as those factors rely on contacts with contiguous salt particles. Further, very thin scaffold cross-sections can be formed due to complexity in removing salt particles deep in the matrix.

With technological advances, microfabrication techniques such as soft lithography, photolithography and microfluidics have gained tremendous impetus in the field of tissue engineering [36]. Nevertheless, many of the patterning techniques utilized early on for the creation of tissues were for two dimensional (2D) applications. However, advances in photolithographic techniques have enhanced the ability to produce 3D structures in a facile and reproducible manner [37]. Techniques such as laser micro-stereo lithography [38-39] have evolved for fabrication of 3D scaffolds. Vozzi and co-workers have demonstrated the use of micro-syringe deposition and micro molding soft lithography techniques for fabricating three dimensional PLGA scaffolds. Their results indicated that both techniques were viable and could be utilized for the preparation of 3D architectures [40]. In recent times, customized scaffolds can be designed with the help of computer aided technologies, which has lead to the establishment of a new field termed as Computer-Aided Tissue Engineering (CATE) [41]. For example, in image-based Bio-CAD modeling the imaging modality is capable of producing three-dimensional views of anatomy, differentiating heterogeneous tissues and displaying the vascular structure; as well as generating computational tissue models which can be utilized for various applications. Computer-aided design (CAD) based bio-tissue informatics models give vital information regarding tissue biological, biophysical, and biochemical properties for modeling, design, and fabrication of complex tissue substitutes [42]. With the advent of additive fabrication technologies, such as solid freeform fabrication (SFF), it is now possible to fabricate scaffolds with fine structures and intricate geometries by using CAD data acquired from medical images of patients. One of the major advantages of SFF is the fact that a variety of biomaterials are suitable for use in various SFF systems [43]. For example, Lu and co-workers developed a sucrose porogen-based solid freeform fabrication system for preparation of scaffolds for bone tissue engineering. They used pressurized extrusion to print biocompatible and water soluble sucrose bone scaffold porogens, while PCL scaffolds were prepared by injecting the molten polymer into the porogens, followed by dissolving those porogens in water. The resultant scaffolds displayed well-defined porous structures designed into the sucrose porogen manufacturing computer-aided design model [44].

Organ printing is another example of rapid prototyping computer-aided 3D printing technology that uses layer by layer deposition of cells or cell aggregates to form 3D gels with sequential maturation of the printed constructs into perfused and vascularized living tissue or organ [45]. A wide variety of printer designs such as jet-based cell printers, cell dispensers or bio-plotters, have been applied. The components of the deposition process have included 3D hydrogels and varying cell lines. For instance, Riley and co-workers demonstrated the use of three-dimensional printing to fabricate phase composite scaffolds from d,l-polylactic-polyglycolic acid (PLGA)/l-polylactic acid (l-PLA) in one phase and a l-PLGA/tri-calcium phosphate mixture in the second phase [46]. Their results indicated a peak polymer/ceramic phase elastic modulus of 450 MPa. In general, if a scaffold is unable to provide a mechanical modulus in the range of 10-1,500 MPa for hard tissue or between 0.4-350MPa for soft tissue, then the engineered tissue construct is not likely to be successful in the long term due to instability caused by deformation [47-48]. Thus the aforementioned osteochondral scaffold designed by 3D printing method, satisfied the elastic modulus requirements for soft tissue constructs.

To develop the next-generation prosthetics and synthetic organs, one of the major issues that scientists need to tackle with is the incorporation of specific sensors that can monitor the specific tissues and stimulate/destimulate them in a similar manner as natural organs. A major breakthrough in this area was recently achieved by Lieber and co-workers [49]. They developed three-dimensional macroporous, gold nanowire based-nanoelectronic hybrid scaffolds (nanoES). Their results indicated that the NanoES displayed excellent electronic properties and could be utilized either by themselves or in combination with other biomaterials as biocompatible extracellular scaffolds for 3D culture of neurons, cardiomyocytes and smooth muscle cells. Additionally, those materials were found to have integrated sensory capability as confirmed by real-time monitoring of the local electrical activity within the 3D nanoES/cardiomyocyte constructs. The three dimensional-nanoES-based neural and cardiac tissue models were responsive toward drugs and pH alterations inside as well as outside tubular vascular smooth muscle constructs.

Overall, there has been stupendous progress in the field of tissue engineering over the past two decades, and new tools for monitoring and assessing engineered tissues and their interactions with the cellular environment have been developed. As new biomaterials with desired mechanical, biological and electrical properties are manufactured, and we get closer to manufacturing a complete organ, there are several factors that still need to be fine-tuned to achieve our final goals. In this review we have discussed the progress made in areas of bone, skin, and cardiac tissue engineering.

BONE TISSUE ENGINEERING

Research toward the development of engineered constructs for musculoskeletal tissues such as bone and cartilage has made incredible progress worldwide. The main function of skeletal tissues is to provide mechanical support. When an injury or disease affects these tissues, repair mechanisms involve reconstruction of the structures involved in proper mechanical and biological environment. After the healing process has taken place, from a clinical stand point, it is desirable to remove the foreign material in order to avoid long term issues related to accumulation of undesired metabolites. Thus, many researchers have focused on the preparation of bone graft substitute materials and biodegradable scaffolds as well as cell and gene therapy methodologies [50]. In particular, biodegradable polymers are progressively being used in bone and cartilage tissue engineering, since they may be implanted and do not need a second surgical event for removal in most cases [51]. For skeletal tissue engineering, one has to take into consideration factors such as durability and mechanical strength in addition to biocompatibility and interactions with living cells. Additionally, the properties of the substrate surface also play an important role. For example, higher hydrophilicity of the substrate allows for increased cell adhesion as well as proliferation [52]. Furthermore, for bone tissue engineering, augmentation in substrate wettability causes an increase in enzymatic activity of alkaline phosphatase (ALP), which essentially proves their osteogenic potential. This phenomenon has been observed in osteoblasts [53] as well as in mesenchymal stem cells (MSCs) [54]. However, there are other reports that have shown that ALP activity may decrease if the hydrophilicity of the material is too high [55]. In general, osteoblast regulation, proliferation, and growth is controlled by various local factors such as bone morphogenetic proteins (BMPs), transcription factors such as core binding factor a-1 (cbfa1) and hedgehog signaling pathway. While BMPs are the major regulators, the transcription factor Cbfa1 is also vital because it has been shown that its absence in knockout mice has resulted in lack of bone formation. Furthermore, it has been reported that BMPs up-regulate Cbfa1 expression [56] while hedgehog signaling pathway modulates BMP function during skeletal formation in vertebrates. In addition to osteoblasts, a group of cells called osteoclasts play a critical role in bone re-sorption [57] ability which can be confirmed by the formation of tartrate-resistant acid phosphatase (TRAP). Thus, it is important to examine the interactions of scaffolds developed for bone tissue engineering applications in the presence of both osteoblasts and osteoclasts.

It has been well documented that diseases such as osteoporosis are primarily caused by loss of calcium and other bone minerals in the matrix. Further, with aging and comparatively lower rates of protein synthesis, collagen production also decreases, making bones more brittle and prone to fracture. In general, calcium phosphate based ceramic biomaterials have been one of the primary choices for researchers working on bone tissue regeneration, primarily because the matrix of bone tissue mainly consists of hydroxyapatite $(Ca_{10}(PO_4)_6(OH)_2)$; calcium carbonate, collagen fibers, and non-collagenous proteins [58]. While the calcium salts provide hardness to bone, the protein collagen facilitates mineralization and gives it tensile strength. In addition, osteocalcin is another bone matrix protein with high affinity for hydroxyapatite and aids in mineralization [59].

In their work, Baslé and co-workers [60] explored the interactions of macroporous calcium-phosphate biomaterials grafted into rabbit bone. They found that the osteoclasts showed characteristic ruffled borders and TRAP results were positive at the surface of both newly formed bone around the implant, as well as inside the macropores. Further, within a week, osteogenesis and re-sorption were observed at the surface of the biomaterials, inside the macropores. In another study, Webster and co-workers reported the formation of re-sorption pits in osteoclast-like cells upon treatment with nanophase alumina and hydroxyapatite (HAp). They found that in comparison with conventional bulk ceramic materials, synthesis of TRAP as well as formation of re-sorption pits were significantly higher in osteoclast-like cells cultured on the nanophase materials. Their results thus indicated the advantages of nanoceramic materials for potential bone tissue generation applications [61]. However, though such bioceramics exhibited encouraging results, the overall mechanical strength of the materials were significantly less than desirable, hence scaffolds functionalized with HAp or calcium phosphate based materials have been developed.

Ellagic acid based microfibrillar assemblies, for instance, were developed as scaffolds for cellular attachment and proliferation of osteoblast cells [62]. The ellagic acid-microfiber composites were prepared by the layer-by-layer (LBL) assembly, in which collagen, poly-arginine, and calcium phosphate nanocrystals were coated on the surface of ellagic acid microfibers. The formed composites were found to be biodegradable and supported the growth of human fetal osteoblast (hFOB) cells *in vitro*. In another study, self-assembled microtubular structures prepared from bis (N-alpha-amido-tyrosyl-tyrosyl-tyrosine)-1,5-pentane dicarboxylate bolaamphiphiles were functionalized with GRGDSP to enhance interactions with ECM. Subsequently, collagen and calcium phosphate nanocrystals were grown on the tubular assemblies in order to mimic the components of bone matrix. The composite microtubes formed were found to be biocompatible and displayed *in vitro* cell-attachment and cell-proliferation in the presence of mouse embryonic fibroblast (MEF) cells [63].

Nanocomposite scaffolds have also been prepared by coalescing bioactive ceramics with biodegradable polymers to enhance their mechanical properties as well as biocompatibility. For example, poly vinyl alcohol (PVA) and HAp nanoparticles were prepared using freeze-drying technique for tissue engineering applications. Their results indicated that porous scaffolds with three dimensional microstructures were formed. Furthermore, *in vitro* studies with osteoblasts showed their ability to support cell growth as well as suitable penetration of the cells into the pores [64]. In a recent study, Lim and co-workers demonstrated the use of air jet spinning (AJS) technique in order to fabricate 3D nanocomposite nanofiber scaffolds of nanohydroxyapatite/ poly(lactic acid) (nHAp/PLA). Their results showed the formation of highly interconnected fibers because of extremely high fabrication rates. Such results are particularly encouraging as the tensile strength of the hybrid nanocomposite nHA/PLA showed improvement compared to that of the PLA casted film. MTT assays in the presence of MC3T3-E1 osteoblast-like cells on the fabricated scaffolds indicated that the nanocomposites were biocompatible and hence could be of potential significance for bone tissue engineering applications [65]. In a separate study, non-toxic degradation products of amino acid ester polyphosphazenes were utilized for the preparation of biomaterials for potential orthopedic applications. Three separate biodegradable polyphosphazenes substituted with side groups of leucine, valine, and phenylalanine ethyl esters were prepared. Amongst the synthesized polymers, the phenylalanine ethyl ester substituted polyphosphazene displayed the highest glass transition temperature and, therefore was utilized for the formation of composite microspheres with nano-hydroxyapatite. Further those composite microspheres were sintered by using dynamic solvent sintering approach. Results showed the formation of three-dimensional (3-D) porous scaffolds with compressive modulus in the range of 46-81 MPa. Additionally, the scaffolds were also found to attach to osteoblasts and proliferate and displayed an increase in ALP activity. Thus, a new biomaterial composed of polyphosphazenes/nHAP was prepared with potential applications in bone tissue engineering [66].

In another study, Kim and co-workers fabricated rapid-prototyped polycaprolactone (PCL)/β-TCP composite scaffolds, and then coated those with a mixture of collagen and HAp. In order to augment coating efficiency, the collagen/HAp mixture was embedded in electrospun PCL nanofibers in the composite scaffold. The results of cell viability, alkaline phosphatase (ALP) activity, and mineralization analyses indicated that, even in presence of small amounts of collagen/HAp the cellular behavior improved substantially [67]. Lu and co-workers designed and fabricated (3D) nanocomposite scaffolds using poly(propylene fumarate) (PPF) and hydroxyapatite (HAp) nanoparticles with controlled internal pore structures that were constructed using computer-aided design (CAD) models and solid freeform fabrication techniques [68]. They also prepared scaffolds with arbitrary pore structures using sodium chloride leaching technique for comparison. *In vitro* biocompatibility studies in the presence of MC3T3-E1 mouse preosteoblast cells showed enhanced cell attachment and proliferation for the PPF/HAp composites with controlled pore sizes, due to increase in inter-connectivity. However the mechanical properties were not found to be considerably dissimilar for the varying pore structures. Fig. (**1a**) shows the scanning electron micrographs of scaffolds with three different internal pore structures, while Fig. (**1b**) represents a comparison of Micro-CT scan and 3D reconstruction images of scaffolds with the three different types of internal pore structures. The SEM images show the morphology of cross-linked PPF and PPF/HAp nanocomposite scaffolds with internal pore structures. Two of the predesigned internal pore structures were found to have smooth surfaces and large-sized pores, which were completely interconnected as indicated in the cross-sectional view. However scaffolds formed using the leaching technique were shown to have uneven, rough surfaces with arbitrary cubic shapes and varying sizes. Overall, it was found that scaffolds with spherical pores had larger pore volumes than those with cylindrical pores. In general, both predesigned pores on the sides were bigger than those on the top and bottom surfaces most likely due to more overlapping pores being created in the sides during the layer-by-layer printing process. Biris and co-workers [69] demonstrated a top-down synthesis process based on a drop-cast method in order to synthesize bionanocomposites comprising of a homogeneous combination of bone minerals. Fig. (**2**) shows the assimilation and integration of HAp, $CaCO_3$, collagen, sodium, and calcium-based polysaccharide or alginate, and citrate in a PCL matrix which resulted in collagen-rich nanofibrous matrix. They reported that the formed 3D scaffold structures were highly porous, with pore size distribution being in the range of 10 to 50μm. A fair degree of interconnectivity was also observed, which is relevant for potential orthopedic applications.

Once the physical, mechanical, and biological aspects of the scaffold materials have been finalized, the next step involves the construction of the scaffold design within a 3D anatomic defect. The ability to create scaffolds layer by layer allows for a computer aided design to be directly translated from a clinical scan (example:

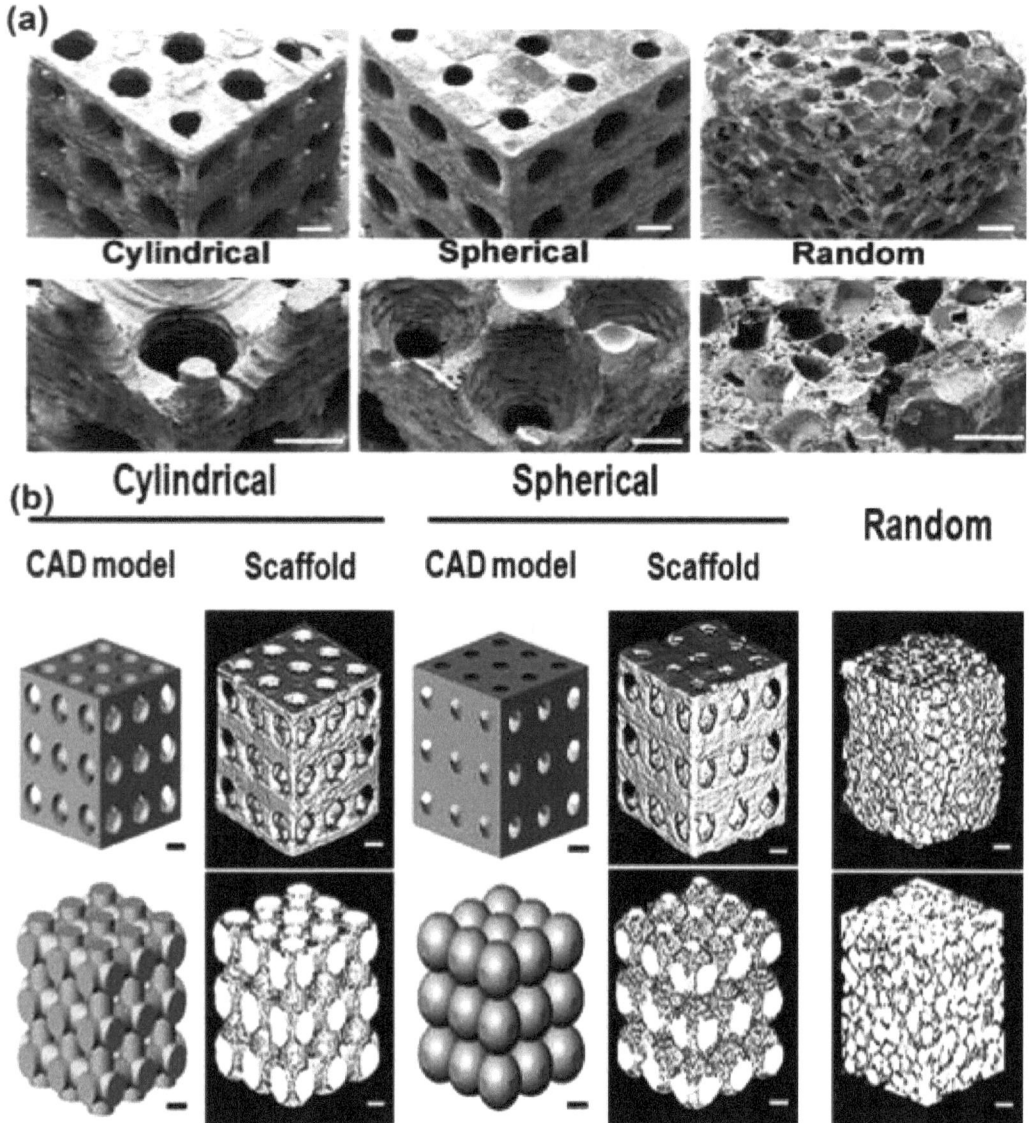

Fig. (1). (**a**) Scanning electron micrographs of scaffolds with three varying structures. Top, 3D view and bottom, high magnification images. Scale bars represent 600 μm (top) and 500 μm (bottom). (**b**) CAD models and 3D reconstruction images of scaffolds obtained from the micro-CT scan: top, solid part; bottom, pore part. Scale bars represent 1 mm (*Ref. 68 Copyright, adapted with permission from the American Chemical Society*).

CT scan) to customized scaffolds that may fit into an anatomical defect site. This step takes into account medical imaging modalities like magnetic resonance imaging (MRI) and computed tomography (CT) obtained from patients. It is to be

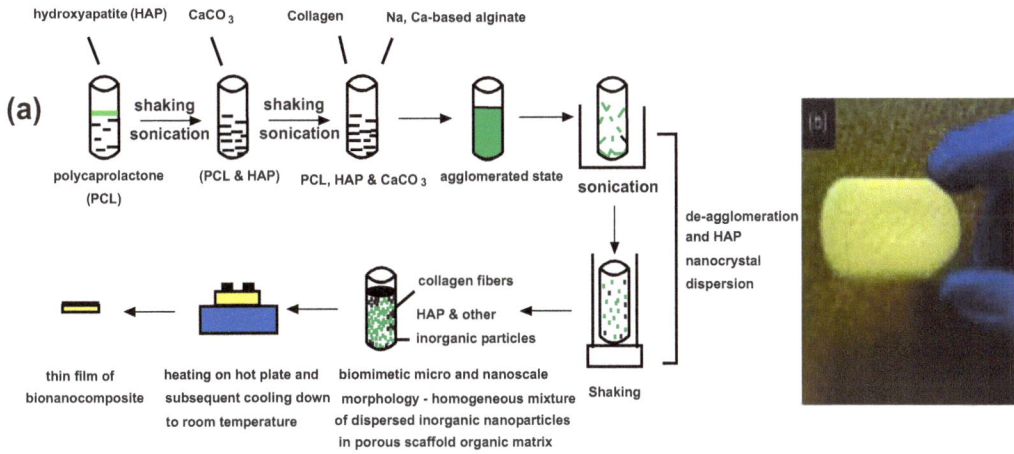

Fig. (2). (**a**) Schematic illustration of the synthesis of a bionanocomposite. (**b**) Photo of the bionanocomposite bone material (length: 2.1 in; width: 1 in; thickness: 5 mm) on a glass slide after heat curing. (*Ref. 69 Copyright, Reproduced with permission from the American Chemical Society*).

noted that CT as well as MRI imaging methods generate structured volumetric pixel (voxel) datasets and anatomical aspects are signified by density distribution. For the actual design process, the voxel database structures may be directly used in image based methods [70]. Alternatively, the data may be converted to geometric models for CAD. The defined anatomic defected shape is then overlapped with the structural design database using boolean techniques, which allows for the final scaffold design. In general scaffolds with preferred anatomical shape and known functional properties may be obtained by putting together global anatomic image data with predefined or optimized unit-cell designs. Fig. (**3**) shows the image-based design method integrated with fabrication to produce a scaffold.

Finally, upon implantation of a scaffold into a bone defect site, constant cell and tissue remodeling is crucial for stable biomechanical conditions and vascularization within the host [71]. The scaffolds should encourage and support initiation and continuance of bone growth as well as bone remodeling and maturation. Furthermore, they must offer adequate mechanical strength to counteract the loss of mechanical function of the injured tissue. It is also vital that the scaffold degrades at a rate which is compatible with new tissue growth and

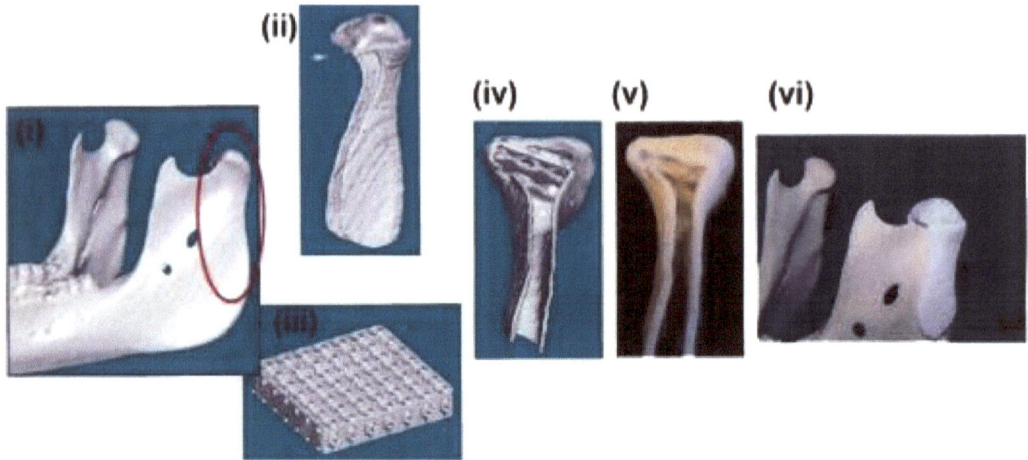

Fig. (3). Image-based method for integrating designed microstructure with anatomical shape. (**i**) A CT or MRI is the starting point for designing scaffold exterior; (**ii**) The scaffold exterior shape is created with additional features for surgical fixation; (**iii**) Architecture image-design is created using CTD; (**iv**), Global anatomic and architecture design are integrated using boolean image techniques; (**v**) SFF or SLS is used to fabricate design from degradable biomaterial; (**vi**) Final fabricated scaffold fits well on the intended anatomic reconstruction site. (*Ref. 70 Copyright, Reproduced with permission from Nature Publishing Group*).

maturation [72]. In general, tissue in-growth does not necessarily mean that it would lead to tissue maturation and remodeling. In other words a defect filled with undeveloped, growing tissue cannot be considered "regenerated". Hence, several scaffolds have not worked in the past as degradation was faster than tissue remodeling and/or maturation [73]. In general, bone displays an intrinsic regenerative capacity following injury or disease. Therefore, a majority of bone defects and fractures heal and may not require surgery. Even though improvements in surgical methods and implant design have enhanced treatment options [74, 75], tissue engineering has opened new doors for regeneration of bone tissue and for combating diseases such as osteoporosis.

SKIN TISSUE ENGINEERING

Skin is the largest organ in vertebrates and at the same time most vulnerable to precarious external influences such as wounds. However, the epidermis, dermis, and hypodermis, three consecutive layers of skin, are functional in protecting it from harm and also assist in the healing process in case it does get affected. The keratinized epidermis is rich in nerve cells, and blood, and has a major role as the first protective barrier of the skin. The dermis which lies below it consists of collagen, elastin, and glycosaminoglycans (GAGs), and is replete with fibroblasts which are extremely important in the wound healing process. The hypodermis, which is just below the dermis, has both fat and connective tissues, and is involved in thermoregulatory and mechanical processes of the skin [76].

Since the introduction of skin grafts by Reverdin in 1871, researchers have constantly been working to improve the process of regenerating skin [77]. Human allografts cover and protect the skin temporarily till autografts are available, but as a result of this, have limited availability. Xenografts are more readily available but are still faced with the problems of rejection in the immune system and failure to completely revascularize [78]. Allografts and xenografts are also often associated with adverse effects such as graft dissolution, encapsulation, foreign body reaction and scarring [79]. Tissue engineering (TE), on the other hand, has shown many advantages [80]. In general, TE replacements serve to treat wounds and replace the damaged or diseased skin tissue. The engineered epidermis should have certain general qualities which include the provision of a functional barrier against water vapor loss and microbial infection. For the substitute dermis, tissue compatibility, sustained adherence to the wound surface, a structure that encourages invasion of granulation tissue and eventual regeneration of normal dermis are attractive qualities [81]. Furthermore, it should be biocompatible, undergo controlled degradation, and evoke minimal inflammatory response and scarring [82]. Being able to facilitate angiogenesis while still being cost-effective is a desirable quality as well. Important steps in skin tissue engineering involve modeling the artificial ECM so that it releases growth factors, bioactive peptides, and cytokines in a timely and targeted manner to encourage effective tissue repair. Some of the current research methods employed in skin tissue engineering are discussed below.

In a recent report, Liu and co-workers explored the potential use of bone marrow mesenchymal stem cells (MSCs) from adult pigs coupled with tissue engineered skin to repair skin defects such as burn wounds [83]. The marrow was aspirated from the iliac crests of pigs and the MSCs were seeded unto collagen-GAG scaffolds. They were later grafted into deep partial thickness wounds created on the back of the pigs. For the grafting procedure, three groups were analyzed: (1) Tissue-engineered (TE) skin containing MSCs, (2) Collagen-GAG scaffolds only, and (3) Control (no graft). The results indicated that TE-MSC as a graft showed better healing, keratinization, less wound contraction, and more vascularization than other groups. This reproducible model could lead to improved performance in clinical attempts at treating burn wounds.

In another study, Han and co-workers have designed a novel asymmetric and porous scaffold system which combines collagen and chitosan and includes fibrin glue to aid cell attachment, migration, and proliferation [84]. To complete the skin substitute, a cell source of human keratinocytes cell line and fibroblasts were used. The scaffolds formed were asymmetric, and hence differed from traditional scaffolds. Their structure possessed two sides with differing pore sizes. The range of pore sizes in the bottom layer was 80-150 μm and on the top layer, 5-20 μm. Their results suggested that the asymmetric scaffolds could provide an ideal environment for cell growth and proliferation. In general, epidermal cells could be seen growing and achieved confluence on the fibrin glue on the upper surface of the scaffold.

To increase the mechanical properties of collagen gels, Kuikui *et al.* [85] have fabricated a compressed collagen gel scaffold through the application of the "Plastic compression" (PC) technique. This technique, first developed by Brown *et al.* [86] and later expanded by others including Bitar *et al.* [87] and Buxton *et al.* [88], serves to reduce collagen gel contraction without affecting its biocompatibility. It involves engineering tissue through the rapid expulsion of fluid from reconstituted gels. It can be applied to collagen because it presents a poro-elastic two-phase system with a loose water-drenched fibrillar lattice structure. PC can eliminate liquid from this gel in minutes so that dense, cellular, and strong scaffolds with improved mechanical properties could be produced. For seeding, dermal fibroblasts were populated inside the compressed collagen gel (CCG), and later, epidermal keratinocyte cells were seeded into the scaffold system to explore the potential application of cellular CCG towards tissue engineering. They also performed control experiments with uncompressed collagen gel. Since compression has been shown to significantly improve the mechanical property of collagen gel, it could potentially be used as a scaffold for tissue engineering. Their results indicated that seeded dermal fibroblasts survived well in the compressed gel and epidermal cells gradually developed into a stratified epidermal later on.

In a separate attempt, Krishnan and co-workers [89] cross-linked biodegradable Xylan/PVA with glutaraldehyde to make nanofibrous scaffolds for treating chronic skin wounds. Xylan is a cost-effective source of polymeric materials [90, 91]. Also, due to the porosity and inherent characteristics of Xylan/PVA, evaporative water loss, great oxygen permeability, and fluid drainage are made possible. Once the Xylan/PVA solution was made and electrospun, the nanofibers were cross-linked with glutaraldehyde to provide a stable environment that encouraged cell adherence, proliferation, and secretion of ECM for wound healing. Tensile properties and mechanical strength were also evaluated. Results showed increases in rate of epitheliazation as well as up to a 72% increase in mechanical properties.

Bioresorbability and infection control are highly desirable characteristics for synthetic biological grafts. Bioresorption prevents the frequent changes during a wound healing process that could harm the underlying vulnerable tissue and cause patient discomfort [92]. Some bioresorbable film dressings in use include those based on lactide-caprolactone copolymers such as Topkin® (Biomet, Europe) and Oprafol® (Lohmann & Rauscher, Germany). However, despite the hydraulic biodegradation of these films, the dressings lack fluid absorbance and are impermeable to water vapor or gases and cause fluid accumulation on larger wounds [93]. Grafts with some form of infection control are also important. They could inhibit exogenous microorganisms as well as wound surface flora and bacteria that could affect the structural integrity of the wounded tissue and lead to complications [94]. In order to avoid this, systemic administration of antibiotics along with skin grafts have been applied. However, issues such as antibiotic resistance and side effects due to high dosage have been associated with it [95]. These drawbacks can be overcome by localized delivery of antibiotics using drug loaded skin grafts that could be dosage-dependent while delivering the drug in a sustained and effective way. In a recent study, composite skin graft loaded with gentamicin was developed to quicken skin regeneration and also fight infections at the wound site [96]. The composite skin graft constituted two components (i)

Component 1-cytomodulin coupled porous PLGA microspheres to function as scaffolds for cell adhesion and growth and, (ii) Component 2- gelatin based gel to deliver the antibacterial drug gentamicin. These two components were formulated in a composite graft cross-linked with glutaraldehyde. Drug release studies suggested higher drug release at initial phases which is attractive for reducing infection at early stages and thereby prevent the wound from further contamination. The composite showed its potential for skin regeneration by supporting cell growth, proliferation and migration and also effectively inhibited microbial growth. Thus a dual functional wound healing, antimicrobial scaffold with skin generation ability was prepared.

The application of poly-3-Hydroxybutaric acid (PHB) and gelatin in the tissue engineering process was explored by Nagiah *et al.* in a recent study [97]. Blended PHB fibers and gelatin were electrospun with glutaraldehyde as the cross-linker. PHB was utilized because its biodegradable surface can be used in devices that require a long half-life *in vivo* [98]. It has also been found to be highly conducive to the growth and proliferation of human keratinocytes [99] making it a suitable candidate for a dermal substitute and is mechanically satisfactory and non-toxic [100, 101]. After PHB-gelatin was electrospun, nanofibers ranging between 90-500nm were obtained. The fibers were thermally stable, and the inclusion of gelatin was found to improve the tensile properties of the fibers as well as surprisingly mask the crystalline nature of PHB. The scaffolds also supported the adhesion and proliferation of dermal fibroblasts and keratinocytes, giving them reliable potential as scaffolds in skin tissue engineering. Thus, skin tissue engineering has shown immense progress over the years, although, researchers are still working to improve long term applications.

CARDIAC TISSUE REGENERATION

According to the WHO (World Health Organization) reports, cardiovascular diseases are considered the number one cause of death globally [102]. Heart ailments such as heart stroke, myocardial infarction, myocardial ischemia [103], or valvular heart diseases, are significant factors in worldwide morbidity [104]. Myocardial infarction, for example, leads to the depletion and eventual obliteration of cardiomyocytes [105], and as a result, fibroblasts and endothelial cells begin to proliferate and a non-functional collagenous scar is formed. This scar tissue affects the contractile function of the myocardium and ultimately leads to heart failure.

In spite of continued efforts and methodological improvements, studies related to myocardial viability and treatment have been plagued by limitations due to factors such as lack of imaging methods or standardized protocols for viability assessment [106]. In most cases, heart transplantation is the foremost method of treatment. However, due to dearth of donors, transplantation is not a highly viable method. Thus, the development of new methods of treatment for heart related diseases has become more crucial than ever. The design and construction of new functional tissues by replacing damaged or failing tissue by tissue engineering methods holds promise. In general, the concept of constructing three-dimensional biodegradable scaffolds and seeding cells that transform their native structure in accordance with the scaffold has found broad acceptance in the field of tissue engineering [107]. Cardiac tissue engineering, however, is a particularly complicated process primarily because the myocardium is incapable of regenerating since cardiomyocytes cannot replicate after damage [108]. The lack of stem cells in the myocardium also complicates matters. Additional factors including elasticity and contractive properties of the heart have to be taken into consideration to avoid complications. In general, for engineering cardiac constructs, it is vital that the cells cultured can overcome limitations of diffusion barriers. The ideal cardiovascular bypass grafts must be durable and resist degradation, and should also be nontoxic, generate optimum tissue reaction to allow healing in long-term use, and provide an adequate surface for seeding. Further, a suitable scaffold for cardiac repair must be adapted to the organ requirements. Hence size, physical properties and topography of the scaffold must match with the architecture of the heart, its mode of action and also provide the relevant cell signals for regeneration [109].

Over the past decade there have been remarkable discoveries in the field of cardiac tissue regeneration methods [110]. Among the various types of scaffolds constructed, polymeric scaffolds have found widespread usage in cardiac tissue engineering. For example, in the path breaking work by Vunjak-Novakovic and co-workers, polyglycolic acid was processed into porous fibrous networks and utilized as scaffolds. Various types of bioreactors were utilized for seeding neonatal rat cardiaomyocytes onto the polymeric scaffolds and cell-polymer constructs were grown. Their results indicated that those cells efficiently formed contractile tissue constructs in the presence of those scaffolds [111]. In a recent study, a biocompatible, degradable, and highly elastic heart patch from poly(glycerol sebacate) (PGS) was prepared. PGS was synthesized at varying temperatures by the polycondensation of glycerol and sebacic acid. The materials formed fulfilled the mechanical requirements for the preparation of three dimensional myocardial tissue engineering constructs [112].

In a separate study by Valence *et al.* [113], two types of bilayered polycaprolactone (PCL) vascular grafts with different porosities were electrospun sequentially and examined *in vivo* in a rat abdominal aorta replacement model. Four types of grafts were set up for study: no-barrier, inside barrier, outside barrier, and only barrier. For the *in vivo* evaluation, rat abdominal aortas were used to test the performance of the inside and outside barrier grafts. The results indicated no de-laminations between the layers or blood leakage for any graft during surgery. All the rats survived and remained healthy throughout the experiment. Compared to using only high porosity grafts, the addition of a lower porosity layer to either the luminal or adventitious side of a high porosity graft served to significantly reduce blood leakage as well as create excellent patency with no thrombosis. Thus, by tailoring the microarchitecture of biodegradable vascular prostheses, scaffolds with reduced blood leakage can be optimized.

Hydrogels such as PVA hydrogels, polythiophene, and polypyrrole [114], make up another group of materials that has been extensively used in combination with the polymer polyaniline (PANI) to obtain nanofibers for cardiac tissue engineering. PANI specifically enhances the modification of various physiochemical properties such as cell attachment, proliferation, migration, because PANI is sensitive to electrical stimulation [115]. For example, researchers have discovered a novel nanobiomaterial through functionalizing polyaniline nanotubes (PANINTs) with highly hydrophilic polyglycerol dendrimers (PGLDs) [116]. PGLD was synthesized by allylation and dihydroxylation reactions and then epoxidized to enhance covalent bonding with PANINTs. The PGLD-PANINT scaffolds were then prepared through electrospinning and then the potential use of the PGLD-PANINTs as scaffolds for cardiac regeneration was evaluated *in vitro* with cardiac myocytes. A schematic for the methodology employed for fabrication of PLGD-PANINTs is shown in Fig. (**4**). The group discovered that combining the electro-activity of PANINTs with the hydrophilicity, swelling ability, and cellular adhesion capabilities of PGLDs encouraged cardiomyocyte infiltration through the dendritic structure. This newly designed biomaterial shows promise in the design of stable 3D scaffolds for cardiac tissue engineering.

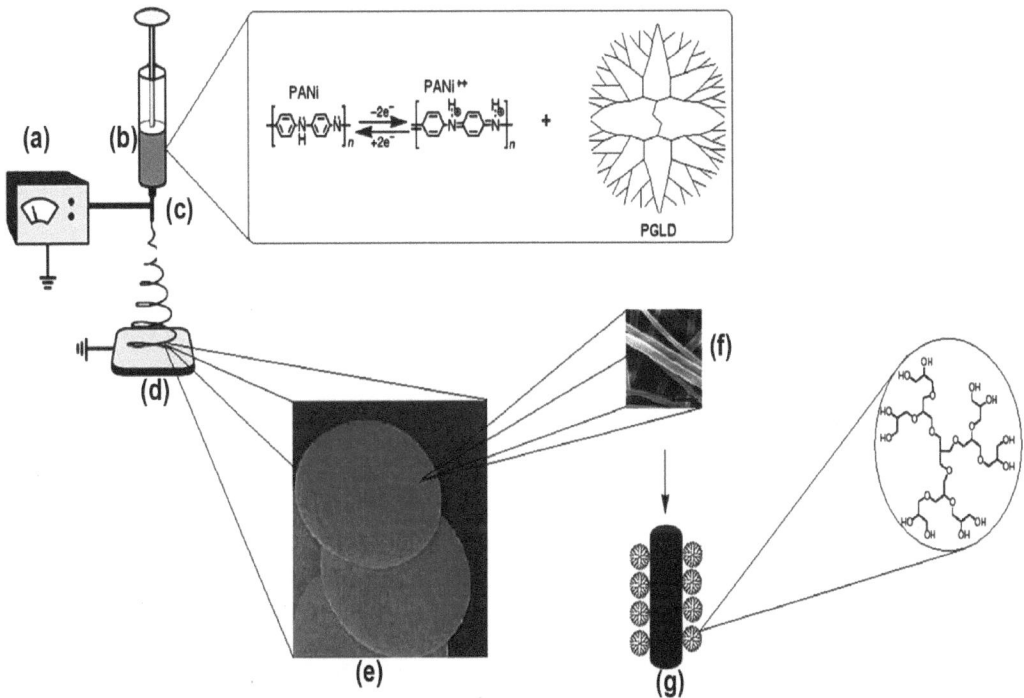

Fig. (4). Schematic fabrication method for the preparation of PGLD-PANINTs nanofibers: (**a**) high voltage power supply (**b**) syringe containing PGLD-PANINTs solution (c) needle (**d**) collector (**e**) formed scaffold (**f**) SEM image (the scale bar = 1 m) (**g**) dendronized PGLD-PANINT. (*Ref. 116 Copyright, Reproduced with permission from Elsevier*).

In another study, Tian and co-workers [117] have indicated that a sustained release scaffold such as those made by encapsulating vascular endothelial growth factor (VEGF) with either dextran or bovine serum albumin (BSA) into the core of poly(L-lactic acid-co-e-caprolactone) nanofibers by emulsion electrospinning, could prove to be a desirable scaffold candidate. Their findings show that emulsion electrospun core-shell structured nanofibers can be applied towards cardiac tissue regeneration involving the sustained release of growth factors. Prosthetic vascular grafts such as expanded polytetrafluoroethylene (ePTFE) and woven polyethyleneterephthalate (Dacron) however have been found to be thrombogenic and poorly compliant. Polyurethane grafts which were used frequently in the past because they overcame these problems, were found to degrade quickly and thus lead to aneurysm [118].

Scaffolds based on natural biomaterials have also been utilized because of their intrinsic natural properties. For example, Leor and co-workers reported that the constructs prepared using alginate scaffolds seeded with fetal cardiac cells and implanted onto rat hearts were found to be vastly vascularized. But, they could not be completely integrated with the host myocardium [119]. Gelatin sponges derived from porcine skin have also been utilized for the construction of 3-D scaffolds and were shown to be successful in creating a new cardiac chamber *in vivo*, due to their softness and flexibility [120]. However, the use of gelatin sponge induced strong inflammatory response. Additionally, it was found that endothelialization developed on the grafts without thrombus formation. In a study conducted by Zimmerman and co-workers, ring shaped engineered heart tissue (EHT) was successfully constructed when cardiac myocytes obtained from neonatal rats were combined with collagen I in addition to other matrix factors. The constructs were cast into circular molds, and subjected to phasic mechanical stretch. It was found that the cardiac cells in EHTs showed morphological similarities with adult myocardial tissue instead of neonatal native tissue. Further, those EHTs showed comparable contractile properties as those of native myocardium [121].

In order to avoid cell toxicity as well as circumvent the problem of introducing foreign materials which non-degradable support structures such as Dacron possess, Berglund *et al.* [122] have designed a construct-sleeve hybrid graft. Fig. (**5**) shows the methodology involved in fabricating such construct-sleeve hybrid grafts. The construct sleeve hybrid was prepared from acid digested Type I rat-tail collagen. For cross linking, the sleeves were subjected to glutaraldehyde, UV, and dehydrothermal treatments. Uniaxial tensile testing and burst testing were done. Results of uniaxial testing of acellular sleeves revealed increased stiffness modulus and tensile stress with the cross linking treatments. A second collagen layer with cells was molded around the sleeve to create a construct sleeve hybrid (CSH). *In vitro* culture showed that CSHs with both un-crosslinked (UnXL) and glutaraldehyde treated (Glut) sleeves exhibited significant increases in mechanical strength compared to unreinforced control constructs. Burst testing also revealed peak pressures of 100 and 650 mmHg in the UnXL and Glut CSHs, respectively. The construct sleeves did not interfere with cell function thus making the construct-sleeve hybrid approach to be a promising method of overcoming graft degradation under hemodynamic pressures of arterial flow.

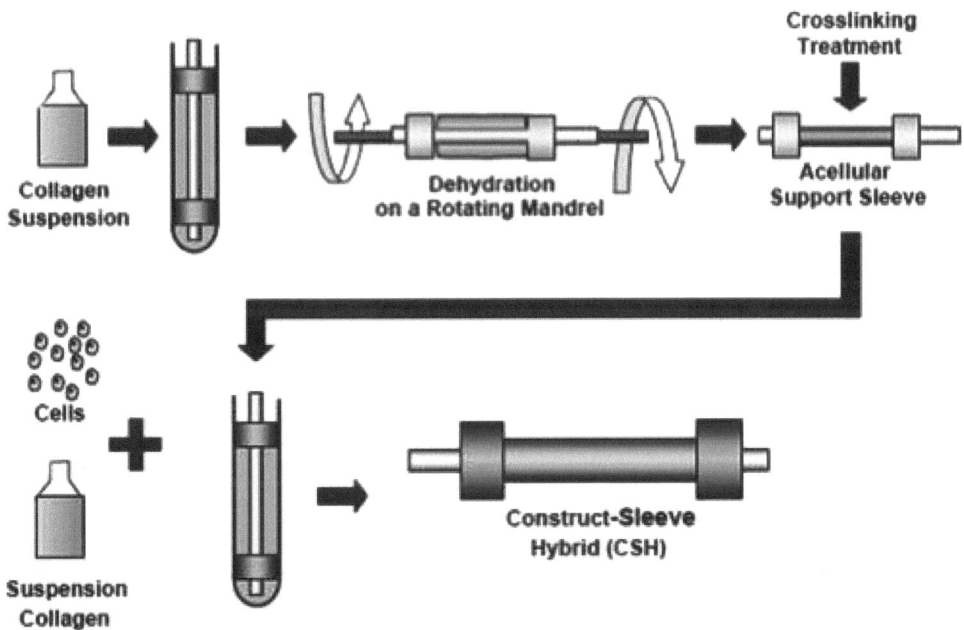

Fig. (5). Fabrication of construct sleeve hybrids (CSH). Gels were constructed from acid soluble, Type I collagen, and dehydrated on a rotating mandrel to form acellular support sleeves. The sleeves were left as such or cross-linked with various cross-linking agents. They were then combined with cells in a second layer of collagen to form CSHs (*Ref. 122 Copyright, Reproduced with permission from Elsevier*).

One of the obstacles in the development of engineered myocardial tissue is the inability to construct functional large vascularized contractile tissue patches as most matrices with preformed porous three dimensional structures lack migratory capacity of cardiomyocytes. In order to overcome this drawback, Dahlmann and co-workers recently developed a hydrogelation system based on alginate and hyaluronic acid, in which their aldehyde and hydrazide-derivatives were cross-linked in the presence of viable myocytes. Their results indicated that the hydrogel allowed for the generation of contractile bioartificial cardiac tissue from cardiomyocyte-enriched neonatal rat heart cells, which resembled the native myocardium. Further, they also reported that a mixture of hyaluronic acid and highly purified human collagen I led to higher active contraction force compared to collagen [123].

A number of injectable materials have been explored for cardiac tissue engineering including those that can mimic the myocardium. For example, Singelin and co-workers used porcine myocardial tissue which was decellularized and processed to form a myocardial matrix that spontaneously formed gels *in vitro* at 37 °C. They then conducted *in vivo* studies by injecting the matrix into rat myocardium. Their results indicated that the myocardial matrix maintained a complex composition, including glycosaminoglycans, and self-assembled into nanofibers. Further it was found that endothelial cells and smooth muscle cells moved toward the myocardial matrix both *in vitro* and *in vivo*, and a substantial enhancement in arteriole formation was seen [124].

While biodegradable scaffolds allow cell-to-cell connections, biodegradation of the scaffolds leads to fibrous tissues containing unwarranted amount of ECM, which is found in pathological conditions such as ischemic heart disease or dilated cardiomyopathy. Thus "cell-sheet engineering technique" was developed in order to allow for a structural balance between cells and to exercise ECM control for the preparation of native cardiac tissues [125]. In this method, three-dimensional functional tissues were constructed by layering two-dimensional cell sheets on poly(*N*-isopropylacrylamide) (PIPAAm) grafted surfaces without the use of biodegradable alternatives for ECM. Further, temperature sensitive culture surfaces were developed for controlling cell-adhesion. Two varied methods were utilized for cell-sheet manipulation based on cell types and objects. In the first method, cell sheets were manipulated directly by the use of forceps or pipetting after the sheets were harvested completely. This method resulted in shrunk and thicker constructs due to active cytoskeletal reorganization. In the second method, support membranes such as tailored poly(vinylidene difluoride) (PVDF) membranes were used for maintaining cell sheet morphology without shrinkage. The methodology utilized for the construction of cell-sheets is shown in Fig. (**6**). Such cell sheet techniques were

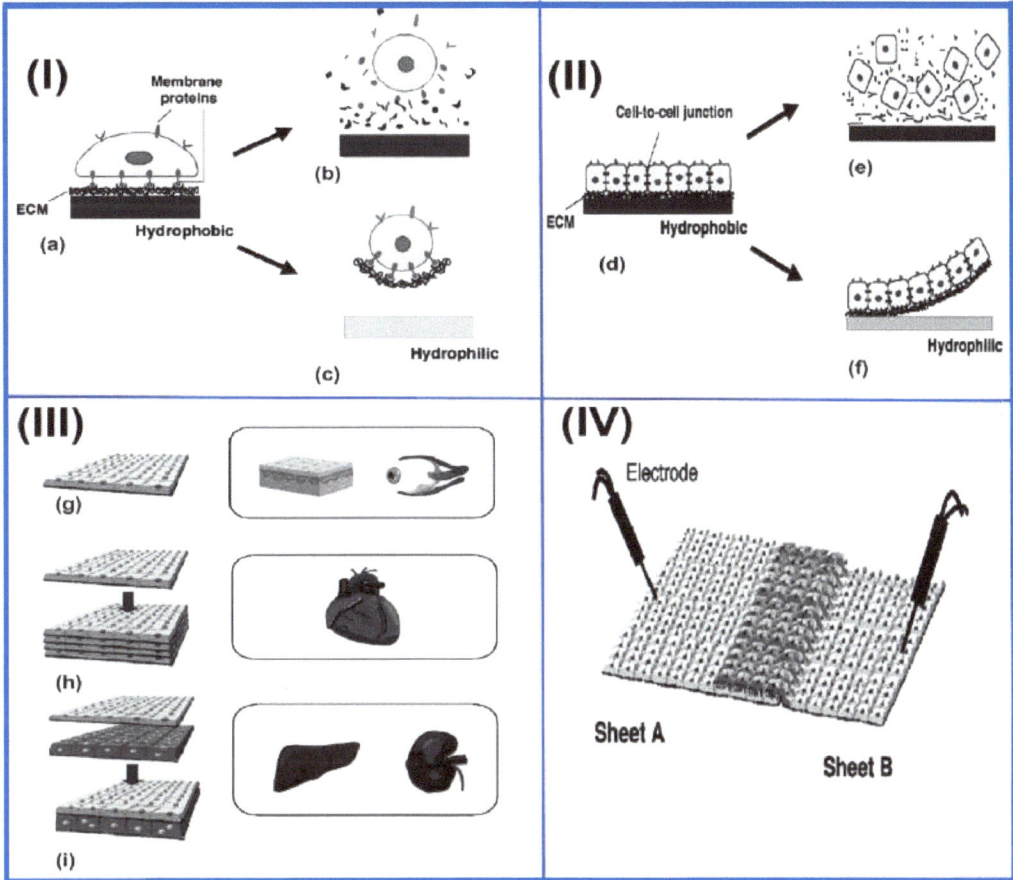

Fig. (6). (I) Cell harvest mechanism by using temperature-responsive culture surfaces. (a) Cells attach to hydrophobic culture surfaces (b) When enzymatic digestion is used, both membrane and ECM proteins are disrupted, resulting in cell detachment. (c) When cells are cultured on temperature-responsive culture surfaces, the interconnection between ECM and hydrophilic culture surfaces is released only by lowering temperature resulting in the detachment of cells together with intact proteins. **(II)** Cell sheet release from temperature-responsive culture surfaces. (d) When cells are cultured confluently, the cells connect to each other *via* cell-to-cell junction proteins; (e) When harvested by protease treatments, cell-to-cell connections are disrupted and cells are released separately; (f) When PIPAAm-grafted surfaces are used, cell-to-cell connections are completely preserved and the cells are released as a contiguous cell sheet. ECM retained underneath the cell sheets play a role as an adhesive agent. **(III)** Three contexts in cell sheet engineering; (g) Single cell sheet is useful for skin or cornea transplantation; (h) Same cell sheets are layered to reconstruct homogeneous 3-D tissues including myocardium; (i) Several types of cell sheets are co-layered to fabricate laminar structures including liver and kidney; **(IV)** Schematic representation of electrical analysis of layered cardiomyocyte sheets. Two cardiomyocyte sheets (A, B) are overlaid partially. Two electrodes are set over monolayer parts of both cell sheets to detect the electrical potentials separately. (*Ref. 125 Copyright, Adapted with permission from Elsevier*).

applied to tissue engineering in transplanting (a) single cell sheet for skin and cornea reconstruction, (b) layered cell sheets for myocardial reconstruction and (c) multilayered cell sheets for liver and kidney reconstruction. Recently, it was also reported that transplantation of such layered myocardial cell sheets onto damaged hearts improved heart function in various animal models [126].

STEM CELLS IN CARDIAC TISSUE REGENERATION

In recent times, utilization of stem cells (both embryonic and mesenchymal) has led to major advances in cardiac tissue engineering [127] and has opened up new prospects within the field of cellular cardiomyoplasty. In particular, MSCs possess distinctive characteristics that may allow for efficient cell therapy, particularly for cardiomyoplasty. In general, MSCs may be applied allogeneically, delivered systemically, and differentiate into a cardiomyocytes when implanted into myocardium [128]. Additionally, MSCs can easily be transduced by a variety of vectors and preserve transgene expression after *in vivo* differentiation [129]. Adult mesenchymal stem cells (MSCs) may be found in a wide variety of tissues such as adipose tissue, synovial membranes, pericytes, blood, bone marrow, and trabecular bone [130-135]. Specifically, bone marrow stroma has been considered to be highly resourceful. For example, Fekuda and co-workers isolated a new cardiomyogenic cell line from bone marrow stroma. Those cells were found to express atrial natriuretic peptide (ANP) and brain natriuretic peptide (BNP). Additionally, an examination of the isoform of contractile protein genes, such as myosin and alpha-actin, revealed that their phenotype was similar to fetal ventricular cardiomyocytes [136]. Transplantation studies have shown that bone marrow-derived mesenchymal stem cells enter the circulation and engraft several tissues, including the artery wall at regions of injury. Reports have also pointed to the fact that artery walls are not only a destination but also a resource for supply of these progenitor cells [137]. Saito and co-workers in their pioneering work showed that MSCs administered intravenously engrafted within areas of myocardial infarction. They found that while most of the engrafting MSCs were positive for cardiomyocyte specific proteins, a subpopulation was also found to be involved in angiogenesis [138]. Although there has been significant progress in the use of MSCs for cardiac tissue regeneration, it has been reported that MSCs used in cell based therapy in post myocardial infarction animal models resulted in limited functional enhancement primarily due to low survival and inept differentiation of MSCs *in vivo*. However, in a recent study, Cho *et al.* demonstrated that *ex vivo* genetic reprogramming of MSCs with glycogen synthase kinase (GSK) 3-beta improved the therapeutic efficiency of MSCs in the post-myocardial infarction heart. This was most likely caused by pre-directing MSCs to cardiomyocyte differentiation and inducing secretion of paracrine factors, including vascular endothelial growth factor A (VEGFA), as the over expression of GSK-3beta induces expression of cardiomyocyte specific genes and proteins [139].

While adult stem cells have been widely utilized for engineered myocardial tissue grafts, embryonic stem cells (though controversial) have also shown promising results. Embryonic stem cells are pluripotent cells derived from the inner cell mass of blastocysts and can differentiate into derivatives of all three germ layers including mesodermal cardiac myocytes. Thus far, embryonic stem cells obtained from varied cell lines from diverse organisms have shown different capacities of differentiation [140]. One of the advantages of using embryonic stem cells is the fact that less immunoreactivity is seen as these cells express less immune-related cell-surface proteins [141]. Min and co-workers have also demonstrated that embryonic stem cell transplantation has resulted in remarkable improvement of cardiac function in rats which were induced with myocardial infarction. The animals were injected with embryonic stem cells in injured myocardium. Compared to the control group of animals, they found that cardiac function in the embryonic stem cell-implanted animals had considerably improved six weeks after cell transplantation. Further, single cells isolated displayed rod-shaped GFP-positive myocytes with characteristic striations. They proposed that the improvement of ventricular function was partly due to cardiogenesis of implanted embryonic stem cells [142]. In another study, Xu and co-workers reported that by using Percoll density centrifugation, functional beating cardiomyocytes could be dissociated and enriched. Further, they found that the enriched cells were proliferative and exhibited desirable expressions of cardiomyocyte markers [143]. Recently it has been reported that stem cells that are multipotent and non-tumorogenic can also be derived from amniotic fluid. Such amniotic fluid-derived stem cells (AFSCs) could potentially provide a resource for cells that may be used in the treatment of congenital defects identified during gestation, largely cardiovascular defects. AFSCs have been shown to effectively differentiate into endothelial cells and can successfully support cardiac tissue engineering [144].

CONCLUDING REMARKS AND FUTURE PERSPECTIVES

Numerous types of biomaterials and fascinating techniques have been investigated over the years in order to form desirable constructs which can be utilized for tissue engineering. Biomaterials from polymers and dendrimers to functionalized peptide nanotubes, carbon nanotubes, and several types of ceramics, have been used in amalgamation or individually. The recent incorporation of sensors into desired scaffolds is a major breakthrough. The ultimate goal is not just to develop methods to construct viable organs in the laboratory, but more importantly to create organs that circumvent problems such as immune response. There has been steady progress as innovative techniques applied towards the reconstruction process have been and are still being designed. Overall, an amalgamation of three dimensional scaffolds, stem cells, along with medical imaging and computer aided techniques have revolutionized the field of tissue engineering and brought the scientific community closer to the development of next generation devices for synthetic organs and clinical use.

ACKNOWLEDGEMENTS

None declared.

CONFLICT OF INTEREST

The authors confirm that this chapter contents have no conflict of interest.

ABBREVIATIONS

AFSCs   = Amniotic fluid-derived stem cells

AJS   = Air jet spinning

ALP   = Alkaline phosphatase

ANP   = Atrial natriuretic peptide

BMP-2   = Bone morphogenetic protein-2

BNP   = Brain natriuretic peptide

BSA   = Bovine serum albumin

CAD   = Computer-aided design

CATE   = Computer-Aided Tissue Engineering

CNT   = Carbon nanotubes

CS   = Chondroitin sulfate

CSH   = Construct sleeve hybrid

CT   = Computer tomography

ECM   = Extra cellular matrix

EHD   = 5-ethyl-5-(hydroxymethyl)-β,β-dimethyl-1,3-dioxane-2-ethanol diacrylate

EHT   = Engineered heart tissue

ePTFE   = Polytetrafluoroethylene

GAGs   = Glycosaminoglycans

Glut   = Glutaraldehyde treated

GSK   = Glycogen synthase kinase

HAp   = Hydroxyapatite

hFOB   = Human fetal osteoblast

hMSCs   = Human mesenchymal stem cells

LbL   = Layer-by-layer

MEF   = Mouse embryonic fibroblast

MPa   = Mega Pascals

MRI   = Magnetic resonance imaging

MSCs = Mesenchymal stem cells

MWCNT = Multiwalled carbon nanotubes

nanoES = Nanoelectronic hybrid scaffolds

NRK cells = Normal rat kidney cells

PCL = Poly(ε-caprolactone)

PEGDA = Poly(ethylene glycol) diacrylate

PIPAAm = Poly(*N*-isopropylacrylamide)

PLA = Poly(L-lactide)

PLGA = Poly (lactide-co-glycolide)

PPF = Poly (propylene fumarate)

PVA = Poly vinyl alcohol

PVDF = Poly(vinylidene difluoride)

SFF = Solid freeform fabrication

SMPs = Shape memory polymers

SWCNTs = Single walled carbon nanotubes

TRAP = Tartrate-resistant acid phosphatase

UnXL = Un-crosslinked

VEGF = Vascular endothelial growth factor

voxel = Volumetric pixel

β-TCP = Beta-tricalcium phosphate

REFERENCES

[1]   Grammatopoulous G, Pandit H, Kamali A, Maggiani F, Glyn-Jones S, Gill HS, Murray DW, Athanasou N. The Correlation of Wear with Histological Features after Failed Hip Resurfacing Arthroplasty. *J. Bone Joint Surg. Am* 2013 June; 95 (12): 81 1-10. doi: 10.2106/JBJS.L.00775

[2]   Wang X, Fan H, Xiao Y, Zhang X. Fabrication and characterization of Porous Hydroxyapatite/Beta-Tricalcium Phosphate Ceramics by Microwave Sintering. *Mater. Lett.* 2006 February; 60 (4): 455-458.

[3]   Hutmacher DW. Scaffolds in Tissue Engineering Bone and Cartilage. *Biomaterials* 2000 December; 21 (24): 2529-2543.

[4]   Park H, Cannizzaro C, Vunjak-Novakovic G, Langer R, Vacanti CA. Nanofabrication and Microfabrication of Functional Materials for Tissue Engineering. *Tissue Eng.* 2007 August; 13(8): 1867-1877.

[5]   Yang S, Leong K-F, Du Z, Chua C-K. The Design of Scaffolds for use in Tissue Engineering Part I: External Factors, *Tissue Eng.* 2001 December; 7 (6): 679-689.

[6]   Mano F, Sousa RA, Boesel LF, Neves NM, Reis RL. Bioinert, Biodegradable and Injectable polymeric matrix composites for hard tissue replacement: state of the art and recent developments. *Compos. Sci. Technol.* 2004 May; 64 (6) 789-817.

[7]   Martina M, Hutmacher DW. Biodegradable Polymers Applied in Tissue Engineering Research: A Review, *Polym. Int.* 2007 February; 56(2): 145-157.

[8]   Cho SH, Park TG. Synthesis and Characterization of Elastic PLGA/PCL/PLGA Tri-Block Copolymers. *J. Biomater. Sci. Polym. Edn.* 2002 July; 13(10): 1163-1173.

[9]   Lendlein A, Langer R. Biodegradable, Elastic Shape-Memory Polymers for Potential Biomedical Applications, *Science* 2002 May; 296 (5573): 1673-1676.

[10]   Liang C, Rogers CA, Malafeew E. Investigation of Shape Memory Polymers and Their Hybrid Composites, *J. Intell. Mater. Syst. Struct.* 1997 April; 8: 380-386.

[11]   Leach JB, Bivens KA, Patrick CW, Schmidt CE. Photocrosslinked Hyaluronic acid Hydrogels: Natural, Biodegradable Tissue Engineering Scaffolds. *Biotechnol. Bioeng.* 2003 June; 82 (5) 578-589.

[12]   Shaoping Z, Wee ET, Xiao Z, Beuerman RW, Ramakrishna S, Yung LY. An Aligned Nanofibrous Collagen Scaffold by Electrospinning and its Effects on *in vitro* Fibroblast Culture. *J. Biomed Mater. Res.* 2006 December; 79A (3): 456-463.

[13]   Ahmed TA, Dare EV, Hinke M. Fibrin: A Versatile Scaffold for Tissue Engineering Applications. *Tissue Eng. Part B.* 2008 June; 14 (2): 199-215.

[14]   Aviv-Gavriel M, Garti N, Füredi-Mihofer H. Preparation of Partially Calcified Gelatin Membrane as a Model for a Soft-to-Hard Tissue Interface. *Langmuir.* 2013 January; 29 (2): 683-689.

[15]   Watthanaphanit A, Supaphol P, Furuike T, Tokura S, Tamura H, Rujiravanit R. Novel Chitosan spotted alignate fibers from wet-spinning of alginate solutions containing emulsified chitosan-citrate complex and their characterization, *Biomacromolecules.* 2009 December 10 (2): 320-327.

[16]   Suekama TC, Hu J, Kurokawa T, Gong JP, Gehrke SH. Double-Network Strategy Improves Fracture Properties of Chondroitin Sulfate Networks. *ACS Macro Lett.* 2013 January; 2 (2): 137-140.

[17]   Lee C-T, Huang C-P, Lee Y-D. Preparation of Amphiphilic poly(L-lactide)-graft Chondroitin Sulfate Copolymer Self-Aggregates and its Aggregation Behavior. *Biomacromolecules.* 2006 March; 7(4): 1179-1186.

[18]   Betz MW, Yeatts AB, Richbourg WJ, Caccamese JF, Coletti DP, Falco EE, Fisher JP. Macroporous Hydrogels Upregulate Osteogenic Signal Expression and Promote Bone Regeneration. *Biomacromolecules.* 2010 March; 11(5): 1160-1168.

[19]   Croll TI, O'connor AJ, Stevens GW, Cooper-White JJ. A Blank State? Layer-by-layer deposition of Hyaluronic acid and Chitosan on Various Surfaces, *Biomacromolecules*. 2006 April; 7 (5): 1610-1622.

[20]   Holmes TH, De Lacalle S, Sus X, Liu GA, Rich S. Zhang, Extensive Neurite Outgrowth and Active Synapse Formation on Self-Assembling Peptide Scaffolds. *PNAS*. 2000 June; 97 (12): 6728-6733.

[21]   Schneider A, Garlick JA, Egles C. Self-Assembling Peptide Nanofiber Scaffolds Accelerate Wound Healing, *PLoS one*. 2008 January; 3 (1) e. 1410, doi: 10.1371/journal.pone.0001410.

[22]   Hsieh P. C. H; MacGillivary, C.; Gannon, J; Cruz, F. U; Lee, R. T. Local controlled intramyocardial delivery of platelet-derived growth factor improves postinfarction ventricular function without pulmonary toxicity, *Circulation*. 2006 August; 114 (7) 637-644.

[23]   Silva GA, Czeisler C, Niece KL, Beniash E, Harrington DA, Kessler JA, Stupp SI. Selective Differentiation of Neural Progenitor Cells by High-Epitope Density Nanofibers, *Science*. February; 2004 303 (5562): 1352-1355.

[24]   Johnson KT, Fath KR, Henricus MM, Banerjee IA. Self-Assembly and Growth of Smart Cell-Adhesive Mucin-Bound Microtubes, *Soft Mater*. 2009 March; 7(1) 21-36.

[25]   Harrison BS, Atala A. Carbon Nanotube Applications for Tissue Engineering. *Biomaterials*. 2007 January; 28 (2): 344-353.

[26]   Abarrategi A, Guitérrez MC, Moreno-Vincente C, Hortiguela MJ, Ramost V, Lopez-Lacomba JL, Ferrer ML, Del Monte F. Multiwall Carbon Nanotube Scaffolds for Tissue Engineering Purposes. *Biomaterials*. 2008 January; 29 (1): 94-102.

[27]   Boccaccini AR, Chicatun F, Cho J, Bretcanu O, Roether JA, Novak S, Chen QZ. Carbon Nanotube Coatings on Bioglass-Based Tissue Engineering Scaffolds, *Adv. Func. Mater*. 2007 October; 17 (15): 2815-2822.

[28]   Yildirim ED, Yin X, Nair K, Sun W. Fabrication, Characterization, and Biocompatibility of Single-Walled Carbon Nanotube-Reinforced Alginate Composite Scaffolds Manufactured using Freeform Fabrication Technique. *J. Biomed. Mater. Res. Part B. Appl. Biomater*. 2008 November; 87 (2): 406-414.

[29]   Mikos AG, Herring SW, Ochareon P, Elisseeff J, Lu HH, Kandel R, Schoen F, Toner M, Mooney D, Atala A, Van Dyke ME, Kaplan D, Vunjak-Novakovic G. Engineering complex tissues. *Tissue Eng*. 2006 December; 12 (12): 3307-3339.

[30]   Harris LD, Kim BS, Mooney DJ. Open Pore Biodegradable Matrices formed with Gas Foaming. *J. Biomed. Mater. Res*. 1998 December; 42 (3): 396- 402.

[31]   Ma PX, Choi JW. Biodegradable Polymer Scaffolds with Well-Defined Inter-Connected Spherical Pore Network. *Tissue Eng*. 2001 February, 7 (1): 23-33.

[32]   Ellis DL, Yannas IV. Recent Advances in Tissue Synthesis *in vivo* by use of Collagen-Glyscosaminoglycan copolymers. *Biomaterials*. 1996 February; 17 (3): 291-299.

[33]   Lo H, Ponticiello MS, Leong KW. Fabrication of Controlled Release Biodegradable Foams by Phase Separation. Tissue Eng. 1995 Spring; 1(1): 15-28.

[34]   Matthews JA, Wnek GE, Simpson DG, Bowlin GL. Electrospinning of Collagen Nanofibers. Biomacromolecules. 2002 March-April; 3 (2): 232-238.

[35]   Zhou WY, Lee SH, Wang M, Cheung WL, Ip WY. Selective Laser Sintering of Porous Tissue Engineering Scaffolds from poly(L-lactide)/Carbonated Hydroxyapatite Nanocomposite Microspheres, J. Mater. Sci. Mater. Med. 2008 July; 19 (7): 2535-2540.

[36]   Khademhosseini HA; Langer R, Borenstein J, Vacanti JP. Microscale Technologies for Tissue Engineering and Biology. PNAS. 2006 September; 103 (8): 2480-2487.

[37]   Lu Y, Mapili G, Suhali G, Chen S, Roy KA. Digital Micro-Mirror Device-Based System for the Microfabrication of Complex, Spatially Patterned Tissue Engineering Scaffolds. J. Biomed. Mater. Res. A. 2006 May; 77 (2): 396-405.

[38]   Lee JW, Lan PX, Kim B, Lim G, Cho D-W. 3D Scaffold Fabrication with PPF/DEF using Micro-Stereolithography. Microelectron. Eng. 2010 May; 84 (5-8): 1702-1705.

[39]   Melchels FP, Bertoldi K, Gabbrielli R, Velders AH, Feijen J, Grijpma DW. Mathematically defined tissue Engineering Scaffold Architectures prepared by stereolithography, Biomaterials. 2010 September; 31 (27): 6909-6916.

[40]   Vozzi G, Flaim CJ, Bianchi F, Ahluwalia A, Bhatia S. Microfabricated PLGA scaffolds: A Comparative Study for Application to Tissue Engineering, Mater. Sci. Eng. C. 2002 May; 20 (1-2): 43-47.

[41]   Taguchi M, Kohsuke C. Computer Reconstruction of the Three-Dimensional Structure of Mouse Cerebral Ventricles. Brain Res. Brain Res. Protoc. 2003 August; 12 (1): 10-15.

[42]   Wang F, Shor L, Darling A, Khalil S, Sun W, Güceri S, Lau A. Precision Extruding Deposition and Characterization of Cellular poly-E-caprolactone Tissue Scaffolds. Rapid Prototyping J. 2004 August; 10 (1): 42-49.

[43]   Seol Y-J, Kang T-K, Cho D-W. Solid Freeform Fabrication Technology Applied to Tissue Engineering with Various Biomaterials. Soft Matter. 2012 December; 8 (6): 1730-1735

[44]   Lu L, Zhang Q, Wootton D, Lekes PI, Zhou J. A Novel Sucrose Porogen-Based Solid Fabrication System for Bone Scaffold Manufacturing, Rapid Prototyping J. 2010 July; 16 (5): 365-376.

[45]   Mironov V, Boland T, Trusk T, Forgacs G, Markwald RR. Organ Printing: Computer Aided Jet-Based 3D Tissue Engineering, Trends Biotechnol. 2003 April; 21 (4): 157-161.

[46]   Sherwood JK, Riley SL, Palazzolo R, Brown SC, Monklouse DC, Coates M, Griffith LG, Landeen LK, Ratcliffe A. A Three-Dimensional Osteochondral Composite Scaffold for Articular Cartilage Repair, Biomaterials 2002 December; 23 (24): 4739-4751.

[47]   Goulet RW, Goldstein SA, Ciarelli MJ, Kuhn JL, Brown MB, Feldkamp LA. The Relationship between the Structural and Orthogonal Compressive Properties of Trabecular Bone. J. Biomech. 1994 April; 27 (4): 375-389.

[48]   Hayashi K. Mechanical properties of soft tissues and arterial walls. In Holzapfel GA, Ogden RW Editors. Biomechanics of Soft Tissue in Cardiovascular Systems. CISM International Centre for Mechanical Sciences: Courses and Lectures No. 441, Berlin: Springer-Verlag GmbH; 2003. P. 15-64.

[49]   Tian B,; Liu J, Dvir T, Jin L, Tsui JH, Qing Q, Suo Z, Langer R, Kohane DS, Lieber CM. Macroporous Nanowire Nanoelectronic Scaffolds for Synthetic Tissues. Nature Mater. 2012 February; 11 (11): 986-994.

[50]   Boyan BD, Lohmann CH, Romero J, Schwartz Z. Bone and Cartilage Tissue Engineering. Clin. Plast. Surg. 1999 October; 26 (4) 629-645.

[51]   Middleton JC, Tipton AJ. Synthetic Biodegradable Polymers as Orthopedic Devices. Biomaterials 2000 December; 21 (23) 2335-2346.

[52]   Kim MS, Shin YN, Cho MH, Kim SH, Kim SK, Cho YH, Khang G, Lee IW; Lee HB. Adhesion Behavior of Human Bone Marrow Stromal Cells on Differentially Wettable Polymer Surfaces. Tissue Eng. 2007 August; 13 (8) 2095-2103.

[53]   Kotobuki N, Hirose M, Funaoka H, Ohgushi H. Enhancement of *in vitro* Osteoblast Potential after Selective Sorting of Osteoblasts with High Alkaline Phosphatase activity from Human Osteoblast-like Cells. Cell Transplant. 2004; 13 (4) 377-383.

[54]   Pittenger MF, Mackay AM, Beck SC, Jaiswal RK, Douglas R, Mosca JD, Moorman MA, Simonetti DW, Craig S, Marshak DR. Multinieage Potential of Adult Human Mesenchymal Stem Cells. Science. 1999 April; 284 (5411): 143-147.

[55]   Jansen EJ, Sladek RE, Bahar H, Yaffe A, Gijbels MJ, Kuijer R, Bulstra SK, Guldemond NA, Binderman I, Koole LH. Hydrophobicity as a Design Criterion for Polymer Scaffolds in Bone Tissue Engineering. Biomaterials. 2005 July; 26 (21): 4423-4431.

[56]   Yamaguchi A, Komori T, Suda T. Regulation of Osteoblast Differentiation Mediated by Bone Morphogenetic Proteins, Hedgehogs and Cbfa1. Endocrine Rev. 2000 August; 21 (4): 393-411.

[57]   Schilling AF, Filke S, Brink S, Korbacher H, Amling M, Rueger JM. Osteoclasts and Biomaterials. Eur. J. Trauma. 2006 April; 32 (2): 107-113.

[58]   Soren O, Martin L, Henning G, Sidsel G, Cody B, Kjeld S. Hydroxyapatite and Fluoroapatite Coatings for Fixation of Weight Loaded Implants. Clin. Orthop. Relat. Res. 1997 March; 336: 286-296.

[59]   Gundberg CM, Lian JB, Gallop PM, Steinbergy JJ. Urinary Gamma-Carboxyglutamic Acid and Serum Osteocalcin as Bone Markers: Studies in Osteoporosis and Paget's Disease. J. Clin. Endocrinol. Metab. 1983 December; 57 (6) 1221-1225.

[60]   Baslé MF, Chappard D, Grizon F, Filmon R, Delecrin J, Daculsi G, Rebel A. Osteoclastic Resorption of Ca-P Biomaterials Implanted in Rabbit Bone. Calcif. Tissue Int. 1993 November; 53 (5): 348-356.

[61]   Webster TJ, Ergun C, Doremus RH, Siegel RW, Bizios R. Enhanced Osteoclast like Cell Functions on Nanophase Ceramics. Biomaterials. 2001 June; 22 (11): 1327-1333.

[62]   Barnaby SN, Fath KR, Nakatsuka N, Sarker NH, Banerjee IA. Formation of Calcium Phosphate-Ellagic Acid Composites by Layer by Layer Assembly for Cellular Attachment to Osteoblasts J. Biomim. Biomater. Tissue Eng. 2012 July; 13: 1-17.

[63]   Spear RL, Tamayev R, Fath KR, Banerjee IA. Templated Growth of Calcium Phosphate on Tyrosine Derived Microtubules and their Biocompatibility. Colloids. Surf. B. Biointerfaces. 2007 November; 60 (2): 158-166.

[64]   Poursamar SA, Azami M, Mozafari M. Controllable Synthesis and Characterization of Porous Polyvinylalcohol/Hydroxyapatite Nanocomposite Scaffolds *via in situ* Colloidal Technique. Colloids Surf. B. Biointerfaces. 2011 June; 84 (2): 310-316.

[65]   Abdal-hay A, Sheikh FA, Lim JK. Air Jet Spinning of Hydroxyapatite/Poly(lactic acid) Hybrid Nanocomposite Membrane Mats for Bone Tissue Engineering. Colloids Surf. B: Biointerfaces. 2013 February; 102 (1): 635-643.

[66]   Nukavarapu SP, Kumbar SG, Brown JL, Krogman NR, Weikel AL, Hindenlang MD, Nair LS; Allcock HR, Laurencin CT. Polyphosphazene/Nano-Hydroxyapatite Composite Microsphere Scaffolds for Bone Tissue Engineering. Biomacromolecules. 2008 June; 9 (7) 1818-1825.

[67]   Yeo MG, Kim GH. Preparation and characterization of 3D composite scaffolds based on rapid-prototyped PCL/ β-TCP struts and Electrospun PCL Coated with Collagen and HA for Bone Regeneration. Chem. Mater. 2012 July; 24 (5): 903-913.

[68]   Lee W, Wang S, Dadsetan M, Yaszemski MJ, Lu L. Enhanced cell ingrowth and proliferation through three dimensional nanocomposite scaffolds with controlled pore structures. Biomacromolecules. 2010 January; 11 (3): 682-689.

[69]   Biswas A, Bayer IS, Zhao H, Wang T, Watanabe F, Biris AS. Design and Synthesis of Biomimetic Multicomponent All-Bone Minerals Bionanocomposites. Biomacromolecules 2010 September 11 (10): 2545-2459.

[70]   Hollister SJ. Porous Scaffold Design for Tissue Engineering. Nature Mater. 2005 July; 4 (7): 518-524.

[71]   Du JZ, Tang YQ, Lewis AL, Armes SP. pH-sensitive Vesicles Based on a Biocompatible Zwitterionic Diblock Copolymer. J. Am. Chem. Soc. 2005 December; 127 (51): 17982-17983.

[72]   Torchilin VP. Recent Approaches to Intracellular Delivery of Drugs and DNA and Organelle Targeting. Annu. Rev. Biomed. Eng. 2006 August; 8: 343-375.

[73]   Moutos FT, Freed LE, Guilak F. A Biomimetic Three-Dimensional Woven Composite Scaffold for Functional Tissue Engineering of Cartilage. Nat. Mater. 2007 January; 6: 162-167.

[74]   Komaki H, Tanaka T, Chazono M, Kikuchi T. Repair of Segmental Bone Defects in Rabbit Tibiae Using a Complex of Beta-Tricalcium Phosphate, Type I Collagen, and Fibroblast Growth Factor-2. Biomaterials. 2006 October; 27 (29): 5118-5126.

[75]   Den Boar, FC, Wippermann BW, Blokhuis TJ, Patka P, Bakker FC, Haarman HJ. Healing of Segmental Bone Defects with Granular Porous Hydroxyapatite Augmented with Recombinant Human Osteogenic Protein-1 or Autologous Bone Marrow. J. Orthop. Res. 2003 May; 21 (3): 521-528.

[76]   Trottier V, Marceau-Fortier G, Germain L, Vincent C, Fradette J. IFATS collection: Using Human Adipose-Derived Stem/Stromal Cells for the Production of New Skin Substitutes. Stem Cells. 2008 October; 26 (10): 2713-2723.

[77]   Horch RE, Kopp J, Kneser U, Beier J, Bach AD. Tissue Engineering of Cultured Skin Substitutes. J. Cell. Mol. Med. 2005 July-September; 9 (3): 592-608.

[78]   Bach FH. Xenotransplantation: Problems and prospects. Annu. Rev. Med. 1998 February; 49: 301-310.

[79]   Xie J, MacEwan MR, Ray WZ, Liu W, Siewe DY, Xia Y. Radially Aligned, Electrospun Nanofibers as Dural Substitutes for Wound Closure and Tissue Regeneration Applications. ACS Nano. 2010 August; 4 (9) 5027-5036.

[80]   Li WJ, Laurencin CT, Caterson EJ, Tuan RS, Ko FK. Electrospun Nanofibrous Structure: A Novel Scaffold for Tissue Engineering. J. Biomed. Mater. Res. Part A. 2002 March; 60 (4): 613-621.

[81]   Gallico GG, O'Connor N. Engineering a Skin Replacement. Tissue Eng. 1995 Fall; 1 (3): 231-240.

[82]   Metcalfe AD, Ferguson MW.J. Tissue engineering of Replacement Skin: the Crossroads of Biomaterials, Wound Healing, Embryonic Development, Stem cells and Regeneration, J. R. Soc. Interface. 2007 June; 4 (14): 413-437.

[83]   Liu P, Deng Z, Han S, Liu T, Wen N, Lu W, Geng X, Huang S, Jin Y. Tissue-Engineered Skin Containing Mesenchymal Stem Cells Improves Burn Wounds. Artif. Organs. 2008 December; 32 (12) 1525-1594.

[84]   Han C, Zhang L, Sun J, Shi H, Zhou J, Gao C. Application of Collagen-Chitosan/Fibrin Glue Asymmetric Scaffolds in Skin Tissue Engineering. J. Zhejiang Univ. Sci. B. 2010 July; 11 (7): 524-530.

[85]   Kuikui H, Hui S, Ji Z, Dan D, Guangdong Z, Wenjie Z, Yilin C, Wei L. Compressed Collagen Gel as the Scaffold for Skin Engineering. Biomed. Microdevices. 2010 August; 12 (4): 627-635.

[86]   Brown RA, Wiseman M, Chuo, CB, Cheema U, Nazhat SN. Ultrarapid engineering of biomimetic materials and tissues: Fabrication of Nano- and Microstructures by Plastic Compression Adv. Funct. Mater. 2005 November; 15 (11): 1762-1770.

[87]   Bitar, M, Brown, R.A, Salih, V, Kidane, G, Knowles, J.C, Nazhat, S.N. Biomacromolecules, 2008, 9, 129

[88]   Buxton PG, Bitar M, Gellynck K, Parkar M, Brown RA, Young AM, Knowles JC, Nazhat SN. Dense Collagen Matrix Accelerates Osteogenic Differentiation and Rescues the Apoptotic Response to MMP Inhibition. Bone. 2008 August; 43 (2): 377-385.

[89]   Krishnan R, Rajeswari R, Venugopal J, Sundarrajan S, Sridhar R, Shayanti M, Ramakrishna S. Polysaccharide Nanofibrous Scaffolds as a Model for *in vitro* Skin Tissue Regeneration. J. Mater. Sci. Mater. Med. 2012 June; 23 (6): 1511-1519

[90]   Dinand E, Vignon MR. Isolation and NMR Characterization of a (4-O-methyl-D-glucorono)-D-xylan from Sugar Beet Pulp. Carbohydr. Res. 2001 January; 330 (2): 285-288.

[91]   Habibi Y, Mahrouz M, Vignon MR. Isolation and Structure of D-Xylans from Pericarp Seeds of Opuntia Ficusindica Prickly Pear Fruits. Carbohydr. Res. 2002 September; 337 (17) 1593-1598.

[92]   Ebringerova A, Alfoldi J, Hromadkova Z, Pavlov GM, Harding SE. Water Soluble p-carboxybenzylated beechwood 4-O-methylglucuronoxylanstructural Features and Properties, Carbohydr. Polym. 2000 June; 42 (2): 123-131.

[93]   Thakur RA, Florek CA, Kohn J, Michniak, BB. Electrospun Nanofibrous Polymeric Scaffold with Targeted Drug Release Profiles for Potential Application as Wound Dressing. Int. J. Pharm. 2008 November; 364 (1): 87-93.

[94]   Elsner JJ, Zilberman M. Antibiotic-Eluting Bioresorbable Composite Fibers for Wound Healing Applications: Microstructure, Drug Delivery and Mechanical Properties. Acta Biomater. 2009 October; 5 (8): 2872-2883.

[95]   Preus HR, Lassen J, Aass AM, Ciancio SG, Bacterial Resistance following Subgingival and Systemic Administration of Minocycline. J. Clin. Periodontol. 1995 May; 22 (5): 380-384.

[96]   Anupama M, Neeraj K. Drug-loaded Polymeric Composite Skin Graft for Infection-Free Wound Healing: Fabrication, Characterization, Cell Proliferation, Migration and Antimicrobial Activity, Pharm Res. 2012 November; 29 (11): 3110-3121.

[97]   Nagiah N, Madhavi L, Anitha R, Srinivasan NT, Sivagnanam UT. Electrospinning of Poly (3-Hydroxybutyric acid) and Gelatin Blended Thin Films: Fabrication, Characterization and Application in Skin Regeneration. Polym. Bull. 2013 August; 70 (8): 2337-2358.

[98]   Piras AM, Chiellini F, Chiellini E, Nikkola L, Ashammakhi N. New Multicomponent Bioerodible Electrospun Nanofibers for Dual-Controlled Drug Release. J. Bioact Compat. Polym. 2008 September; 23 (5): 423-443.

[99]   Li X, Zhang Y, Chen G. Nanofibrous Polyhydroxyalkanoate Matrices as Cell Growth Supporting Materials. Biomaterials. 2008 September; 29 (27): 3720-3728.

[100] Lee SY. Bacterial polyhydroxyalkanoates. Biotechnol. Bioeng. 1996 January; 49 (1): 1-14.

[101] Williamson DH, Mellanby J, Krebs HA. Enzymic Determination of D (-)-Beta-Hydroxybutyric acid and Acetoacetic acid in Blood. Biochem. J. 1962 January; 82 (1): 90-96.

[102] Global Status Report on Noncommunicable Diseases 2010. World Health Organization Editors. Geneva, April; 2011.

[103] Mazzadi AN, Andre-Fouet X, Costes N, Croisille P, Revel D, Janier MF. Mechanisms leading to Reversible Mechanical Dysfunction in Severe CAD: alternatives to myocardial stunning. Am. J. Physiol. Heart. Circ. Physiol. 2006 December; 291: H2570 -H2582.

[104] Zimmermann, W, Melynchenko, I, Eschenhagen T. Engineered Heart Tissue for Regeneration of Diseased Hearts. Biomaterials. 2004 April; 25 (9): 1639-1647.

[105] Zhang M, Methot D, Poppa V, Fujio Y, Walsh K, Murry CE. Cardiomyocyte Grafting for Cardiac Repair: Graft Cell Death and Anti-Death Strategies. J. Mol. Cell. Cardiol. 2001 May; 33 (5): 907-921.

[106] Wu KC, Lima JA. Noninvasive Imaging of Myocardial Viability: Current Techniques and Future Developments. Circ. Res. 2003 December; 93 (12): 1146 -1158.

[107] Moroni L, De Wijn JR, Van Blitterswijk CA. 3D Fiber-Deposited Scaffolds for Tissue Engineering: Influence of Pores Geometry and Architecture on Dynamic Mechanical Properties. Biomaterials. 2006 March; 27 (7): 974-985.

[108] Soonpaa MH, Field LJ. Survey of Studies Examining Mammalian Cardiomyocyte DNA synthesis. Circ. Res. 1998 July; 83 (1): 15-26.

[109] Karam JP, Muscari C, Montero-Menei, CN. Combining Adult Stem Cells and Polymeric Devices for Tissue Engineering Infracted Myocardium. Biomaterials. 2012 August; 33 (23): 5683-5695.

[110] Battler A, Granot Y, Cohen S, Leor J, Aboulafia-Etzion S, Dar L. Shapiro, A, Barbash, I.M. Bioengineered Cardiac Grafts: A New Approach to Repair the Infarcted Myocardium? Circulation, 2000 November; 102 Suppl. III: 56-61.

[111] Carrier RL, Papadaki M, Rupnick M, Schoen FJ, Bursac N, Langer R, Freed LE, Vunjak-Novakovic, G. Cardiac Tissue Engineering: Cell Seeding, Cultivation Parameters and Tissue Construct Characterization. Biotechnol. Bioeng. 1999 September; 64 (5): 580 -589.

[112] Chen Q-Z, Bismarck A, Hansen U, Junaid S, Tran MQ, Harding SE, Ali, NN, Boccaccini AR. Characterization of Soft Elastomer poly(glycerol sebacate) Designed to Match the Mechanical Properties of Myocardial Tissue. Biomaterials. 2008 January; 29 (1): 47-57.

[113] De Valence S, Tille J-C, Giliberto J-P, Mrowczynski W, Gurny R, Walpoth BH, Möller, M. Advantages of Bilayered Vascular Grafts for Surgical Applicability and Tissue Regeneration. Acta Biomater. 2012 November; 8 (11): 3914-3920.

[114] Pana L, Yub G, Zhaia D, Leec HR, Zhaod W, Liue N, Wangd H, Teec B-K, Shia Y, Cuid Y, Baob Z. Hierarchical Nanostructured Conducting Polymer Hydrogel with High Electrochemical Activity, PNAS. 2012 June; 109 (24): 9287-9299.

[115] Pedrotty DM, Koh J, Davis BH, Taylor DA, Wolf P, Niklason, LE. Engineering Skeletal Myoblasts: Roles of Three Dimensional Culture and Electrical Stimulation. Am. J. Physiol. Heart Circ. Physiol. 2005 April; 288 (4): H1620-H1626.

[116] Moura RM, Alencar de Queiroz, AA. Dendronized Polyaniline Nanotubes for Cardiac Tissue Engineering. Artif. Organs. 2011 May; 35: 471-477.

[117] Tian L, Prabhakaran MP, Ding X, Kai D, Ramakrishna, S. Emulsion Electrospun Vascular Endothelial Growth Factor Encapsulated poly(L-lactic acid-co-e-caprolactone) Nanofibers

for Sustained Release in Cardiac Tissue Engineering. J. Mater. Sci. 2012 April; 47 (7): 3272-3281.

[118] Tai NR, Salacinski H, Edwards A, Hamilton G, Seifalian AM. Compliance Properties of Conduits used in Vascular Reconstruction. Br. J. Surg. 2000 November; 87 (11): 1480-1488.

[119] Amir G, Miller L, Shachar M, Feinberg MS, Holbova R, Cohen S, Leor J. Evaluation of a Potential Peritoneal-Generated Cardiac Patch in Rat Model of Heterotopic Heart Transplantation. Cell Transplant. 2009 March; 18 (3): 275-282.

[120] Sakai T, Li RK, Weisel RD, Mickle DA, Kim ET, Jia ZQ, Yau TM. The Fate of a Tissue-Engineered Cardiac Graft in the Right Ventricular Outflow Tract of the Rat. J. Thorac. Cardiovasc. Surg, 2001 May; 121 (5): 932-942.

[121] Zimmerman WH, Schneiderbanger K, Schubert P, Didié M, Munzel F, Heubach JF, Kostin S, Neuhuber WL, Eschenhagen T. Tissue Engineering of a Differentiated Cardiac Muscle Construct. Circ. Res. 2002 February; 90 (2): 223-230.

[122] Berglund JD, Mosheni MM, Nerem R, Athanassios S. A Biological Hybrid Model for Collagen-Based Tissue Engineered Vascular Constructs. Biomaterials. 2003 March; 24 (7): 1241-1254.

[123] Dahlmann J, Krause A, Möller L, Kenash G, Möwes M, Diekmann A, Martin U, Kirschning A, Gruh I, Dräger G. Fully Defined *in situ* cross-linkable Alginate and Hyaluronic acid Hydrogels for Myocardial Tissue Engineering. Biomaterials. 2013 January; 34 (4): 940-951.

[124] Singelyn JM, DeQuach JA, Seif-Naraghi SB, Littlefield RB, Schup-Magoffin PJ, Christman KL. Naturally Derived Myocardial Matrix as an Injectable Scaffold for Cardiac Tissue Engineering. Biomaterials. 2009 October; 30 (29): 5409-5416.

[125] Shimizu T, Yamato M, Kikuchi A, Okano T. Cell Sheet Engineering for Myocardial Tissue Reconstruction. Biomaterials. 2003 June; 24 (13) 2309-2316.

[126] Masuda S, Shimizu T, Yamato M, Okano, T. Cell Sheet Engineering For Heart Tissue Repair. Adv. Drug Deliv. Rev. 2008 January; 60 (2): 277-285.

[127] Le Huu A, Xu PL, Prakash S, Shim-Tim D. Recent Advances in Tissue Engineering for Stem Cell-Based Cardiac Therapies. Ther. Deliv. 2013 April; 4 (4): 503-516.

[128] Pittener MF, Martin BJ. Mesenchymal Stem Cells and their Potential as Cardiac Therapeutics. Circ. Res. 2004 July; 95 (1): 9-20.

[129] Mosca JD, Hendricks JK, Buyaner D, Davis-Sproul J, Chuang LC, Majumdar MK, Chopra R, Barry F, Murphy M, Thiede MA, Junker U, Rigg RJ, Forestell SP, Bohnlein E, Storb R, Sandmaier, BM. Mesenchymal Stem Cells as Vehicles for Gene Delivery. Clin. Orthop. Relat. Res. 2000 October; 379 Suppl: S71-S90.

[130] Zuk, PA, Zhu M, Mizuno H, Huang J, Futrell JW, Katz AJ, Benhaim P, Lorenz HP, Hedrick, MH. Multilineage cells from Human Adipose Tissue: Implications for Cell-based Therapies. Tissue Eng. 2001 April; 7 (2): 211-228.

[131] De Bari C, Dell'Accio F, Tylzanowski P, Luyten FP. Multipotent Mesenchymal Stem Cells from Adult Human Synovial Membrane. Arthritis Rheum. 2001 August; 44 (8): 1928-1942.

[132] Diefenderfer DL, Brighton CT. Microvascular Pericytes express Aggrecan Message which is Regulated by BMP-2. Biochem. Biophys. Res. Commun. 2000 March; 269 (1): 172-178.

[133] Zvaifler NJ, Marinova-Mutafchieva L, Adams G, Edwards CJ, Moss J, Burger JA, Maini RN. Mesenchymal Precursor Cells in the Blood of Normal Individuals. Arthritis Res. 2000 August; 2 (6): 477-488.

[134] Green DE, Adler BJ, Chan ME, Rubin CT. Devastation of Adult Stem Cell pools by Irradiation precedes Collapse of Trabecular Bone Quality and Quantity. J. Bone Mineral Res. 2012 April; 27(4): 749-759.

[135] Noth U, Osyczka AM, Tuli R, Hickok NJ, Danielson KG, Tuan RS. Multilineage Mesenchymal Differentiation Potential of Human Trabecular Bone-derived Cells. J. Orthop. Res. 2002 September; 20 (5): 1060-1069.

[136] Fukuda K. Development of Regenerative Cardiomyocytes from Mesenchymal Stem Cells for Cardiovascular Tissue Engineering. Artif. Organs. 2001 March; 25 (3): 187-193.

[137] Abedin M, Tintut Y, Demer LL. Mesenchymal Stem Cells and the Artery Wall. Circ. Res. 2004 October; 95 (7): 671-676.

[138] Saito T, Kuang JQ, Bittira B, Al-Khaldi A, Chiu RC. Xenotransplant Cardiac Chimera: Immune Tolerance of Adult Stem Cells. Ann Thorac Surg. 2002 July; 74 (1): 19-24.

[139] Cho J, Zhai P, Maejima Y, Sadoshima J. Myocardial injection with GSK-3beta-overexpressing Bone Marrow-derived Mesenchymal Stem Cells Attenuates Cardiac Dysfunction after Myocardial Infarction. Circ. Res. 2011 February; 108 (4) 478-489.

[140] Zimmermann, W-H, Didié, M, Döker, S, Melnychenko, I, Naito, H, Rogge, C, Tiburcy, M, Eschenhagen, T. Heart Muscle Engineering: An update on Cardiac Muscle Replacement Therapy. Cardiovasc. Res. 2006 August; 71 (3): 419-429.

[141] O'Shea KS. Embryonic Stem Cell Models of Development. Anat. Rec. 1999 February; 257 (1): 32-41.

[142] Min JY, Yang Y, Converso KL, Liu L, Huang Q, Morgan JP, Xiao YF. Transplantation of Embryonic Stem Cells Improves Cardiac Function in Postinfarcted Rats. J. Appl. Physiol. 2002 January; 92 (1): 288-296.

[143] Xu C, Police S, Rao N, Carpenter MK. Characterization and Enrichment of Cardiomyocytes Derived from Human Embryonic Stem Cells. Circ. Res. 2002 September; 91 (6): 501-508.

[144] Petsche CJ, Camci-Unal G, Khademhosseini A, Jacot JG. Amniotic Fluid derived Stem Cells for Cardiovascular Tissue Engineering Applications. Tissue Eng. Part B. Rev. 2013 August; 19 (4): 368-379.

CHAPTER 3

Nanocrystalline Diamond Films for Biomedical Applications

Cristian Pablo Pennisi[*] and María Alcaide

Department of Health Science and Technology, Aalborg University, Aalborg, Denmark

Abstract: Nanocrystalline diamond films, which comprise the so called nanocrystalline diamond (NCD) and ultrananocrystalline diamond (UNCD), represent a class of biomaterials possessing outstanding mechanical, tribological, and electrical properties, which include high surface smoothness, high corrosion resistance, chemical inertness, superior electrochemical behavior, biocompatibility, and nontoxicity. These properties have positioned the nanocrystalline diamond films as an attractive class of materials for a range of therapeutic and diagnostic applications in the biomedical field. Consequently, the interaction of nanocrystalline diamond films with biomolecules and cells has been focus of intense research during the last years, with many studies focused in tailoring the properties of the films for the control of their biological performance. In this chapter, the current knowledge regarding the biological performance of nanocrystalline diamond films is reviewed from an application-specific perspective, covering topics such as enhancement of cellular adhesion, anti-fouling coatings, non-thrombogenic surfaces, micropatterning of cells and proteins, and immobilization of biomolecules for bioassays. In order to better understand the terminology used in the literature, which is related to the fabrication and surface functionalization of this class of materials, some of the most common approaches for synthesis and modification of CVD diamond films is introduced. Although many challenges still remain, it is envisioned that the application of this unique class of materials will significantly influence the next generation of biomedical devices.

Keywords: Antifouling surfaces, biocompatibility, bionanotechnology, biosensors, blood compatibility, cell adhesion, cell growth, cell-material interface, chemical vapor deposition, diamond films, differentiation, immobilization, implant, micropatterning, nanocrystalline diamond, protein adsorption, surface functionalization, synthetic diamonds, ultrananocrystalline diamond, wettability.

---

*Corresponding Author Cristian Pablo Pennisi: Laboratory for Stem Cell Research, Department of Health Science and Technology, Aalborg University, Fredrik Bajers Vej 3B, DK-9220, Aalborg Ø, Denmark; Tel: +45 9940 2419; Fax: +45 9940 7816; E-mail: cpennisi@hst.aau.dk

1. INTRODUCTION

The nanocrystalline diamond films constitute a unique class of materials within the group of synthetic diamonds. Although these films span a wide range of morphologies and properties, they can be essentially defined as a thin continuous layer of nanometer-sized diamond crystallites (smaller than 100 nm), which are synthesized by using the chemical vapor deposition (CVD) technique [1]. These kind of diamond films possess some unique mechanical, tribological, and electrical properties, which combined with their surface smoothness, high corrosion resistance, chemical inertness, absence of toxicity, and biocompatibility have positioned them as an attractive class of materials for both therapeutic and diagnostic applications in the biomedical field. There are many proposed biomedical applications for which nanocrystalline diamond films hold an unprecedented potential, such as orthopedic and dental implants [2-4], cardiovascular and ophthalmologic devices [5, 6], neural prostheses [7-9], and biosensors [10, 11].

In this chapter, we will review the current knowledge about the biological performance of nanocrystalline diamond films from an application-specific perspective. In order to better understand the terminology used in the different studies, some of the most common approaches for synthesis and modification of CVD diamond films will be introduced. Also, the synthesis of diamond particles will be briefly described in the context of the historical development of synthetic diamonds and due to their application in the process of CVD growth of nanocrystalline diamond films. We do not include here studies involving diamond-like carbon (DLC) films, which are a class of amorphous carbon materials that find widespread application in the biomedical field [12].

2. DIAMOND SYNTHESIS

2.1. General Overview

The exploitation of naturally occurring diamonds for industrial applications is not practically viable, not only due to their scarcity but also for technical reasons. Therefore, for many years, methods for the fabrication of artificial diamonds were investigated. Nowadays, it is possible to obtain synthetic diamonds in form of particles and films with various sizes and qualities, which are readily available from various commercial sources. In the following sections, the most relevant methods in the context of fabrication of nanocrystalline diamond films for biomedical applications will be introduced. Fig. (**1**) illustrates the main types of synthetic diamonds of biomedical interest.

Synthetic diamonds of biomedical interest

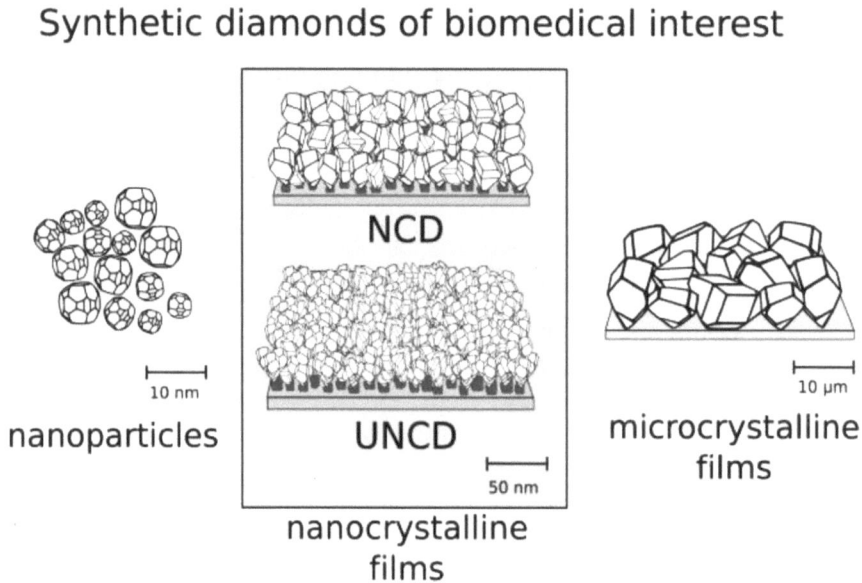

Fig. (1). Types of synthetic diamonds of biomedical interest. Nanoparticles comprise diamond particles with size smaller than 100 nm, which are obtained either by processing HPHT diamond or by detonation synthesis (DND). Polycrystalline diamond films are synthetized by CVD onto non-diamond substrates. They are primarily classified according to the average crystallite size in microcrystalline diamond films (size > 100 nm) and nanocrystalline diamond films (average size <100 nm). The nanocrystalline diamond films are further subdivided in NCD (10 to 100 nm) and UNCD (<10 nm).

2.2. High-Pressure High-Temperature Diamonds

Bundy *et al.* announced the first successful approach for reproducible diamond synthesis in 1955 [13]. The process was inspired in the nature's method for creating diamond, subjecting graphite to elevated pressures and temperatures (approx. 60000 atm and 1000-1400 °C) in presence of a catalyst. This technology constitutes the basis for the current production of the so-called high-pressure-high-temperature (HPHT) diamonds. HPHT diamonds consist of single crystalline diamond particles ranging in size from few nanometers to millimeters, which find many diverse industrial applications, such as cutting tools and abrasives in the mechanical industry, optical components, *etc.* HPHT diamonds have been applied in the fabrication of CVD substrates for the assessment of cell compatibility of single crystalline [9] and polycrystalline diamond films [14, 15].

2.3. Detonation Nanodiamonds

Scientists from the former USSR discovered an alternative method for the fabrication of synthetic diamonds in the 1960's [16]. The approach basically consists in the conversion of a carbon containing explosive (such as trinitrotoluene, TNT) to diamond nanoparticles under a controlled detonation taking place inside a closed container. This class of synthetic diamonds is known as detonation nanodiamond (DND), which have raised tremendous interest during the last years due to their outstanding mechanical, chemical, electronic and optical properties [17]. In particular, DNDs are subject of intense research in the biomedical field for application as drug delivery agents, markers for bioimaging, and components of composite biomaterials. This topic is covered by several detailed reviews in the literature [17-22]. In the context of fabrication of nanocrystalline diamond films, similarly to the HPHT nanoparticles, DNDs are used as seeds for the CVD growth of polycrystalline diamond films onto non-diamond substrates [23, 24].

2.4. Diamond Films

2.4.1. Growth by Chemical Vapor Deposition

Another approach for the synthesis of diamond consists in the thermal decomposition of a carbonaceous gas, such as methane, in presence of hydrogen. The carbon atoms derived from the chemical reactions taking place in the gas phase are deposited onto a solid surface; thereby the process is called chemical vapor deposition. This process was initially developed by the Union Carbide Corporation in the 1950's [25]. One of the major limitations of the original method was its low rate of growth. A major breakthrough in the technique was achieved by researchers from the Japanese Institute for Research in Inorganic Materials (NIRIM) in the 1980's, who were able to obtain good quality diamond films at reasonably high rates [26]. Since then, the interest in the CVD synthesis has grown tremendously and significant development in the technique has been reported [27, 28]. Several methodologies are currently available that allow growing nanocrystalline diamond films on a variety of substrates. These methods share in common the fact that all require a source of energy to activate the chemical reactions in the gas phase. Based on the source used for the activation, the most common methods comprise the hot filament-assisted CVD (HF-CVD) [26], the microwave plasma-enhanced CVD (MP-CVD) [29-31], and the radiofrequency-assisted CVD (RF-CVD) [32]. A detailed review and a comparative analysis of the different modalities can be found in the literature [28].

2.4.2. Types of CVD Diamond Films

By adjusting the growth environment used in the CVD process, it is possible to obtain a range of films with distinct microstructure and physical properties [1]. Two basic forms of diamond films can be synthesized according to the substrate material: single-crystalline diamond (SCD) and poly-crystalline diamond (PCD). SCD films are grown on HPHT substrates and natural diamond. These films are said to be homoepitaxial, since no lattice mismatch exist between the substrate and the newly deposited material. Although the quality of the SCD films produced by CVD is quite high, the need for a monocrystalline diamond substrate makes this procedure rather expensive and also limits the range of applications for which the films can be employed. The cost is reduced and the range of possibilities is expanded when films are grown on non-diamond substrates, such as silicon, titanium or quartz. In this situation the resulting films are polycrystalline, and said to be heteroepitaxial.

PCD films can be divided in categories according to the final crystallite size. Typically, if the crystallites possess an average size that exceeds 100 nm, the films are defined as microcrystalline diamond (MCD). Although MCD films preserve most of the properties of monocrystalline diamonds, they suffer from several disadvantages that limit their application in the biomedical field. The most critical is the very large surface roughness, which not only leads to poor tribological properties but also hinders the homogeneous deposition of films on substrates with surface topographies smaller than the crystallite size. The application of MCD films is therefore limited to the fabrication of abrasive and cutting tools used in dentistry and orthopedic surgery [33, 34]. However, it is expected that the nanocrystalline films, those in which crystallite size is below 100 nm, will reach a much larger impact within the biomedical field. Nanocrystalline diamond films are further subdivided in nanocrystalline diamond (NCD) or ultrananocrystalline diamond (UNCD) according to a criterion that will be discussed in the following section. Fig. (**2**) presents scanning electron micrographs displaying the typical morphology of PCD films. As previously mentioned, nanocrystalline diamond films and their biomedical applications constitute the main focus of this chapter.

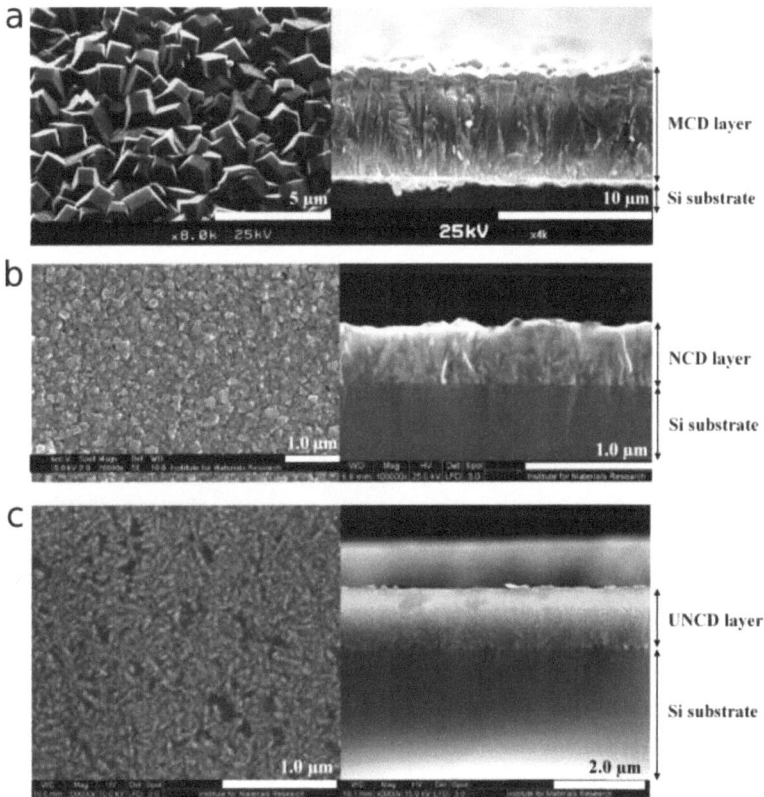

Fig. (2). Typical morphology of the polycrystalline diamond films grown by CVD. Top and cross sectional view scanning electron micrographs of different types of polycrystalline diamond films grown on Si substrates. (**a**) MCD film displaying clearly visible micrometer-sized grains and columnar growth. (**b**) NCD film of approx. 400 nm of thickness grown from hydrogen rich plasma. (**c**) UNCD film of approx. 1 μm in thickness grown from Ar rich plasma. Modified from ref. [11], by Vermeeren *et al.*

2.4.3. Process of Formation of Polycrystalline Diamond Films

There are basically three steps involved in the synthesis of PCD films by CVD: nucleation, formation of a continuous film, and competitive crystal growth [35]. A schematic diagram of the process is depicted in Fig. (**3**). Nucleation corresponds

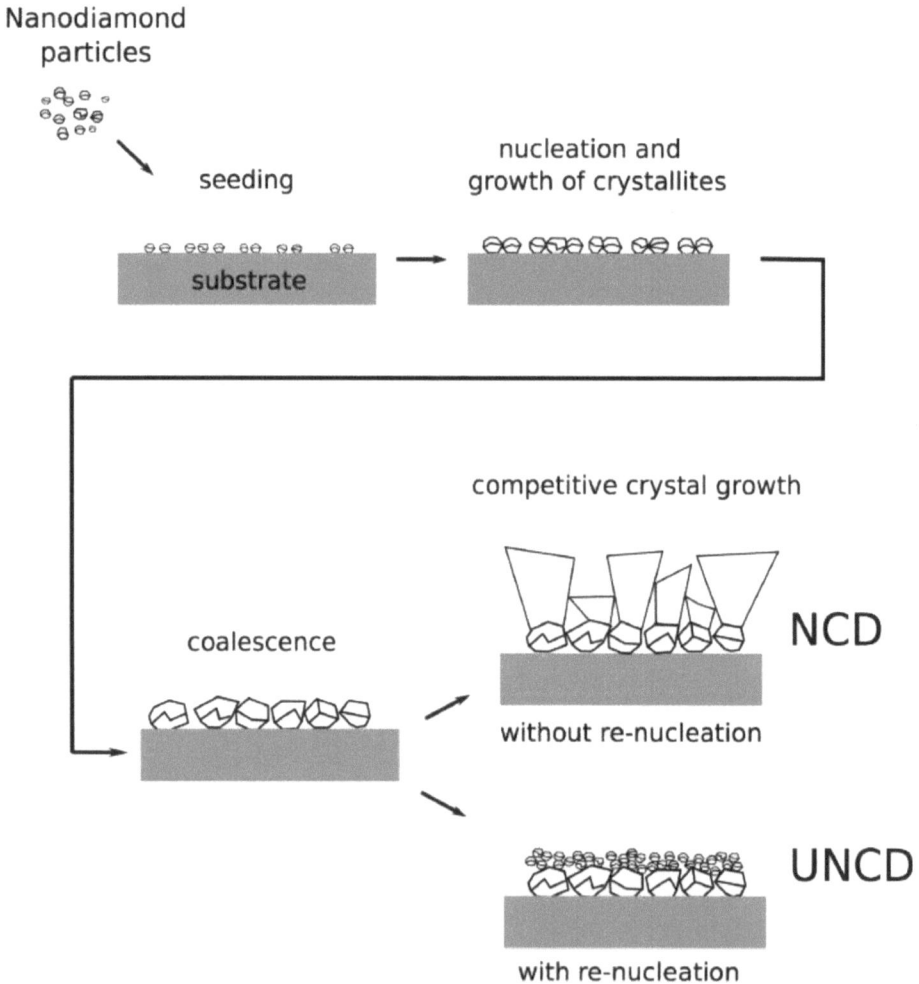

Fig. (3). CVD growth of nanocrystalline diamond films on non-diamond substrates. The process is usually started by seeding the substrate with nanocrystalline diamond particles. Under growth conditions, the seeds are converted to the nuclei of crystalline diamond and begin to grow. Some crystals grow faster and swallow their neighbors. When the crystals coalesce into a continuous film, they start to competitively grow in a vertical direction. Depending on the suppression or enhancement of re-nucleation, the resulting material is called NCD or UNCD.

to the formation of the smallest thermodynamically stable diamond nuclei at the substrate surface. Since this initial step could take prohibitively long time in non-diamond substrates due to the absence of initial sites for a stable carbon binding, diverse strategies have been employed to provide a template for the diamond film [36]. One of the most useful strategies consists in the use of diamond nanoparticles (DND or HPHT), which are pre-adsorbed in the substrate to facilitate the nucleation [37]. Depending on the growth conditions, the nuclei will grow into larger grains and eventually coalesce onto a continuous film, in which some of these grains have fused together. Subsequently, the grains start to grow in a direction perpendicular to the substrate, leading to a columnar structure in which faster growing structures overgrow the slower ones. Diverse parameters, such as initial seeding density, growth chemistry and surface temperature will determine the relative growth rate of the columns and the final mechanical, morphological and chemical properties of the film [23]. Films that are grown with a very high initial nucleation density, in a conventional diamond growth process (in which the ratio of hydrogen to methane is high), and whose thickness does not typically exceed few microns, tend to have grains smaller than 100 nm and are designated as nanocrystalline diamond (NCD) [38]. Other types of films, which are grown in Ar-rich plasma with little or no hydrogen content, display a significant interruption of the crystal formation process. This is caused by the appearance of new nucleation sites, meaning that grain coarsening does not occur. This type of diamond films, in which a high re-nucleation rate keeps the grain size in the range of few nanometers independently of the film thickness, are denominated ultrananocrystalline diamond (UCND) [39].

3. CONTROLLING THE PROPERTIES OF NANOCRYSTALLINE DIAMOND FILMS

3.1. Surface Termination

Surface properties such as wettability, reactivity, and surface conductivity of a material are strongly dependent on the surface termination. As-grown nanocrystalline diamond films present a hydrogen-terminated surface, which is stable under atmospheric conditions and displays a contact angle around 93° [40]. In addition, H-terminated diamond surfaces display a high surface conductivity

[41]. Upon appropriate physical or chemical treatment, the surface termination can be changed by several functional groups. Thus, O-terminated diamond surfaces can be obtained by exposure to an O_2 rich plasma [4, 24, 42, 43] or by UV oxidation [44]. Upon oxidation diamond surfaces are rendered hydrophilic and the surface potential vanishes. Depending on the oxidation level, the water contact angle can be reduced below 5°. On the contrary, by exposing the diamond surface to fluorine radicals, such as by using CF_4 plasmas, superhydrophobic diamond surfaces can be obtained [45].

The primary aim of surface modification is to tailor the surface properties of the diamond. As a general principle, as it will be shown later, hydrophilic surfaces are preferred to promote cell attachment while hydrophobic and superhydrophobic surfaces are used to prevent biofouling of the material. However, modification of the diamond surface termination is also desired when the aim is to promote the covalent attachment of a variety of molecules such as proteins, DNA, or macromolecular complexes, as it will be described in the following sections.

3.2. Surface Functionalization

Covalent grafting of diverse organic or bioorganic molecules can extend the functionalities offered by the different surface termination groups described in the previous section. Molecular monolayers grafted to the diamond surfaces can provide the moieties for the covalent coupling of a wide variety of biomolecules, such as DNA or proteins [46]. In addition, the presence of an intermolecular layer between the material and the bioorganic molecules can help preventing non-specific adsorption. Most of the approaches for the covalent grafting of organic molecular layers on diamond have been developed for H-terminated surfaces. The most common method consists in photochemical grafting of alkene-based molecules [47]. Functionalization can also be induced by means of simple chemical or electrochemical reactions, grafting the organic layers *via* reaction with diazonium salts [48, 49]. For the functionalization of O-terminated diamond surfaces, some of the primary functionalization methods include silanization [50] and esterification [51], both dependent on the reaction with surface hydroxyl groups present in the surface upon oxidation.

The molecular monolayers grafted on the diamond surface provide specific reactive groups to which the bioorganic molecules can covalently attach. For the covalent attachment of proteins, the reactive groups are usually selected to react with the amine of surface lysine residues or the thiol of surface cysteine residues [52].

3.3. Doping

The crystalline structure of diamond is constituted by a three dimensional lattice of carbon atoms forming very strong C-C bonds, displaying a with a wide 5.5 eV band gap. This makes diamond an excellent electrical insulator, with a typical conductivity above 10^9 $\Omega \cdot cm$. Polycrystalline CVD films are also insulating in nature, though conductivity is increased due to the presence of graphitic carbon, impurities and lattice defects. Extrinsic conductivity can be induced by means of doping, which can produce diamond CVD films displaying a wide range of electrical properties, from semiconductor to semi-metallic behavior depending on the level of doping [23, 27].

NCD films can achieve a p-type semiconductor behavior by means of boron doping. Boron doping is realized by addition of a boron containing gas such as diborane or trimethylboron during the CVD process. Heavily boron doped NCD films represent an attractive material for use as electrode in bioelectrochemical applications [53, 54]. The main advantages of this type of electrodes are the low and stable capacitive background current, which allows larger sensitivities, and the very wide potential window for water stability (up to 3.2 V in water, in contrast to 1.3 V for platinum). Although the synthesis and characterization of boron doped NCD films has been extensively studied, the fabrication of n-type doped diamond films remains a challenge [53, 55, 56].

In the case of UNCD films, doping is achieved by incorporation of nitrogen in the gas mixture during the CVD deposition [57]. Nitrogen does not act as conventional dopant, but it is believed that nitrogen atoms are incorporated into the grain boundaries, giving rise to graphitic grain boundary conduction [58].

4. BIOMEDICAL APPLICATIONS OF NANOCRYSTALLINE DIAMOND FILMS

4.1. Surfaces Supporting Cellular Adhesion

In the context of cell material interactions, adhesion is the process involving the development of anchorage contacts between the cells and material surface. Although in the absence of serum proteins cells can adhere by nonspecific interactions on surfaces, here we only consider relevant to discuss approaches in which integrin mediated anchorage is involved, since interaction between integrins and cell adhesion molecules regulates cell behaviours like proliferation, migration, and differentiation [59-61]. As it will be described in the following sections, nanocrystalline diamond films provided by appropriate chemistries or cell-adhesion ligands seem to be an optimal approach for a variety of applications in which cell adhesion to a material surface is desired, both *in vitro* and *in vivo*.

4.1.1. Interfacing Bone Tissue for Orthopaedic Applications

As mentioned before, nanocrystalline diamond films seem to be well suited for orthopaedic applications due to their superior properties, such as hardness, durability, and wear resistance. Thus, nanocrystalline diamond has been envisioned as an ideal interface for bone implants, based on a number of studies that have investigated the adhesion, proliferation, metabolic activity, and differentiation of bone-derived cells [3, 62-66]. Several studies investigated the behaviors of the MG63 human osteoblast-like cell line on NCD films grown on silicon substrates by MP-CVD [62, 64, 67]. These studies have shown that cells on hydrophilic O-terminated NCD surfaces displayed mature cytoskeletons, as evidenced by a large amount of actin filaments and focal adhesions. Other studies, using osteoblasts cultured for up to two weeks on NCD films, have shown that cells displayed increased differentiation levels, supported by higher alkaline phosphatase (ALP) activity, protein synthesis, and mineral deposition (calcium and phosphate) [3, 68, 69]. As an example, Amaral *et al.* have investigated the behavior of osteoblasts on HF-CVD films grown on Si_3N_4 substrates, showing that these coatings elicited an enhanced cell proliferation and the stimulation of differentiation markers, such as ALP activity and matrix mineralization (see Fig. 5). In agreement with these findings, other studies have shown that bone marrow-derived mesenchymal stem cells also increase their metabolic activity on NCD films, even though their adhesion is similar to polystyrene control surfaces [70]. From these studies, it appears to be a correlation between surface properties (specific topography and chemistry) of the nanocrystalline diamond films and osteoblast functions, since cells show enhanced cell functions on O-terminated and NH$_3$-terminated surfaces rather than H-terminated surfaces [4, 68]. In addition, it has also been suggested that osteoblast functions may be enhanced on NCD surfaces presenting a surface topography similar to that of the bone [70].

The effect of boron doping on the behavior of osteoblasts has been also subject of a recent investigation [71]. The authors have employed NCD films grown on silicon substrates by MP-CVD, which were doped with various levels of boron. After assessing the number of osteoblasts after 7 days in culture, they observed a higher growth in all boron-doped samples in contrast to the intrinsic films. Immunofluorescent analysis of focal adhesion complexes by talin staining revealed that this protein was better organized in boron-doped NCD films than in the undoped controls (see Fig. **4**). Cells displayed a viability that was close to 100%, a clear increase in the number of focal adhesions, and higher levels of collagen I, ALP and osteocalcin, which suggests that surface charge may have an important effect in the cellular behavior.

A promising approach for increasing the biocompatibility of nanocrystalline diamond films in the context of orthopedic implants consists in the immobilization of bioactive molecules that influence the process of bone healing. Thus, NCD films grown on titanium surfaces have been efficiently functionalized with bone morphogenetic protein-2 (BMP-2) by simple physisorption [72]. BMP-2 appears firmly bound to the surface and fully active, especially when interacting with O-terminated NCD surfaces, as shown by the fact that cells in contact with the biomaterial strongly up-regulate ALP [72]. NCD coated implants were further tested *in vivo* in a sheep model [73]. The results confirmed the *in vitro* observations, demonstrating improved osseointegration outcomes for the O-terminated BMP-adsorbed surfaces after 4 weeks of implantation. Interestingly, when comparing the results regarding surface termination alone, O-terminated surfaces outperformed the H-terminated ones [73].

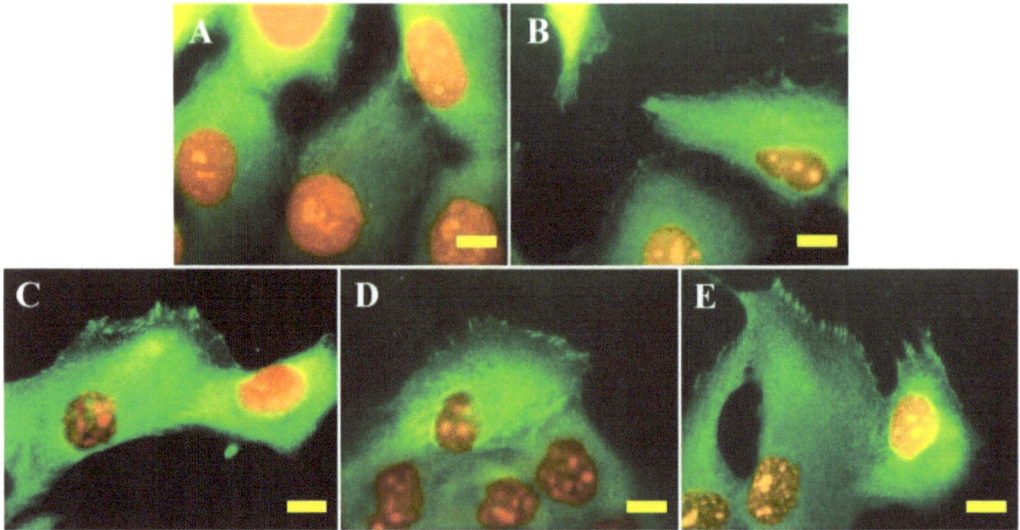

Fig. (4). Effect of boron doping on cell adhesion. Immunofluorescence staining of talin in MG 63 osteoblast-like cells on day 3 after seeding on: (A) glass coverslips, (B) undoped NCD, (C) NCD films doped with boron in concentrations of 133 ppm, (D) 1000 ppm, and (E) 6700 ppm. The cell nuclei are counterstained with propidium iodide. Calibration bar = 10 μm. Modified from ref. [69], ©2011 by Grausova *et al*.

In summary, surface properties of the NCD films such as chemistry, topography and charge have a strong influence on the fate of cultured osteoblasts, which reflects the fact that cell behavior is highly dependent on the microenvironmental conditions. As previously mentioned, the surface properties of NCD films can be easily tailored, which could be used to modulate osteoblast proliferation and bone growth in orthopedic implants and other bone tissue engineering applications.

4.1.2. Interfacing Soft Tissue

NCD films also represent an attractive alternative for biomedical implants in which an improvement of soft-tissue attachment is required, such as in the transmucosal part of osseointegrated dental implants. In these applications, the aim is to create a soft tissue seal to prevent infections and implant loosening [74]. Since the tissue seal involves both epithelial and connective tissue components, several studies have investigated *in vitro* the adhesion of epithelial cell types and fibroblasts on nanocrystalline films.

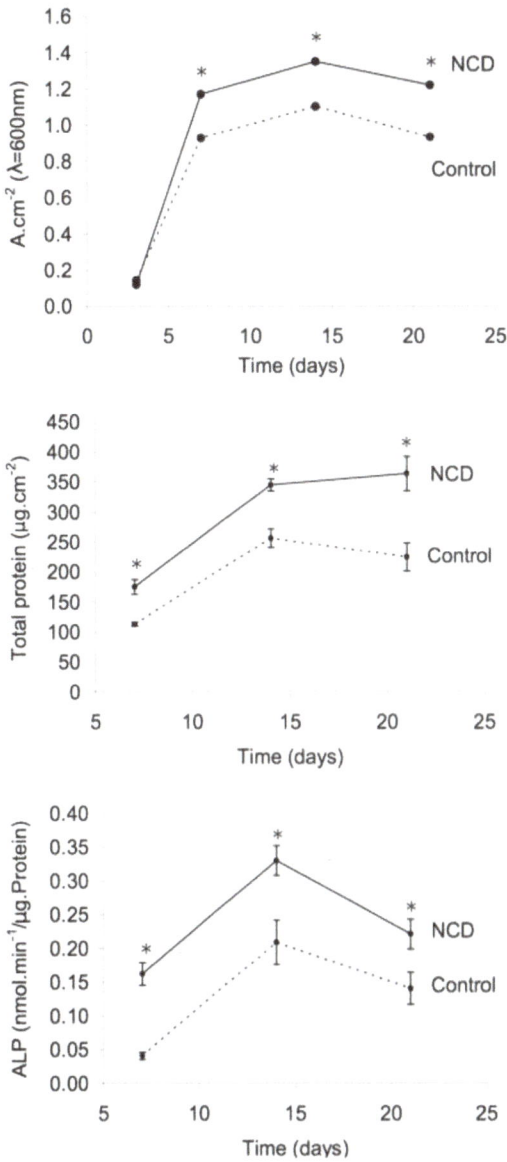

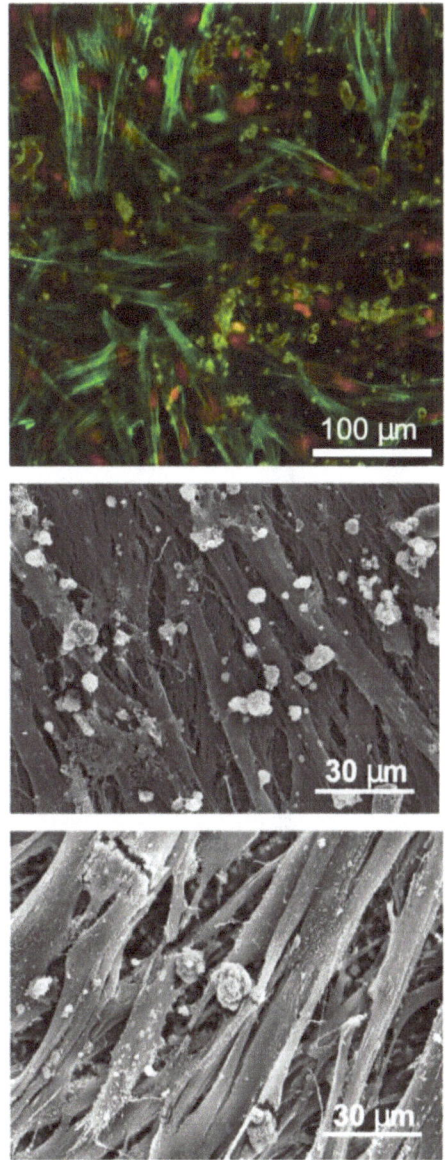

Fig. (5). Responses of osteoblasts cultured on NCD films. (a) Cell viability/proliferation, **(b)** total protein content, and **(c)** ALP activity of human bone marrow osteoblast cells grown on NCD-coated Si_3N_4 substrates for 21 days. Asterisk denotes statistically different from the control. The images to the right display: **(d)** immunofluorescent staining of osteoblast cultures after 21 days on NCD films (phalloidin, propidium iodide, and calcein staining), and scanning electron micrographs of cells on **(e)** NCD and **(f)** tissue culture polystyrene, showing the morphology and the presence of mineral deposits. Modified from ref [3], ©2008 by Margarida Amaral *et al*.

Bajaj and coworkers have compared cell adhesion, proliferation, and growth of HeLa cells and fibroblasts on UNCD films. They have found an increased attachment and proliferation of cells on UNCD films, when comparing to other substrates like platinum or silicon [75]. Accordingly, other studies have found that primary fibroblasts displayed the maximum cytoplasmic and nuclear area on UNCD films, indicating a greater affinity of the cells for the material [44]. Studies by Lechleitner *et al.* have shown the importance of surface termination in controlling epithelial cell adhesion to NCD surfaces. They have shown that attachment and proliferation of these cells is enhanced on O-terminated surfaces, in contrast to H- terminated surfaces, suggesting that the lack of functional polar groups prevents adherent cells from settling on the NCD surface [76]. On the other hand, Amaral *et al.* have assessed the behavior of L929 fibroblasts and human gingival fibroblasts cultured on NCD films grown on Si_3N_4 ceramic substrates by HF-CVD [77]. After analyzing cell adhesion, viability, and proliferation for 8 days, they have shown that cell proliferation is slightly higher for both cell types compared to polystyrene controls. NCD coatings offered a suitable surface for cell attachment, spreading and proliferation and were completely covered with continuous cell layers after few days. Remarkably, their films were used "as prepared", which indicates that cell adhesion to the NCD surface was enhanced even without a hydrophilic treatment or surface functionalization. Smisdom *et al.* have assessed the growth and viability of Chinese hamster ovary (CHO) cells cultured on H- and O-terminated MP-CVD MCD and NCD films [78]. They have shown absence of toxicity and an equivalent growth of cells on all surfaces irrespective of the topography or surface termination. This apparent lack of effect from surface chemistry and topography might be explained by recent studies from Klauser and coworkers. They have assessed the behavior of epithelial cells on O-terminated NCD coatings, showing that cells are able to attach after 24 to 72 hours with and without addition of fetal bovine serum (FBS) to the growth medium. Remarkably, the experiments performed on hydrophobic surfaces (H-NCD and F-NCD) have shown that cell-adhesion is only possible in the presence of FBS, suggesting that the proteins contained in the serum are important mediators of cell adhesion, independently of their chemical termination [24].

One of the first reports of the *in vivo* biocompatibility of NCD films has been carried out using a subcutaneous implantation rat model [79]. This study aimed to assess the tissue responses to implanted titanium discs in which NCD was grown by HF-CVD. Their results show that hydrophilicity has a positive influence on the tissue healing at the implant surfaces, revealed by an increase in the number of cells and the attachment of connective tissue to the O-terminated implant surfaces. Interestingly, the inflammatory response was also reduced in the peri-implant area of the O-terminated implants.

4.1.3. Neural Interfacing Applications

Nanocrystalline diamond films are also being investigated as promising materials to improve the stability of neural interfaces, for applications ranging from *in vitro* platforms used for neurophysiologic studies to implantable neural prosthesis [6, 9, 80]. The interaction of neural cells with nanocrystalline diamond films and particles has been primarily studied *in vitro* using neural cell lines. These studies have demonstrated that cells are able to attach, display high viability, low content of reactive oxygen species, and lack of alteration of the mitochondrial membrane [81-83]. Ariano *et al.* have also observed that neural cell lines can adhere and maintain their functionality when cultured on H-terminated NCD substrates despite its hydrophobic nature, revealing the spontaneous electrical activity by capacitive coupling with the cell membrane [9]. Other studies investigated the behavior of primary neurons on functionalized NCD films, assessing parameters such as neuronal morphology, outgrowth, synaptic activity, ion channel availability, and calcium signals during stimulation [84, 85]. These studies have shown that primary neurons can be successfully cultured for several days on the NCD films, displaying neurite extensions, and keeping their electrical properties, including spontaneous action potentials. However, unlike transformed cell lines or other primary cell types such as fibroblasts, surface functionalization was needed to successfully promote neural cell attachment.

UNCD films also represent promising substrates for neural applications, since it has been shown that they are able to spontaneously induce neuronal differentiation of neural stem cells [8]. Using MP-CVD UNCD films grown on quartz substrates, both H- and O- terminated, it was found that stem cell differentiation is promoted even in absence of differentiation reagents. In the case of H-terminated samples, the mechanism seems to be mediated by the absorption of fibronectin, which activates an integrin β1-Fak-Erk signaling pathway. Furthermore, the different terminations, -H or -O, possess different neural differentiation abilities towards neurons and oligodendrocytes respectively [7, 8]. These observations suggest that UNCD could be used as a potential material for central nervous system applications in tissue engineering or cell transplantation

4.2. Antifouling Surfaces

The progress on implant technologies requires special attention to possible surface colonization by microorganisms. It is estimated that around 60% of all microbial infections are caused by biofilms that create a reservoir for immunologically quiet bacteria, release toxic substances and can cause high resistance to antibiotics. Bacterial adhesion and biofilm formation are both mediated by proteins adsorbed onto the material surface. In this direction, several studies have focused on the analysis of biomaterial susceptibility to bacterial adhesion and infection and their capacity to reduce colonization and formation of biofilms. Observations on the bactericide and bacterial anti-adhesive properties of different materials when incubated with *E. Coli* cells, with and without pre-treatment with proteins, have evidenced that bacterial colonization depends on the previous adhesion of proteins and that CVD-NCD surfaces present the highest resistance to it, even in the presence of plasma proteins, compared to other materials such as stainless steel, and very similar to titanium [94]. Furthermore, Medina *et al.* have analysed the ability of *Pseudomona aeruginosa* to colonize different surfaces, including H-terminated HF-CVD NCD [86]. NCD exhibits bactericidal effects within 24 hours and shows the lowest bacterial colonization density after Cu. Surface roughness and free energy are parameters expected to influence the rate of bacterial colonization of the different surfaces. However, not all data show a correlation between them and the anti-adhesive activity of the materials and, even though it is generally believed that hydrophobic surfaces with a large contact angle favour anti-bacterial properties, results here are contradictory, with cases when a decrease of bacterial adhesion is correlated by a reduction in the hydrophobicity. As previously mentioned, interaction of cells with NCD is favoured by O-terminated surfaces and bacteria require similar conditions for their survival, it is expected that H-terminated NCD substrates will not favour their colonization. It appears to be an association of the anti-bacterial properties of NCD and its semiconductivity, so that the electrically active surface of NCD interacts with the bacterial membrane altering its morphology and avoiding adhesion and colonization [86].

Another major problem of the adhesion of surface-active materials, such as proteins, is the interference with working electrodes that lead to alterations and even suppression of the recording signals. The resistance of diamond electrodes to protein adhesion has been evidenced by voltammetry measurements in the presence of various proteins and surfactants showing that, specifically in the case of boron-doped diamond films, this material displays insignificant fouling effects and is very resistant to surfactant interferences, making it ideal for electro analytical applications [87].

4.3. Patterning of Cells and Proteins

Micropatterning of living cells on solid substrates has recently attracted much attention due to its extensive range of applications, especially for cell-based bioassays, tissue-engineering and fundamental studies of cell biology [88-90]. Micrometer-sized patterns allow the study of cell sensitivity for fine spatial cues and thus enable more complex investigations of morphogenesis, cell polarity, and cell division axis. Most cell micropatterning methods focus on how interactions between cells and surfaces control cell adhesion.

A variety of techniques have been developed for patterning cellular growth. The most commonly used methods include micro-contact printing (MCP), photolithography, inkjet printing and stencil-assisted patterning techniques. These techniques generally involve patterning proteins or factors that either attract (extra-cellular matrix proteins, such as poly-lysine) or repel cellular attachment (anti-biofouling agents), although some techniques have focused on the direct placement of cells. MCP has been used to produce patterns of laminin and poly-lysine for spatially directing the growth of primary hippocampal and cortical neurons on many different substrates, including glass, polystyrene and diamond [81]. Inkjet printing has been widely used for depositing patterns of liquids and suspensions onto surfaces at micrometer-scale resolutions. Laser micromachining uses a high-power focused laser beam to directly write patterns into the substrate surface, or into the polymer adhesion layer upon which the cells subsequently grow. UV-directed light micropatterning has been recently introduced for its ability either to oxidize surface coatings, and thus destroy their anti-adhesive properties, or to de-protect or activate photosensitive linkers [91].

Most of these techniques are being used in central nervous system applications, where the aim is to direct neuronal growth in an ordered manner while reducing glial scarring, thus improving the recorded signal quality to increase the long-term performance of devices such as brain computer interfaces (BCI) [80]. Electrodes fail very often when implanted into the central nervous system because of the glial encapsulation, known as glial scarring, that limits their long-term functionality.

Due to its excellent properties, CVD diamond has attracted much attention as a base material for neural implant coatings to achieve reduced levels of glial scarring and spatially control growth of neurons on different surfaces. Its mechanical and chemical properties make it very suitable for improving the long-term performance of the invasive electrodes systems used in BCIs, as it does the fact that can be modified with dopants. In the case of boron doping, it increases the electrical conductivity of diamond making it more suitable for electrode applications. Therefore boron-doped NCD has been tested in a number of studies for spatially directing neural cell growth and limiting the attachment of cells involved in the immune response and foreign body reaction. May *et al.* have successfully cultured neurons on H- and O- terminated boron-doped NCD surfaces by laser micro machining, achieving a spatially directed neuronal growth along predesigned pathways. Cells grow well across the coatings avoiding crossing over the etched areas and forming a spatially defined surface [92]. Regan *et al.* have tried different micropatterning techniques including inkjet printing and laser micro-machining to control neural adhesion and modify inflammatory cell attachment onto boron-doped NCD surfaces resulting in an improvement in neural connectivity [80]. Marcon *et al.* report a new method using UV-directed light to pattern cells in a spatially controlled manner exploiting the superhydrophobic/superhydrophilic wetting contrast of chemically functionalized boron- doped NCD nanowires that has a great impact on cell adhesion. This approach enables the production of single-cell arrays without any geometrical constraints, opening a wide range of possible applications in the development of cell-based biological assays in well-controlled and biologically relevant environments [91].

Although most work has been done with neural cells, some other studies have used other cells, like osteoblasts, showing a selective adhesion and arrangement of these cells on NCD grown on silicon substrates by CVD, which was microscopically patterned with H- and O- terminated regions (see Fig. **6**) [93]. Control of cellular density and serum concentration in the cell medium influences colonization of the substrates with preference for O-terminated regions and a lower evolution of cell morphology in H-terminated areas. In this case, to reach an optimal status, cells communicate and secrete ECM, modifying the surface. This mechanism enables to overgrow electrically conductive H-terminated surfaces when surrounded by O-terminated regions at small dimensions, making it very attractive for bio-electronic applications [93]. Although this area of research is still in development, the results obtained so far indicate that microtailored NCD substrates could provide great benefits for applications in bioelectronics, tissue engineering and biotechnology.

4.4. Development of Non-Thrombogenic Coatings

Hemocompatibility is a characteristic of great importance for a biomaterial, since blood is usually the first body fluid contacting with implants or other medical devices. The interaction of blood with biomaterials includes, primarily, adsorption of plasma proteins on their surfaces right after implantation followed by platelet adhesion that contributes to a surface-induced thrombosis. An inflammatory reaction takes place as well, with the recruitment of leukocytes, fibroblast proliferation and collagen synthesis. Thus, a long exposure to blood can cause embolization, calcification and changes in the biomaterial properties that can compromise the stability and functionality of the implanted devices.

To reduce clotting, materials and surfaces with high protein-resistant properties have been investigated. Some strategies have developed strongly hydrophilic and

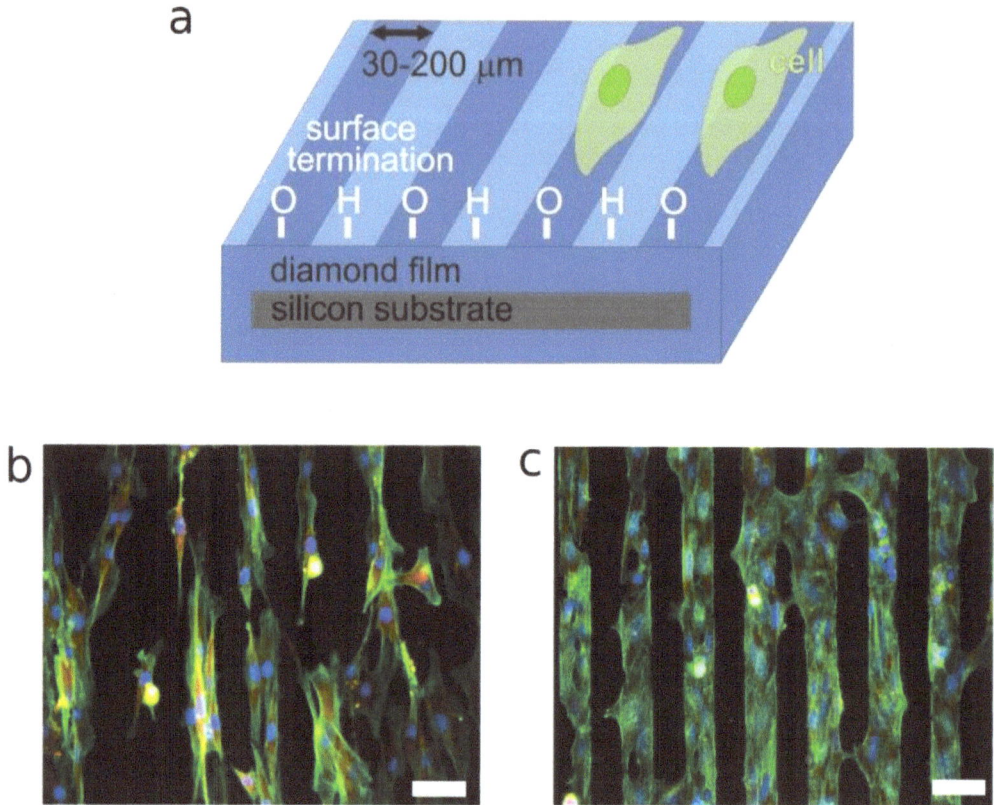

Fig. (6). Micropatterning of NCD films. (a) Schematic picture of micropatterned substrates consisting of silicon hermetically coated with NCD. The micro-stripes possessed either H- or O-surface termination. Cell adhesion on the O-terminated region is also schematically illustrated. The fluorescence micrographs depict (b) human periodontal fibroblasts and (c) HeLa cells cultivated on 30 μm H-/O-micropatterns. The cells aligned on the O-terminated regions, some of them forming bridges across H-terminated regions. Scale bar 50 μm. Modified from ref [91], © 2009 by Rezek *et al.*

strongly hydrophobic surfaces, other are based in the immobilization of bioactive molecules such as heparin or urokinase, coating with albumin or the attachment of endothelial cells as an attempt of mimicking the internal surface of blood vessels and their fibrinolytic activity.

One of the first studies reporting the biocompatibility of NCD films was performed by Tang *et al.* in 1995 [94], who have assessed the adsorption of fibrinogen, the *in vitro* adhesion of polymorphonuclear cells (PMN), and the inflammatory responses after 1 week of implantation in a mice model. The amount of adsorbed fibrinogen to NCD films was similar than to other biomaterials, including stainless steel and titanium. The adhesion of PMN to plasma pre-incubated samples was similar to that on stainless steel but 40% lower than that on titanium. Similar to the other biomaterials, minimal inflammatory responses were found on the implanted NCD samples [94].

Okroj *et al.* have shown that NCD-coated steel exhibits a higher level of resistance to blood platelet adhesion and thrombus formation than the bare material, presenting a practically free-of adhered platelets surface after 1 hour incubation with whole blood. In addition, the NCD coating can also prevent ion release [95]. These observations correspond well with other *in vitro* studies showing that NCD films cause reduced plasma protein adsorption [96] and that aggregation of proteins or platelets barely occurs on the surface of the films [97]. Further indication of the excellent hemocompatibility of NCD films has been recently provided by an *in vivo* study, which has shown that NCD coated stents are able to significantly reduce the neointimal hyperplasia in a pig coronary artery model [98]. In perspective, it is expected that NCD films will be established as blood contacting material for use in cardiovascular applications such as heart valves and vascular stents.

4.5. Immobilization of Biomolecules for Biosensing Applications

A biosensor is a device that uses biological receptors for the detection of an analyte that usually is a biological substance too. In general, the detection is performed by selective, biological receptors such as enzymes, antibodies, nucleic acids, membranes or cells, whereas biomimetic sensors use synthetic receptors, such as molecularly imprinted polymers. Biosensors are devices designed to detect or quantify biochemical molecules, and they have been widely used as powerful analytical tools in areas such as medical diagnostics, food industry, and environmental monitoring. A biosensor is usually fabricated by immobilizing a biological receptor material on the surface of a suitable transducer that converts the biochemical signal into quantifiable electronic signals, which can be used to detect proteins, nucleic acids or antigen-antibody interactions. An ideal biosensor should combine nature's sensitivity and specificity with the advantages of modern microelectronics [10, 99, 100].

Thanks to its dual role as a substrate for bio-functionalization, presenting high strength of C-C bonds, and as an electrode, with the capacity to promote different electron transfer reactions, its low background current and its large electrochemical potential window, nanocrystalline diamond films are particularly attractive substrates for biosensor applications. Recent advances in the synthesis of highly conducting NCD thin films have led to an entirely new class of electrochemical biosensors and bioinorganic interfaces. Diamond nanowires as well can be a new approach towards next generation electrochemical gene sensor platforms.

The role of NCD has been investigated in the fabrication of biosensors binding very different molecules. Studies assessing different substrates for DNA immobilization have demonstrated that NCD films have superior properties to those of other materials such as glass, gold or silicon [99]. The general principle of the diamond-based DNA sensor research is to develop a prototype biosensor for diagnostic purposes based on DNA covalently attached to CVD diamond with the same sensitivity and specificity as the commonly used methods, such as blotting techniques and microarrays, but with the particular benefits of allowing real time and label-free measurements for optical, electronic and acoustic read-out [101, 102]. Other studies have tried to immobilize RNA and proteins in order to determine RNA-protein and RNA-RNA interactions on NCD surfaces [103]. The aim is to apply these experimental conditions based on RNA biosensor systems for a variety of biotechnological applications, such as screening approaches for early diagnosis of cancer.

Diamond films are also excellent platforms for studies using supported lipid bilayers to investigate physiological processes such as ligand-receptor interactions, membrane disruption and cell signaling. Optically transparent diamond films offer a unique combination of transparency and surface conductance, allowing detection of permeation events based on optical and field-effect properties, which have been used to investigate the effects of an antimicrobial peptide on the permeability of supported artificial lipid bilayers [104]. Other approach for highly sensitive measurement of peptide-induced membrane disruption consists in the use of conducting boron-doped diamond films, which are employed as active electrodes for the electrochemical impedance spectroscopy measurements [105].

Other biosensors that have been around for many years involve the use of many different types of enzymes, immobilization chemistries and substrates. Thus, glucose sensors for example, work using this principle, and the covalent immobilization of glucose oxidase or similar enzymes forms the basis for commercial devices. Garrido *et al*. have analyzed the immobilization of the enzyme catalase on diamond, showing promising results for the use of this material also for enzyme-based biosensors [99]. Another interesting application of nanocrystalline diamond films in the field of biosensors is that of linking antibodies to diamond surfaces (UNCD) for the detection of bacterial pathogens [106]. The UNCD film minimizes the desorption of antibody from the surface due to the strong chemical bond, while the activity is maintained due to reduced water density and reduced antibody-surface interactions. The ability to selectively capture bacterial cells can be kept stable even after exposure to buffer solutions at 37 °C for periods up to 2 weeks [106].

5. SUMMARY

In this chapter, the interaction of nanocrystalline diamond films with biomolecules and cells, as well as approaches to control these interactions, have been reviewed. It has been shown that properties such as wettability, electric conductivity, and surface chemistry have a significant impact in the control of these interactions. Accordingly, it has been shown that the properties of nanocrystalline diamond films can be tailored to facilitate the control of biological responses such as adsorption and immobilization of proteins, cellular adhesion, and thrombogenicity. Although many correlations have been clearly established, some discrepancies still remain, as for instance regarding the effect of surface wettability on the protein and cellular attachment. These discrepancies are probably caused by the diversity in growth conditions, substrate preparation methods, surface pretreatment, and biological models that are employed by each research group. Therefore, one of the focus areas for further research will be related to standardization of the conditions for film growth and modification. For some of the intended applications the full potential of nanocrystalline diamond films will be revealed only when appropriate proof-of-concept experiments are carried out, including relevant *in vitro* and *in vivo* assays.

ACKNOWLEDGEMENTS

We are grateful to Andy Taylor for critically reading the manuscript and providing helpful comments. Also, we thank Veronique Vermeeren, Margarida Amaral, and Bohuslav Rezek for providing the original images reproduced in this work. This work was supported by the EU through the project MERIDIAN (Micro and Nano Engineered Bi-Directional Carbon Interfaces for Advanced Peripheral Nervous System Prosthetics and Hybrid Bionics), contract n. 280778-02.

CONFLICT OF INTEREST

The authors confirm that this chapter contents have no conflict of interest.

ABBREVIATIONS

CVD	=	Chemical vapor deposition
DND	=	Detonation nanodiamond
HF-CVD	=	Hot filament chemical vapor deposition
HPHT	=	High-pressure high-temperature diamond
MCD	=	Microcrystalline diamond
MP-CVD	=	Microwave plasma enhanced chemical vapor deposition
NCD	=	Nanocrystalline diamond
PCD	=	Poly-crystalline diamond
RF-CVD	=	Radiofrequency-assisted chemical vapor deposition
SCD	=	Single-crystalline diamond
UNCD	=	Ultrananocrystalline diamond

REFERENCES

[1]   Williams OA. Nanocrystalline diamond. *Diam Relat Mater* 2011; 20: 621-40.

[2]   Yang L, Sheldon BW, Webster TJ. Orthopedic nano diamond coatings: Control of surface properties and their impact on osteoblast adhesion and proliferation. *J. Biomed. Mater. Res.* 2008; 91: 548-56.

[3]   Amaral M, Gomes PS, Lopes MA, Santos JD, Silva RF, Fernandes MH. Nanocrystalline Diamond as a Coating for Joint Implants: Cytotoxicity and Biocompatibility Assessment. *J Nanomater* 2008; 2008: 1-9.

[4]   Yang L, Li Y, Sheldon BW, Webster TJ. Altering surface energy of nanocrystalline diamond to control osteoblast responses. *J. Mater. Chem.* 2011; 22: 205.

[5]   Xiao X, Wang J, Liu C, Carlisle JA, Mech B, Greenberg R, *et al*. *In vitro* and *in vivo* evaluation of ultrananocrystalline diamond for coating of implantable retinal microchips. *J. Biomed. Mater. Res.* 2006; 77: 273-81.

[6]   Hadjinicolaou AE, Leung RT, Garrett DJ, Ganesan K, Fox K, Nayagam DAX, *et al*. Electrical stimulation of retinal ganglion cells with diamond and the development of an all diamond retinal prosthesis. *Biomaterials* 2012; 33: 5812-20.

[7]   Chen YC, Lee DC, Hsiao CY, Chung YF, Chen HC, Thomas JP, *et al*. The effect of ultra-nanocrystalline diamond films on the proliferation and differentiation of neural stem cells. *Biomaterials* 2009; 30: 3428-35.

[8]   Chen YC, Lee DC, Tsai TY, Hsiao CY, Liu JW, Kao CY, *et al*. Induction and regulation of differentiation in neural stem cells on ultra-nanocrystalline diamond films. *Biomaterials* 2010; 31: 5575-87.

[9]   Ariano P, Budnyk O, Dalmazzo S, Lovisolo D, Manfredotti C, Rivolo P, *et al*. On diamond surface properties and interactions with neurons. *Eur Phys J E Soft Matter* 2009; 30: 149-56.

[10]   Wenmackers S, Vermeeren V, Vandeven M, Ameloot M, Bijnens N, Haenen K, *et al*. Diamond-based DNA sensors: surface functionalization and read-out strategies. *Physica Status Solidi A Appl Res* 2009; 206: 391-408.

[11]   Vermeeren V, Wenmackers S, Wagner P, Michiels L. DNA sensors with diamond as a promising alternative transducer material. *Sensors* 2009; 9: 5600-36.

[12]   Roy RK, Lee K-R. Biomedical applications of diamond-like carbon coatings: A review. *J. Biomed. Mater. Res.* 2007; 83B: 72-84.

[13]   Bundy FP, Hall HT, Strong HM, Wentorf RH. Man-made diamonds. *Nature* 1955; 176: 51-5.

[14]   Liu YL, Sun KW. Protein Functionalized Nanodiamond Arrays. *Nanoscale Res Lett* 2010; 5: 1045-50.

[15]   Girard HA, Perruchas S, Gesset C, Chaigneau M, Vieille L, Arnault J-C, *et al*. Electrostatic grafting of diamond nanoparticles: a versatile route to nanocrystalline diamond thin films. *ACS Appl Mater Interfaces* 2009; 1: 2738-46.

[16]   Danilenko VV. On the history of the discovery of nanodiamond synthesis. *Phys Solid State* 2004; 46: 595-9.

[17]   Mochalin VN, Shenderova O, Ho D, Gogotsi Y. The properties and applications of nanodiamonds. *Nature Nanotech* 2011; 7: 11-23.

[18] Lam R, Ho D. Nanodiamonds as vehicles for systemic and localized drug delivery. *Expert Opin. Drug Deliv.* 2009; 6: 883-95.

[19] Schrand AM, Suzanne A, Hens C, Shenderova OA. Nanodiamond particles: properties and perspectives for bioapplications. *CRC Cr Rev Sol State* 2009; 34: 18-74.

[20] Krueger A. Beyond the shine: recent progress in applications of nanodiamond. *J. Mater. Chem.* 2011; 21: 12571-8.

[21] Zhu Y, Li J, Li W, Zhang Y, Yang X, Chen N, *et al.* The biocompatibility of nanodiamonds and their application in drug delivery systems. *Theranostics* 2012; 2: 302.

[22] Krueger A, Lang D. Functionality is Key: Recent Progress in the Surface Modification of Nanodiamond. *Adv. Funct. Mater.* 2012; 22: 890-906.

[23] Williams OA, Nesládek M, Daenen M, Michaelson S, Hoffman A, Osawa E, *et al.* Growth, electronic properties and applications of nanodiamond. *Diam Relat Mater* 2008; 17: 1080-8.

[24] Klauser F, Hermann M, Steinmüller Nethl D, Eiter O, Pasquarelli A, Bertel E, *et al.* Direct and Protein-Mediated Cell Attachment on Differently Terminated Nanocrystalline Diamond. *Chem Vapor Depos* 2010; 16: 42-9.

[25] Eversole WG. Synthesis of Diamond. USPTO; 3, 030, 187, 1958.

[26] Matsumoto S, Sato Y, Tsutsumi M, Setaka N. Growth of diamond particles from methane-hydrogen gas. *J Mater Sci* 1982; 17: 3106-12.

[27] Butler JE, Sumant AV. The CVD of nanodiamond materials. *Chem Vapor Depos* 2008; 14: 145-60.

[28] Gracio JJ, Fan QH, Madaleno JC. Diamond growth by chemical vapour deposition. *J Phys D Appl Phys* 2010; 43: 374017.

[29] Kamo M, Sato Y, Matsumoto S, Setaka N. Diamond synthesis from gas phase in microwave plasma. *J Cryst Growth* 1983; 62: 642-4.

[30] Bachmann PK. Microwave plasma CVD and related techniques for low pressure diamond synthesis. In: Thin Film Diamond. Dordrecht: *Springer Netherlands*; 1994; pp. 31-53.

[31] Taylor A, Fendrych F, Fekete L, Vlcek J, Rezacova V, Petrak V, *et al.* Novel high frequency pulsed MW-linear antenna plasma-chemistry: Routes towards large area, low pressure nanodiamond growth. *Diam Relat Mater* 2011; 20: 613-5.

[32] Meyer DE. Radio-frequency plasma chemical vapor deposition growth of diamond. *J. Vac. Sci. Technol. A* 1989; 7: 2325.

[33] Trava-Airoldi VJ, Corat EJ, Leite NF, do Carmo Nono M, Ferreira NG, Baranauskas V. CVD diamond burrs — Development and applications. *Diam Relat Mater* 1996; 5: 857-60.

[34] Amar M, Ahmed W, Sein H, Jones AN, Rego CA. Chemical vapour deposition of diamond coatings onto molybdenum dental tools. *J Phys: Condens Matter* 2003; 15: S2977-82.

[35] May PW. Diamond thin films: a 21st-century material. *Philos T Roy Soc A* 2000; 358: 473-95.

[36] Liu H, Dandy DS. Studies on nucleation process in diamond CVD: an overview of recent developments. *Diam Relat Mater* 1995; 4: 1173-88.

[37] Das D, Singh RN. A review of nucleation, growth and low temperature synthesis of diamond thin films. *Int. Mat. Rev.* 2007; 52: 29-64.

[38] Philip J, Hess P, Feygelson T, Butler JE, Chattopadhyay S, Chen KH, *et al.* Elastic, mechanical, and thermal properties of nanocrystalline diamond films. *J. Appl. Phys.* 2003; 93: 2164.

[39] Gruen DM. Nanocrystalline diamond films. *Annu. Rev. Mater. Sci.* 1999; 29: 211-59.

[40]   Ostrovskaya L, Perevertailo V, Ralchenko V, Saveliev A, Zhuravlev V. Wettability of nanocrystalline diamond films. *Diam Relat Mater* 2007; 16: 2109-13.

[41]   Maier F, Riedel M, Mantel B, Ristein J, Ley L. Origin of Surface Conductivity in Diamond. *Phys. Rev. Lett.* 2000; 85: 3472-5.

[42]   Michalikova L, Rezek B, Kromka A, Kalbacova M. CVD diamond films with hydrophilic micro-patterns for self-organisation of human osteoblasts. *Vacuum* 2009; 84: 61-4.

[43]   Kromka A, Grausova L, Bacakova L, Vacik J, Rezek B, Vanecek M, *et al.* Semiconducting to metallic-like boron doping of nanocrystalline diamond films and its effect on osteoblastic cells. *Diam Relat Mater* 2010; 19: 190-5.

[44]   Chong KF, Loh KP, Vedula SRK, Lim CT, Sternschulte H, Steinmüller D, *et al.* Cell Adhesion Properties on Photochemically Functionalized Diamond. *Langmuir* 2007; 23: 5615-21.

[45]   Freedman A, Stinespring CD. Fluorination of diamond (100) by atomic and molecular beams. *Appl. Phys. Lett.* 1990; 57: 1194.

[46]   Szunerits S, Boukherroub R. Different strategies for functionalization of diamond surfaces. *J Solid State Electr* 2008; 12: 1205-18.

[47]   Hamers RJ, Butler JE, Lasseter T, Nichols BM, Russell JN Jr., Tse K-Y, *et al.* Molecular and biomolecular monolayers on diamond as an interface to biology. *Diam Relat Mater* 2005; 14: 661-8.

[48]   Kuo T-C, McCreery RL, Swain GM. Electrochemical Modification of Boron-Doped Chemical Vapor Deposited Diamond Surfaces with Covalently Bonded Monolayers. *Electrochem Solid St* 1999; 2: 288-90.

[49]   Wang J, Firestone MA, Auciello O, Carlisle JA. Surface Functionalization of Ultrananocrystalline Diamond Films by Electrochemical Reduction of Aryldiazonium Salts. *Langmuir* 2004; 20: 11450-6.

[50]   Notsu H, Fukazawa T, Tatsuma T, Tryk DA, Fujishima A. Hydroxyl groups on boron-doped diamond electrodes and their modification with a silane coupling agent. *Electrochem Solid St* 2001; 4: H1-H3.

[51]   Delabouglise D, Marcus B, Mermoux M, Bouvier P, Chane-Tune JRM, Petit J-P, *et al.* Biotin grafting on boron-doped diamond. *Chem. Commun.* 2003; 99: 2698-9.

[52]   Garrido JA. Biofunctionalization of Diamond Surfaces: Fundamentals and Applications. In: Sussmann/CVD Diamond for Electronic Devices and Sensors. Chichester, UK: *John Wiley & Sons, Ltd*; 2009; pp. 399-437.

[53]   Vanhove E, de Sanoit J, Mailley P, Pinault MA, Jomard F, Bergonzo P. High reactivity and stability of diamond electrodes: The influence of the B-doping concentration. *Physica Status Solidi A Appl Res* 2009; 206: 2063-9.

[54]   Wei JJ, Li CM, Gao XH, Hei LF, Lvun FX. The influence of boron doping level on quality and stability of diamond film on Ti substrate. *Appl Surf Sci* 2012; 258: 6909-13.

[55]   Kraft A. Doped diamond: a compact review on a new, versatile electrode material. *Int. J. Electrochem. Sci* 2007; 2: 355-85.

[56]   Luong JHT, Male KB, Glennon JD. Boron-doped diamond electrode: synthesis, characterization, functionalization and analytical applications. *Analyst* 2009; 134: 1965-79.

[57]   Bhattacharyya S, Auciello O, Birrell J, Carlisle JA, Curtiss LA, Goyette AN, *et al.* Synthesis and characterization of highly-conducting nitrogen-doped ultrananocrystalline diamond films. *Appl. Phys. Lett.* 2001; 79: 1441.

[58] Birrell J, Gerbi JE, Auciello O, Gibson JM, Gruen DM, Carlisle JA. Bonding structure in nitrogen doped ultrananocrystalline diamond. *J. Appl. Phys.* 2003; 93: 5606.

[59] Giancotti FG, Ruoslahti E. Integrin signaling. *Science* 1999; 285: 1028-33.

[60] Cavalcanti-Adam EA, Micoulet A, Blümmel J, Auernheimer J, Kessler H, Spatz JP. Lateral spacing of integrin ligands influences cell spreading and focal adhesion assembly. *Eur J Cell Biol* 85: 219-24.

[61] Pennisi CP, Dolatshahi-Pirouz A, Foss M, Chevallier J, Fink T, Zachar V, *et al.* Nanoscale topography reduces fibroblast growth, focal adhesion size and migration-related gene expression on platinum surfaces. *Colloids and Surfaces B: Biointerfaces* 2011; 85: 189-97.

[62] Bacakova L, Grausova L, Vacik J, Fraczek A, Blazewicz S, Kromka A, *et al.* Improved adhesion and growth of human osteoblast-like MG 63 cells on biomaterials modified with carbon nanoparticles. *Diam Relat Mater* 2007; 16: 2133-40.

[63] Grausova L, Kromka A, Bacakova L, Potocky S, Vanecek M, Lisa V. Bone and vascular endothelial cells in cultures on nanocrystalline diamond films. *Diam Relat Mater* 2008; 17: 1405-9.

[64] Kalbacova M, Michalikova L, Baresova V, Kromka A, Rezek B, Kmoch S. Adhesion of osteoblasts on chemically patterned nanocrystalline diamonds. *Phys Status Solidi B Basic Solid State Phys* 2008; 245: 2124-7.

[65] Rezek B, Ukraintsev E, Kromka A, Ledinský M, Broz A, Nosková L, *et al.* Assembly of osteoblastic cell micro-arrays on diamond guided by protein pre-adsorption. *Diam Relat Mater* 2010; 19: 153-7.

[66] Bacakova L, Filova E, Parizek M, Ruml T, Svorcik V. Modulation of cell adhesion, proliferation and differentiation on materials designed for body implants. *Biotechnol. Adv.* 2011; 29: 739-67.

[67] Babchenko O, Kromka A, Hruska K, Kalbacova M, Broz A, Vanecek M. Fabrication of nano-structured diamond films for SAOS-2 cell cultivation. *Physica Status Solidi A Appl Res* 2009; 206: 2033-7.

[68] Kalbacova M, Broz A, Babchenko O, Kromka A. Study on cellular adhesion of human osteoblasts on nano-structured diamond films. *Phys Status Solidi B Basic Solid State Phys* 2009; 246: 2774-7.

[69] Yang L, Sheldon BW, Webster TJ. The impact of diamond nanocrystallinity on osteoblast functions. *Biomaterials* 2009; 30: 3458-65.

[70] Broz A, Baresova V, Kromka A, Rezek B, Kalbacova M. Strong influence of hierarchically structured diamond nanotopography on adhesion of human osteoblasts and mesenchymal cells. *Physica Status Solidi A Appl Res* 2009; 206: 2038-41.

[71] Grausova L, Kromka A, Burdikova Z, Eckhardt A, Rezek B, Vacik J, *et al.* Enhanced growth and osteogenic differentiation of human osteoblast-like cells on boron-doped nanocrystalline diamond thin films. *PLoS ONE* 2011; 6: e20943.

[72] Steinmüller-Nethl D, Kloss FR, Najam-Ul-Haq M, Rainer M, Larsson K, Linsmeier C, *et al.* Strong binding of bioactive BMP-2 to nanocrystalline diamond by physisorption. *Biomaterials* 2006; 27: 4547-56.

[73] Kloss FR, Gassner R, Preiner J, Ebner A, LARSSON K, Hächl O, *et al.* The role of oxygen termination of nanocrystalline diamond on immobilisation of BMP-2 and subsequent bone formation. *Biomaterials* 2008; 29: 2433-42.

[74] Berglundh T, Lindhe J, Ericsson I, Marinello CP, Liljenberg B, Thornsen P. The soft tissue barrier at implants and teeth. *Clin Oral Implants Res* 1991; 2: 81-90.

[75]   Bajaj P, Akin D, Gupta A, Sherman D, Shi B, Auciello O, *et al.* Ultrananocrystalline diamond film as an optimal cell interface for biomedical applications. *Biomed Microdevices* 2007; 9: 787-94.

[76]   Lechleitner T, Klauser F, Seppi T, Lechner J, Jennings P, Perco P, *et al.* The surface properties of nanocrystalline diamond and nanoparticulate diamond powder and their suitability as cell growth support surfaces. *Biomaterials* 2008; 29: 4275-84.

[77]   Amaral M, Gomes PS, Lopes MA, Santos JD, Silva RF, Fernandes MH. Cytotoxicity evaluation of nanocrystalline diamond coatings by fibroblast cell cultures. *Acta Biomater* 2009; 5: 755-63.

[78]   Smisdom N, Smets I, Williams OA, Daenen M, Wenmackers S, Haenen K, *et al.* Chinese hamster ovary cell viability on hydrogen and oxygen terminated nano-and microcrystalline diamond surfaces. *Physica Status Solidi A Appl Res* 2009; 206: 2042-7.

[79]   Kloss FR, Steinmüller Nethl D, Stigler RG, Ennemoser T, Rasse M, Hächl O. *In vivo* investigation on connective tissue healing to polished surfaces with different surface wettability. *Clin Oral Implants Res* 2011; 22: 699-705.

[80]   Regan EM, Taylor A, Uney JB, Dick AD, May PW, McGeehan J. Spatially controlling neuronal adhesion and inflammatory reactions on implantable diamond. *IEEE J. Emerg. Sel. Topics Power Electron.* 2011; 1: 557-65.

[81]   Specht CG, Williams OA, Jackman RB, Schoepfer R. Ordered growth of neurons on diamond. *Biomaterials* 2004; 25: 4073-8.

[82]   Schrand AM, Huang H, Carlson C, Schlager JJ, Ōsawa E, Hussain SM, *et al.* Are Diamond Nanoparticles Cytotoxic? *J. Phys. Chem. B* 2007; 111: 2-7.

[83]   Frewin CL, Jaroszeski M, Weeber E, Muffly KE, Kumar A, Peters M, *et al.* Atomic force microscopy analysis of central nervous system cell morphology on silicon carbide and diamond substrates. *J. Mol. Recognit.* 2009; 22: 380-8.

[84]   Ariano P, Baldelli P, Carbone E, Gilardino A, Giudice Lo A, Lovisolo D, *et al.* Cellular adhesion and neuronal excitability on functionalised diamond surfaces. *Diam Relat Mater* 2005; 14: 669-74.

[85]   Thalhammer A, Edgington RJ, Cingolani LA, Schoepfer R, Jackman RB. The use of nanodiamond monolayer coatings to promote the formation of functional neuronal networks. *Biomaterials* 2010; 31: 2097-104.

[86]   Medina O, Nocua J, Mendoza F, Gómez-Moreno R, Ávalos J, Rodríguez C, *et al.* Bactericide and bacterial anti-adhesive properties of the nanocrystalline diamond surface. *Diam Relat Mater* 2012; 22: 77-81.

[87]   Shin D, Tryk DA, Fujishima A, Merko i A, Wang J. Resistance to Surfactant and Protein Fouling Effects at Conducting Diamond Electrodes. *Electroanalysis* 2005; 17: 305-11.

[88]   Chen CS, Mrksich M, Huang S, Whitesides GM, Ingber DE. Micropatterned Surfaces for Control of Cell Shape, Position, and Function. *Biotechnol. Prog.* 1998; 14: 356-63.

[89]   Kane RS, Takayama S, Ostuni E, Ingber DE, Whitesides GM. Patterning proteins and cells using soft lithography. *Biomaterials* 1999; 20: 2363-76.

[90]   Shen CJ, Fu J, Chen CS. Patterning cell and tissue function. *Cel. Mol. Bioeng.* 2008; 1: 15-23.

[91]   Marcon L, Addad A, Coffinier Y, Boukherroub R. Cell micropatterning on superhydrophobic diamond nanowires. *Acta Biomater* 2013; 9: 4585-91.

[92]   May PW, Regan EM, Taylor A, Uney J, Dick AD, McGeehan J. Spatially controlling neuronal adhesion on CVD diamond. *Diam Relat Mater* 2012; 23: 100-4.

[93]   Rezek B, Michalikova L, Ukraintsev E, Kromka A, Kalbacova M. Micro-pattern guided adhesion of osteoblasts on diamond surfaces. *Sensors* 2009; 9: 3549-62.

[94]   Tang L, Tsai C, Gerberich WW, Kruckeberg L, Kania DR. Biocompatibility of chemical-vapour-deposited diamond. *Biomaterials* 1995; 16: 483-8.

[95]   Okroj W, Kamińska M, Klimek L, Szymański W, Walkowiak B. Blood platelets in contact with nanocrystalline diamond surfaces. *Diam Relat Mater* 2006; 15: 1535-9.

[96]   Walkowiak B, Jakubowski W, Okroj W, Kochmanska V, Kroliczak V. Interaction of body fluids with carbon surfaces. 2001; pp. 75-6.

[97]   Narayan RJ, Wei W, Jin C, Andara M, Agarwal A, Gerhardt RA, *et al.* Microstructural and biological properties of nanocrystalline diamond coatings. *Diam Relat Mater* 2006; 15: 1935-40.

[98]   Kocka V, Jirasek T, Taylor A, Fendrych F, Rezek B, Simunkova S, *et al.* Novel Nanocrystalline Diamond Coating of Coronary Stents Reduces Neointimal Hyperplasia in Pig Model. *Exp Clin Cardiol* 2014; 20: 65-76.

[99]   Härtl A, Schmich E, Garrido JA, Hernando J, Catharino SCR, Walter S, *et al.* Protein-modified nanocrystalline diamond thin films for biosensor applications. *Nat Mater* 2004; 3: 736-42.

[100] Qureshi A, Gurbuz Y, Howell M, Kang WP, Davidson JL. Nanocrystalline diamond film for biosensor applications. *Diam Relat Mater* 2010; 19: 457-61.

[101] Vermeeren V, Bijnens N, Wenmackers S, Daenen M, Haenen K, Williams OA, *et al.* Towards a Real-Time, Label-Free, Diamond-Based DNA Sensor. *Langmuir* 2007; 23: 13193-202.

[102] Vermeeren V, Wenmackers S, Daenen M, Haenen K, Williams OA, Ameloot M, *et al.* Topographical and Functional Characterization of the ssDNA Probe Layer Generated Through EDC-Mediated Covalent Attachment to Nanocrystalline Diamond Using Fluorescence Microscopy. *Langmuir* 2008; 24: 9125-34.

[103] Popova B, Kulisch W, Popov C, Hammann C. Immobilization of RNA and Protein Biomolecules on Nanocrystalline Diamond for the Development of New Biosensors. In: Functional Properties of Nanostructured Materials. *Springer*; 2006; pp. 515-20.

[104] Ang PK, Loh KP, Wohland T, Nesladek M, Van Hove E. Supported Lipid Bilayer on Nanocrystalline Diamond: Dual Optical and Field-Effect Sensor for Membrane Disruption. *Adv. Funct. Mater.* 2009; 19: 109-16.

[105] Petrak V, Grieten L, Taylor A, Fendrych F, Ledvina M, Janssens SD, *et al.* Monitoring of peptide induced disruption of artificial lipid membrane constructed on boron-doped nanocrystalline diamond by electrochemical impedance spectroscopy. *Physica Status Solidi A Appl Res* 2011; 208: 2099-103.

[106] Radadia AD, Stavis CJ, Carr R, Zeng H, King WP, Carlisle JA, *et al.* Control of Nanoscale Environment to Improve Stability of Immobilized Proteins on Diamond Surfaces. *Adv. Funct. Mater.* 2011; 21: 1040-50.

Frontiers in Biomaterials, Vol. 1, 2014, 101-128   101

CHAPTER 4

Bioceramics-Design, Synthesis and Biological Applications

A.C. Jayalekshmi and Chandra P. Sharma[*]

Division of Biosurface Technology, Biomedical Technology Wing, Sree Chitra Tirunal Institute for Medical Sciences and Technology, Poojappura, Thiruvananthapuram 695012, Kerala, India

Abstract: This chapter discusses in detail the design and synthetic strategies of ceramics for biomedical application, the biocompatibility as well as new emerging trends towards the application of ceramic materials in the biomedical field. Ceramics are a promising group of materials having potential applications in various fields such as engineering, technology, medicine *etc.* They are inorganic materials and can be prepared by high temperature as well as low temperature processes. The porosity, crystallinity, composition *etc.* are the features which determine the property of ceramics. These characteristics were tuned to get a desired property at the molecular level for the intended application by appropriate modification in the synthesis process of ceramics as well as functionalization with other materials. They could be designed from bulk materials to nano level materials. They usually fall in the category of bioinert, bioactive as well as resorbable ceramics. Based on their activity they find application in biomedical field. In the biomedical field ceramic materials were used as substitute materials for bone and teeth as well as coatings for metallic implants. Advanced research is going on in the molecular level modification of ceramic materials for developing artificial transplantation materials, drug release materials as well as materials for tissue engineering and gene therapy applications.

Keywords: Artificial implants, biocompatibility, bioglass, ceramics, calciumphosphate, drug delivery, gene delivery, hydroxyapatite, synthesis of ceramics, tissue engineering.

INTRODUCTION

Ceramic materials have wide range of applications, from building materials such as flooring materials to materials used in aero planes and space shuttles. They are

*Corresponding Author Chandra P. Sharma: Division of Biosurface Technology, Biomedical Technology Wing, Sree Chitra Tirunal Institute for Medical Sciences and Technology, Poojappura, Thiruvananthapuram 695012, Kerala, India; Tel: +91 471 2520294; Fax: +91 471 2341814; E-mail: drcpsharma@rediffmail.com

inorganic nonmetallic solid materials. They are often processed at high temperature and cooled to room temperature. Ceramic materials used for biological application fall into three major groups: Bioinert, Bioactive and Bioresorbable. Table **1** shows the classification of ceramic materials based on the performance in biological environment.

Table 1.   **Classification of Ceramic Materials Based on their Bioactivity**

Classification	Examples
Bioinert	Alumina Zirconia Crystalline Carbon (Diamond like) Calcium aluminates Silica ceramics
Bioactive	Hydroxyapatite Bioglass
Bioresorbable	Calcium phosphate group materials Hydroxyapatite Bioglass

Ceramic materials can also be classified into oxide ceramics and non-oxide ceramics. The oxide ceramics such as alumina, zirconia are bioinert ceramics. These ceramics were used for developing acetabular cavities, plates and screws for bone repair and also for hip replacement. Ceramic materials containing phosphate group have high bioactivity, biocompatibility and bone integration and they possess similar composition as that of inorganic fraction of bone. The remarkable bioactivity and biocompatibility of phosphate glasses make them suitable materials for biomedical applications and controlled drug release. Calcium phosphates (CAP) group ceramics comprises: Monocalcium phosphate monohydrate (Ca $(H_2PO_4)_2$. H_2O), Dicalcium phosphate dihydrate (CaHPO$_4$. $2H_2O$), Dicalcium phosphate anhydrous (CaHPO$_4$), Octacalcium phosphate (Ca$_8$ (PO$_4$)$_6$.5H$_2$O), Amorphous calcium phosphate (ACP) (Ca$_3$ (PO$_4$)$_2$, α-tricalcium phosphate (α-TCP) (α-Ca$_3$ (PO$_4$)$_2$), β-tricalcium phosphate (β-Ca$_3$ (PO$_4$)$_2$), tetracalcium phosphate (Ca$_4$ (PO$_4$)$_2$O) and hydroxyapatite (Ca$_{10}$ (PO$_4$)$_6$(OH)$_2$). Scaffolds can be prepared from calcium phosphates, which support bone formation, osteoblast adhesion and proliferation [1]. Calcium phosphate group materials form a functional interface with the host tissue when implanted in contact with biological environment and protein and cell adhesion occur on the CAP surface forming a calcified matrix. The one unit cell of Hydroxyapatite (HA) ($Ca_5 (PO_4)_3(OH)$) comprises two entities and denoted as $Ca_{10} (PO_4)_6 (OH)_2$. The OH^- can be replaced with F^-, Cl^- or CO_3^{2-}. The mineral part of bone and teeth is comprised of HA and is commonly used as a filler to replace damaged bone. Prosthetic implants were coated with HA to promote bone growth. Hydroxyapatite (HA) also promote calcification *in vitro* and *in vivo*, but the process is slow and addition of substituents in the HA matrix increases the bioactivity [2-4]. Bioactive nanoceramics are useful for bone replacement and drug delivery. Their size, meso-porosity, pore volume, tunable surface, apatite forming ability *etc.* make them suitable for hard tissue regeneration. 45S5 bioglass powder could be used as a bioactive and biodegradable scaffold material [5]. Under optimum sintering conditions they produce fine crystals of $Na_2Ca_2Si_3O_9$, which upon immersion in simulated body fluid get converted into bioactive amorphous calcium phosphate within 28 days of immersion period. The crystallinity of the bioactive glass has a prominent role in determining this transformation kinetics.

Ceramic Materials were used in hard tissue replacement, drug delivery and tissue engineering in the field of dentistry, orthopaedics and plastic surgery. They were used as components of dental implants, hip implants, middle ear implants and heart valves. They were generally more chemically stable and inert than most metals due to their chemical bonding. There is considerable difference between normal bone and ceramics. Ceramic materials were used for bone filling because they can maintain porosity and inter connecting pore system. Ceramic based materials were considered ideal scaffolds if they provide good mechanical stability along with bioactivity as well as show degradation at a later stage in a tunable manner. 45S5 bioglass is such type of an ideal scaffold. Ceramic materials were used for implant applications for more than three decades because these materials have similar surface composition as that of bioactive materials and the mineral phase of bone. They were used for drug release because the controlled release makes efficient utilization of the drug and produce minimum side effects.

Ceramic materials have a promising future in biomedical materials field because some of them were conductors, some others were insulators and they can be made magnetic. They have piezo electric properties as well as they can be made photosensitive by incorporating suitable inorganic materials. Based on these properties ceramic materials and its composites were modified for various applications. The molecular level modifications of ceramic materials with functional additives will result in new variety of biomedical materials. The design and development of ceramic materials have great influence on the biomedical applications. The present chapter discusses how the design and synthesis of ceramic materials were carried out for specific biomedical applications as well as their present and future applications.

DESIGN OF CERAMIC MATERIALS FOR BIOMEDICAL APPLICATIONS

The design of ceramic materials for specific biomedical application was carried out by controlling the particle size, porosity, surface area, tensile strength, elasticity *etc.* The influence of these parameters is discussed in detail here.

Particle Size

Particle size has great importance in the properties of ceramics. The nanoceramics have unique properties due to their size in the nanoscale regime. The particle size could be controlled by adding inhibitors during the sintering process of ceramics. The inhibitors can reduce the activity occurring in particle boundary and it can inhibit particle growth [6]. An example of this is seen in the preparation of bioactive nanotitania ceramics. When hydroxyapatite was used as particle growth inhibitor it enhanced the biomechanical compatibility of nanotitania ceramics, while magnesium oxide as inhibitor reduced the biomechanical compatibility of nanotitania [7]. HA and TCP particles having diameter in between 0.5-1.0 mm promote bone development by transplantation of human bone marrow stromal cells (BMSCs). Particles having diameter in the range of 0.1-0.25 mm show enhanced bone growth, and the reason may be the difference in cell attachment with difference in surface area [8]. The cellular response of ceramics inside the body and the expression of genes by the release of active ions were influenced by its particle size [9].

Porosity

The properties of ceramics were determined to a large extent by the porosity of the surface. By controlling the processing parameters of ceramics the porosity, pore size and shape could be controlled [10]. The volatile by-products water and alcohol, formed during the low-temperature sol-gel process introduces porosity in ceramic matrix produced by such processes. But the drying step degrades the thermo-labile substances, which could be overcome by room temperature evaporation by applying uni-axial pressure. The uniaxial pressure method can also be used for preparing drug loaded ceramic particles with maximum drug loading efficiency since the drugs which were affected by high temperature loading and preparation process remain unaffected during the low temperature sol-gel process. The behaviour of bioglass in tissue formation is largely dependent on chemical composition and its textural property such as pore size and pore volume [11, 12]. Spherical nano-bioglass having 80-90 nm with mesopores having 3-5 nm were produced by a sono-reacted sol-gel process. They exhibit excellent apatite forming ability and low cellular toxicity when subjected to *in vitro* test. Macropores contribute large porosity while micropores contribute small porosity in the total percentage porosity of ceramics [13]. Macro-porous ceramics contain large number of micro-pores and such type of ceramics exhibit bone formation after three months of implantation [14]. Mesoporous bioactive glasses possess improved surface area and nanopore volume, and it enhances bioactivity and degradation and also increases the rate of drug delivery [15, 16]. Small drug molecules and gene (small interfering RNA, siRNA) could be delivered *via* such type of mesoporous ceramics [17]. siRNA nanoparticles are taken up by cells and thus nano bioglass could be made as suitable carriers for gene delivery.

The poor mechanical strength makes porous ceramics non-favourable for load bearing (implant) applications. The traditional porous sintered ceramics must be replaced by bioresorbable macroporous ceramic scaffold for implantation purpose.

Surface Area

The surface area and surface roughness greatly influences the properties of ceramics. Nanocrystalline ceramic powders have greater surface area and it improves fracture toughness and mechanical property of hard tissue implants [18]. Acid etching was used to create micro-roughness on the surface of the bioglass and this result in a greater area for cell-material interaction. The increase in microroughness did not reduce the mechanical strength [19]. The selective adsorption of serum proteins cause the osteoblast cell attachment and mineralization as surface roughness increases [20]. Tubular shaped bioactive glass has greater bioactive surface area capable of forming hydroxyapatite and it is effective for drug loading, whereas bioactive glass fibers have only mineralization on their surface. In tubular structures mineralization occurs on the inner and outer side of the tube. It has great potential for gene delivery, drug delivery and tissue engineering [21].

Tensile Strength and Elasticity

The measure of stiffness of an elastic material is termed Young's modulus and is the ratio of stress to strain along an axis. Ceramic materials have higher Young's modulus than that of metals since they have covalent as well as ionic bonding. They are hard because of their well-ordered structure and dislocations were difficult along the atomic lattices. But glasses have less hardness because they have an amorphous structure and low modulus of elasticity. Ductile polymer matrix when reinforced with bioactive fillers such as ceramics, Young's modulus, yield strength and binding strength increases. Reinforcement of glass-ceramic-apatite-wollastonite in polyethylene is an example of this [22]. Ceramic materials may sometimes fail due to slow crack growth [23]. For structural implants mechanical stability is a favourable property. Incorporation of zirconia to hydroxyapatite ceramics improves the mechanical property [24]. Freeze casting method can be applied for producing ceramic materials with high compressive strength. The parameters influencing the porosity and compressive strength are the initial slurry composition [25]. Whisker orientation has importance on the mechanical properties of composite ceramics. The parallel tensile strength and normal shearing stress to the hot-pressing plane gives favourable mechanical properties to the material. But normal tensile strength and parallel shearing stress with the hot pressing plane gives worse mechanical properties [26].

Functionally graded ceramics with a transition in porosity from the outer surface towards the inner were developed to improve the mechanical strength of HA for orthopaedic applications and to improve the cellular penetration. These gradient structures were prepared based on multiple tape casting method in a slurry containing polybutylmethacrylate (PBMA) spheres with diameters ranging from 100 μm to 300 μm. The PBMA was burnt out and then the pore diameter reduces to 70-200 μm. The HA ceramics having graded structure and 50% pore-volume fraction have high binding strength [27].

Biochemical compatibility and biomechanical compatibility were achieved by structural and molecular tailoring of the bioactive composite and its surface chemistry [28]. Presence of ceramics (bioglass) in Poly (lactic-co-glycolic) (PLA) polymers delay the degradation rate of the polymer compared to polymer without any ceramic content [29]. The high processing temperature make ceramics mechanically stressed. Stress or thermally activated transformations results in plasticity or transformation toughening. Transformation toughening improves the reliability and structural integrity of ceramics [30].

Composition

Incorporation of nanoparticles in the ceramic matrix improves its biocompatibility. Grain boundaries were the starting points for dissolution *in vitro* and incorporation of nanoparticles create such grain boundaries. Silicate incorporated HA is more soluble than HA alone because silicate induces dissolution at grain boundaries [31]. Sintering additives such as $CaO-P_2O_5-Na_2O$ were added into HA ceramics to improve failure strength under compressive loading [32]. Maximum compressive strength occurs by adding 2.5wt% CaO as filler. A low temperature sintering and crystallization process was used to produce a monophasic glass ceramic akermanite from a Ca-mica and wollastonite. The sintering behaviour can be improved by adding P_2O_5. The additive increases the stability of glass against crystallization at the sintering start up temperature. The glass-apatite formed by this sintering process is suitable for biological application because it had good *in vitro* acceptance from osteoblasts and moderate bioactivity due to the enrichment of the glass phase with Ca and Si [33].

Inter-layers were provided in the ceramics by means of inorganic oxides. By providing a silica-calcium oxide interlayer make softening and spreading of silica-alumina-flourapatite glass ceramic outer layer and avoid the crystallization of undesired phases and results in good bioactive properties [34]. Increasing bioactive fillers and ductile polymer matrix increases Young's modulus, yield strength and decreases strain to failure [22].

Coating of Ceramics on Metals and Alloys

Metals and metallic alloys were corrosive in the physiological environment and the corrosion can be prevented by providing ceramic coatings on the metallic substrate. Hydroxyapatite coating can be made on titanium substrate by making the surface of titanium (Ti) porous by H_2O_2 treatment and then the coating was transformed into a carbonate and calcium deficient HA layers with a bone like crystallinity by immersion in simulated body fluid [35]. Electrodeposition in modified simulated body fluid (SBF) at 60 °C for 1 hour by maintaining cathodic potentials of -1.5 V, -2 V & -2.5 V (*vs* saturated calomel electrode (SCE)) produced calcium phosphate coating on Ti. The calciumphosphate converted into apatite during immersion in SBF at 36.5 °C for 5 days. The coating electrodeposited at -2.0 V in the modified SBF containing CO_3^{-2} ions was bioactive and transforms into carbonate apatite similar to bone apatite [36]. Suitable electrochemical parameters were selected for producing a homogeneous coating of HA, amorphous calcium phosphate (ACP) or other intermediate phases having different solubility and morphology [37].

The ceramic materials were designed based on their application. By controlling the processing parameters during the synthesis of ceramic, they can be designed in the favourable manner. The following part discusses the various methods of synthesis of ceramic materials for getting the desired application and suitable biocompatibility.

SYNTHESIS OF CERAMICS

Ceramic materials were synthesized by high temperature as well as low temperature processes. High temperature processing methods were usually applied for preparing ceramic materials for hard tissue repair applications. Low temperature synthesis methods were particularly suitable for *in situ* incorporation of certain drugs and biological components in the ceramic matrix.

High Temperature Processes

Ceramic materials were prepared by high temperature sintering and calcination process. Bioactive glass (BG) ceramics were prepared by mixing inorganic oxide materials such as SiO_2, CaO, Na_2O, P_2O_5 in suitable proportions at temperatures > 1500 °C. The bioactivity of BG depends on the proportion of the oxide precursors used in the preparation process. Sinterability of the ceramics could be increased by adding small amounts of CaF_2. The substitution with F^- and OH^- ions forming flour-hydroxyapatite solid solution during the sintering process suppresses the decomposition of HA to ß-TCP. This results in a dense ceramic which has high flexural strength and fracture toughness. It also showed *in vitro* bioactivity similar to hydroxyapatite [38]. Oxide materials can be used for reinforcing with hydroxyapatite prepared through liquid phase sintering process [39]. A Na_2O-CaO-P_2O_5-SiO_2 system in combination with bioglass have a reduced tendency to crystallize and it can be sintered at 750 °C, and this low sintering temperature helps to preserve the amorphous nature of the bioactive glass and this amorphous nature improves bioactivity [40]. The mixture of HA-BG powders were prepared by calcinations at 600 °C resulting in particles in the nanometer range of 40-70 nm [41].

Ceramic agglomerated powder was prepared by air plasma spray or high velocity oxy fuel spray. By developing ceramic materials by these methods nanozones could be developed on ceramic powders which have influence on the bioactivity and mechanical behaviour of the powder [42]. Thermally induced solid-liquid phase separation and subsequent solvent sublimation produces porous composite scaffolds of poly (lactic-co-glycolic acid) (PLGA) containing varying amount of bioglass. Addition of more amounts of bioglass decreases the pore volume of the scaffolds and this improves the mechanical properties of polymer materials. But the presence of bioactive glass in the polymer matrix delays the degradation of the polymer [29].

High temperature methods were used for providing ceramic coating on metallic substrate. The techniques used to obtain HA coating on Ti were physical vapour deposition [43], chemical vapour deposition [44], pulsed laser deposition [45, 46] and sol-gel based dip-coating [47, 48]. The coating thickness and crystallinity of phase could be controlled by some of the preparation techniques. Radiofrequency magnetron sputtering is one method to coat ceramics on metals and plastics [49]. The high temperature coating methods of HA on the Ti substrates suffer from some major problems such as instability of HA at high temperature and the phase transition of Ti at 1163 K. Hence low temperature methods were adopted for providing coating on metallic substrates.

Low Temperature Processes

Low temperature preparation method such as sol-gel process was used to prepare biologically active ceramic materials. This process allows the incorporation of biologically active components in the ceramic matrix, making the material suitable for drug and growth factor incorporation. A biologically active hydroxyl carbonate apatite layer on the bioglass surface make it suitable for bonding with living tissues. Bioglass developed by sol-gel method allows bone tissue growth from the surface towards the inner side of the implant and allows the penetration of bone inside the implants. On implantation bioglass got resorbed by a slow process. The poor mechanical property of bioglass limits its application in load bearing implants [5, 50, 51]. But its resorption in the body results in integration of the implant with the living tissue. Ceramics formed by biological means are nanodimensional and nanocrystalline [52] and were similar to the nanocrystalline apatite found in human bone.

Mechanical mixing processes were also used to make ceramic materials. An example is the ball milling process used for the production of HA-ultra high molecular weight polyethylene. After the wet ball milling process, the swelling sintered HA particles were ground in ethanol. The nano-HA was mechanically mixed with Ultra High Molecular Weight Polyethylene (UHMWPE) in the ball mill and then compression molded into solid slabs. The process of swelling in pharmaceutical grade paraffin oil enhances the chain mobility of UHMWPE. This also enhances HA/UHMWPE interface adhesion before hot final press. The resultant composite has two zone network structure formed by a homogeneous HA-rich phase and a UHMWPE-rich phase [53]. Polymer ceramic microspheres can be prepared by dispersion polymerization technique. Hydroxyapatite and gelatin microspheres were produced by this method [54]. Spherical nano hydroxyapatite particles were synthesized by a wet chemical approach in the presence of small amount of chitosan and the chitosan modulated HA crystallization and aided the self-assembly of nano HA particles.

A two-step acid catalyzed self-assembly process combined with hydrothermal treatment was used for the synthesis of well-ordered mesoporous bioactive glass with high specific surface area [15]. Bioglass was surface functionalized with 3-amino-propyl-triethoxysilane (APTS) and then proteins were immobilized on the surface. This method was used as an efficient method for incorporation of growth factors for local delivery [55]. Alginate cross linking with calcium ions results in mesoporous bioactive glass [56]. Reproducible micro-roughness could be produced on the surface of bioactive glass and atomic force microscopy (AFM) and back scattered electron imaging were used to characterize such rough surface [57]. A two-step process namely one foaming and subsequent hydrolysis was used for the preparation of an α-tricalcium phosphate cement phase into an apatite phase. The foaming agent used was hydrogen peroxide, which decomposes into water and oxygen gas [10].

Suspending the ceramic raw materials in water and homogenizing and dropping the resulting slurry on to a hot plate results in micro porous alumina. Thus produced alumina has a hollow-sphere like shape with a central opening to allow the in-growth of vascularized tissues. This can be used as cell carriers [58]. Hot isostatic pressing method produces reusable zirconia molds for implants. Nanotitania ceramics were reinforced with HA for biomechanical compatibility and bioactivity [59].

BIOMEDICAL APPLICATIONS

The biomedical applications of ceramic materials can be classified as follows.

Tissue Engineering Applications

The process of reconstruction of living tissues with the help of biodegradable scaffolds for replacing a damaged or lost tissue is termed tissue engineering [60]. Portions/whole tissue is repaired or replaced in the process, since the tissues require certain mechanical and structural properties for proper functioning. Synthetic ceramics such as calcium phosphate and the combination of HA and TCP were used as scaffold materials for tissue engineering. The degradation of these bioactive ceramics is slow and they are brittle in nature. The scaffolds provide favourable physicochemical environment as well as structural integrity for bone regeneration. Ceramic scaffolds which release growth factors in a controlled manner is suitable for tissue engineering applications. Bioactive glass has the ability to bond with soft tissue as well as hard tissue and they can form hydroxyapatite layer in contact with simulated body fluid. Ionic dissolution products from bioactive glass could increase the growth of genes found in osteoblasts and it promote osteogenesis. Calcium orthophosphates are most important inorganic constituent of hard tissue [61]. They are chemically similar to the inorganic components of bone and teeth. Enamel matrix protein embedded bioactive glass stimulates the expression of major phenotypic markers and this promotes the osteoblast differentiation and support the growth of osteoblast like cells *in vitro* [62]. Bioactive glass-silk fibroin could release adPDGF-b and adBMP-7 into osteoporotic critical-sized femur defects in ovariectomized rats in a treatment period of 2 & 4 weeks. These growth factors recruit mesenchymal stem cells into the defect sites and cures osteoporotic diseases [63]. The osteoinductive properties of ceramic materials make them suitable for tissue engineering applications. But its high density and slow biodegradability is unfavourable for tissue engineering applications. By making ceramic materials macroporous they can be made suitable for tissue engineering applications [64].

Drug Delivery Applications

Drug delivery is the process of release of therapeutic components in a controlled manner in a localized area for a particular period. Drug delivery minimizes the problems of drug overdose and associated toxicity. Calcium phosphate group of ceramics as well as bioactive glass were used as drug delivery matrix. These ceramics have *in vitro* bioactivity in simulated body fluid. They deposit apatite layer in a selective manner when immersed in simulated body fluid [65]. They can safely deliver the therapeutic agent without causing adverse effect to the surrounding tissues. Ceramics alone or in combination with polymeric matrix were used for developing drug delivery matrix. The polymeric content in the ceramics minimize the rapid drug delivery by minimizing the burst effect seen with hydrophilic content in ceramics [66].

Ceramic particles containing macropores could deliver growth factors and show bioactivity for weeks with osteoconductive and osteoinductive properties [67]. The porosity in the ceramics provide a large surface area for loading the drug and also its controlled degradation results in slow and controlled release of drug. Ceramic microspheres can be made from polymer-ceramic combinations. Hydroxyapatite-gelatin microspheres were used for the release of gentamicin. The microspheres have both acidic and basic groups [54].

Mesoporous matrices were also suitable for drug delivery applications. Supra molecular templating method produces mesoporosity in the silica coating and produces biocompatibility and it work as a carrier system for drugs [68]. Silica-hydroxypatite hybrid matrix is bioactive under *in vitro* conditions.

Antibiotic loaded bone cements were produced from borate bioactive glass. It releases an antibiotic teicoplanin in a sustained manner while supporting bone ingrowth [69]. Drug delivering implants can be used to treat osteomyelitis as well as osteoporosis. Implants having the drug delivery property could be made from ceramic coatings. Anodization process can be used to prepare titania nanotubes. These nanotubes could load a large amount of drugs and can release it in a controlled manner and could be used as a drug eluting coating for implantable medical devices [70].

Self-setting bioactive cement based upon $CaO-SiO_2-P_2O_5$ glass can load Eudragit coated cephalexin. Initial drug release is 30% and thereafter drug release becomes slow. The initial burst release is due to the homogeneous nature of the system. The heterogeneity make the system a slow releasing one [71]. Bioactive glass scaffold coated with chitosan was used as a drug delivery system. The release profile of the drug depends upon the particle size and concentration of drug in the system [72]. Bioactive glass is also used as a controlled release device for tetracycline hydrochloride and inclusion complex formed by tetracycline and ß-cyclodextrin at 1:1 molar ratio. Cyclodextrin slow down the release of tetracycline for a long period of time without affecting the bioactivity of bioglass [73].

Zirconia (ZrO_2) based ceramics have potential biomedical applications [74]. Zirconiumphosphate can intercalate high loads of doxorubicin between their layers and these were good carriers for drug delivery [75]. Alumina nanoparticles have toxicity towards bacterial cells, *i.e.*, near neutral pH, positive surface charge of alumina nanoparticles interacts with the negatively charged bacterial cells and an electrostatic interaction occurs there leading to the adhesion of bacterial cells on the alumina particles and the cells get destroyed [76]. The surface functionalization of diopside ($CaMgSi_2O_6$) with polymer enhances and control drug loading and release ability. The porosity and size were the determining factor of the microspheres size. The modification of diopside microspheres with PLGA on the surface resulted in an enhanced drug loading and release ability. These microspheres can be used as bioactive filling materials for bone regeneration [77].

Ciprafloxacin loaded hydroxyapatite and zinc doped hydroxyapatite have good antimicrobial activity. The presence of zinc increases the drug release percentage and the drug was released in a controlled manner [78]. Electrostatic binding of an aquated species of cis-diamminedichloroplatinum to the nano-CaP in a chloride free solution results in the formation of nano CAP conjugated cis-platin.

Calciumphosphate-PEG-insulin-casein (CAPIC) based oral insulin delivery system was developed and its functional activity was tested in a non-obese diabetic mice model. The biological activity of insulin was retained in the formulation and displays a prolonged hypoglycemic effect after oral administration than free insulin. The formulation was unaffected in acidic environment of the gastro intestinal (GI) tract and insulin was released in less acidic environment of the intestine and then it was absorbed in to the body [79]. PEG functionalized calciumphosphate nanoparticles were synthesized by surface modification of CAP having particle size of 47.9 nm with poly ethylene glycol (PEG) and the developed particle showed zero zeta potential. The system is protected in acidic gastric environment and insulin was released in mild alkaline pH of the intestine [80]. Zinc-calcium-phosphorous oxide (ZCAP) was developed and it maintained normoglycemia for 3 weeks in rats [81].

Malignant bone tumours result in bone defects as well as bone loss. In such cases the cavity formed was filled with some bone regenerative material. If the material used is capable of osteogenesis and at the same time can treat further spread of the bone tumour growth, then it is effective for prevention of the disease. Ceramic materials were used for filling such bone defects. Localized drug delivery prevents further spreading of the disease. Ceramic materials having drug delivery property along with a local temperature increase around the tumour cells may better cure the disease. The use of increased temperature to treat malignant cells is termed as hyperthermia. Cancer cells are destroyed at temperature > 43 °C. In the case of normal cells a temperature dissipation mechanism exists in the cells and it can transfer heat to the surrounding cells. But in tumour cells such temperature dissipation mechanism is absent because of poor vascular system in the cells [82]. Calcium phosphate ceramics and bioglasses can be made hyperthermic by incorporating magnetic materials into the tumours and usually iron oxide based materials were used for hyperthermia therapy [83-85]. Hyperthermia treatment is effective against tumour cells and it does not affect normal cells and the possible side effects are avoided [86]. Ferrous ion incorporated hydroxyapatite particles were magnetic and when they were mixed with phosphate buffered saline solution and injected into tumour in mice with high frequency alternating magnetic field showed a dramatic reduction in tumour volume. The magnetic particles were bioactive and showed less toxicity [83].

Glass microspheres for drug delivery were approved by Food and Drug Administration (FDA) and are used in hospitals in US. The microspheres were inserted into the tumour with the help of a catheter and radiation is focused on tumors. Malignant cells were destroyed and no harm occurs to normal tissue. The serious side effects of chemotherapy can also be eliminated.

Radiotherapy is an effective method for the treatment of cancer, but external irradiation may provide small doses of radiation to deep seated tumors inside the body and hence injectable microspheres that can provide a large localized dose of radiation was used for the effective treatment. $17Y_2O_3$-$19Al_2O_3$-$64SiO_2$ glass microspheres are developed and activated to provide large doses of beta radiation. Y_2O_3 and YPO_4 having high chemical stability are effective for radiotherapy [87]. Alumina ceramics in tumors are effective for the combination of chemotherapy and radiotherapy [88].

Gene Delivery Applications

Gene therapy process releases high concentrations of endogeneous growth factors in a cost effective and controllable manner at a physiological spatiotemporal fashion [89]. This was an effective method for the treatment and prevention of osteoporosis. Osteoporosis is a chronic condition in which there is an imbalance between osteoclasts and osteoblasts. The osteoporotic related fractures have to be repaired by recruiting mesenchymal stem cells to the defect site by delivering growth factors and gene therapy. Ceramics were a promising group of materials for growth factor delivery [63]. Mesoporous bioglass/silk fibrin scaffolds containing PDGF-b and BMP-7 into some osteoporotic femur defects showed new bone formation after treatment for 2 to 4 weeks. Gene therapy for clinical treatment is in its infancy stage. Patients suffering from osteoporotic fractures may get benefit by the delivery of growth factors for recruitment of mesenchymal stem cells. By designing low temperature synthesis methods, the hydroxyapatite ceramics can be used for gene delivery [90].

Artificial Implants

Hydroxyapatite when used in implants favoured the growth of normal bone with bone marrow. Bicalcium phosphate (BCP) ceramics also has a similar behaviour. Bone like tissues were formed inside the pores of the ceramic implant. The induced bone in both HA and BCP ceramics remain and grow in a controlled fashion for a period of 2.5 years when the study was carried out in dog models [91]. Hydroxyapatite-bariumtitanate mixture has piezoelectric property and when they are implanted in the jawbones of dogs, they increased the growth and repair of bones. It also increased the direction depended tissue-growth around the implants resulting in an ordered arrangement of collagen and increased the efficiency of osteogenesis around the implanted ceramics [92]. The composite of

HA-BG has high bioactivity and is suitable for hard-tissue repair applications [41]. Ceramics when used as implants should have the properties of wear resistance, corrosion resistance and long-term stability.

The calcium phosphates which have a Ca/P ratio higher than 1 could be used for hard tissue implants because those CAP with Ca/P ratio less than 1 dissolves easily in human body due to its high solubility and acidity. But they can be combined with other calciumphosphates for implantation purpose.

Pure tricalcium phosphate has lower cell proliferation rate compared with HA or HA/TCP mixture. Messenger-RNA (mRNA) expression of osteonectin and osteocalcin were similar in HA, TCP and HA/TCP mixture [93]. The porous carbon lattices possessing little inherent strength developed interfacial strength after the growth of cortical bone [94]. Heart muscle cells can be developed on TiO_2 ceramics. The micromechanical properties of TiO_2 ceramics helped to maintain tissue-like structural organization of the cardiac cells *in vitro* and coat the cell surface with fine grained TiO_2 ceramics [95]. Cell carriers developed from microporous alumina were implanted into the abdominal wall of Zur:SIV rats. There is no inflammation or capsule formation was observed on the unirritated muscle tissue into which the surface of the hollow alumina carriers were in touch with. Loose connective tissues grow into the hollow cell carrier and no inflammation and scar tissue formation as well as the vitality within the hollow cavity indicate that the microporous hollow alumina carrier were suitable for cell transplantation devices [58]. In order to increase the fatigue endurance property CaPinver glasses ($CaO-P_2OTiO_2-Na_2O$) was coated on Ti alloy to increase the adherence of the coating to the substrate [96].

When wollastonite-tricalcium phosphate was immersed in simulated body fluid, the material exhibited high reactivity with two well differentiated zones of hydroxyapatite and a pseudomorphic transition of tricalcium phosphate to hydroxyapatite. The morphology of hydroxyapatite formed by this method is similar to that of porous bone [34]. Precipitates formed on glass ceramics immersed in biological fluid have strong adherent nature with a needle like morphology [97].

Ceramic materials can be coated on metals. A strong coating of calciumphosphate-invert glass ceramic can be formed on ß-type titanium alloy [98]. Diamond like carbon coatings were provided on metal surface for producing wear resistant surfaces and for preventing metal ion leaching from the surface.

Flourapatite-anorthite could exhibit biocompatibility and no Al^{+3} ions were dissoluted when they were subjected to *in vitro* tests [99]. ß-TCP and ß-calcium silicate when implanted in rabbit calvarial defects exhibited better resorption of calcium silicate. On the surface of ß-calcium silicate, TRAp-positive multi nucleated cells were observed indicating that a cell mediated process is involved in the in-vivo resorption. Better bone growth was shown in ß-calcium silicate than ß-TCP [100]. Bioglass microspheres reinforced PLGA scaffold were used in bone tissue engineering and also it is a good bone replacement material [101]. Hydroxypatite reinforced PMMA bone cement have increased biological response and the HA increases the anchorage of human osteoblast cells on the surface [102].

Alumina hip- implants retrieved after a period of 8.6 years show three types of wear, low wear in one case and stripe wear in 6 cases and severe wear in 4 cases. In stripe wear, the worn area on the head showed 150 μm deep crack, while the rest of the area was intact with low wear. In severe wear cases, there is a huge loss of volume on both head and cups [103]. Femoral implants of macroporous biphasic calcium phosphate when implanted in rabbit femoral bones showed new bone formation around peripheral and deep pores in implants with 565 μm pore size than implants with 300 μm pore size [104]. Macroporosity of implants have great effect on bone ingrowth than macroporosity percentage. Yao *et al.* studied the influence of PLGA-30%BG microspheres based porous scaffolds for bone tissue engineering, because PLGA has controllable bioresorption and ease of processing, while bioglass stimulate osteoblasic differentiation of osteoprogenitor cells. The PLGA-BG composite has the ability to promote osteogenesis of marrow stromal cells [100]. Polymethyl methacrylate (PMMA) is used as bone cement, and it forms a strong bond with implant. But there is the growth of fibroblasts around the implant site and it loosens the implant from the bone. Hydroxyapatite incorporation in the PMMA bone cement increases biological response of the cement. It increases the synergy between focal contact formation, cytoskeletal organization, cell proliferation and expression of phenotype [102]. Incorporation of wollastonite into polycaprolactum improves the hydrophilicity of the composite and it could be used for hard tissue repair applications [105].

Combining chitosan and ß-glycero phosphate salt formulations with bioactive glass nanoparticles results in an injectable thermoresponsive hydrogel. The initial rheological properties and the gelation points of the organic-inorganic thermosetting system were adequate for intra corporal injection. It forms bone like apatite and the bioactivity increased with increasing BG content [106].

Perioglas is a synthetic absorbable osteoconductive bone graft substitute composed of a calcium orthophospho-silicate bioactive glass commercialized under the trade name NOVABONE. The device is in a particulate form of size range 90-710 μm. The device is intended for dental, intraosseous, oral and cranio/ maxillofacial bony defects [107].

Zirconia was used for hip replacements, shoulders, knee joints, spinal implants *etc.* In dentistry zirconia group materials can be used as porcelain crowns and bridges. Crystalline zirconia is a biocompatible material.

FUTURE APPLICATIONS

The physiological processes going on inside the body were not completely understood by scientists. However the harsh physiological condition results in the rejection of foreign materials by the body. Ceramics were a particular group of materials which were less rejected by the body. By proper design of biocompatible ceramics, various unmet problems in biomedical field can be tackled. Gene delivery is one of the emerging fields which have immense therapeutic applications. By designing biocompatible synthesis methods the calcium phosphate group of biomaterials can be studied for gene delivery applications [90]. A new generation of light, tough and high strength material for bone implantation purpose can be made by coating bioactive glass with biomorphic silicon carbide ceramics [16]. Here the osteoconducting property of bioactive glass is combined with the excellent mechanical property and low density of bioactive glass. Alumina-zirconia composites were used as an alternative to monolithic alumina and zirconia [108].

Piezoelectric materials are those which produce voltage by the application of stress. Piezo electric ceramics have great future in biomedical applications. By selecting suitable designing methods, structures can be made that bend, expand or contact. Hydrogel-hydroxyapatite can be made which has mineral to organic matrix ratio as that of bone.

Magnesia partially stabilized zirconia (MgPSZ) and Ceria stabilized tetragonal zirconia (CeO$_2$-TZP) have shape memory properties [109, 110]. Presently ceramics were used for shape memory devices at high temperature applications. In some transition metal oxides magnetic transitions such as paramagnetic-ferrimagnetic, paramagnetic-antiferro magnetic and reversible transitions occur by recoverable lattice distortions. The orbital ordered and disordered phases co-exist in a wide range of temperature and Jahn-Teller transitions may take place and the effect of magnetic field on the transformation have to be studied for understanding the shape memory effect. Alumina and zirconia have chemical stability under physiological condition, but the long term radiation effect of zirconia must be eliminated for making it as an implant. ZrO$_2$ have high fracture strength, toughness and low modulus of elasticity than alumina.

Electronic sensors, cardiac pacemakers, defrillators, cochlear implants, hearing devices, drug delivery and neuro stimulatory devices can be developed from ceramics. Ceramic Freed-Thru are produced by placing metal pins between ceramic components. Ceramic component acts as insulators and charge is passed through the metal pins. By controlling the voltage pass time, drug release can be maintained in a suitable manner. Material scientists and ceramics engineers have great opportunity to engineer and develop new varieties and combinations of ceramic materials for potential biomedical applications.

ACKNOWLEDGEMENTS

The authors are thankful to the Director, Sree Chitra Tirunal Institute for Medical Sciences and Technology, Thiruvananthapuram, for providing facilities to carry out this work. One of the authors, Jayalekshmi A. C. expresses her gratitude to Kerala State Council for Science, Technology and Environment (KSCSTE) for providing Post Doctoral Research Fellowship to carry out this work.

CONFLICT OF INTEREST

The authors declare that this chapter has no conflict of interest.

ABBREVIATIONS

ACP	=	Amorphous calcium phosphate
APTS	=	3-amino-propyl-triethoxysilane
AFM	=	Atomic force microscopy
BCP	=	Bicalcium phosphate
BG	=	Bioactive glass
BMSCs	=	Bone marrow stromal cells
CAP	=	Calcium phosphate
CAPIC	=	Calciumphosphate-PEG-insulin-casein
FDA	=	Food and Drug Administration
GI tract	=	Gastro intestinal tract
HA	=	Hydroxyapatite
MgPSZ	=	Magnesia partially stabilized zirconia
mRNA	=	Messenger-RNA
PBMA	=	Polybutylmethacrylate
PEG	=	Poly ethylene glycol
PLA	=	Poly (lactic-co-glycolic)
PLGA	=	Poly (lactic-co-glycolic acid)

PMMA = Polymethyl methacrylate

SBF = Simulated body fluid

SCE = Saturated calomel electrode

siRNA = Small interfering - RNA

Ti = Titanium

TZP = Ceria stabilized tetragonal zirconia

UHMWPE = Ultra High Molecular Weight Polyethylene

ZCAP = Zinc-calcium-phosphorous oxide

REFERENCES

[1]   Anselme, K., Osteoblast adhesion on biomaterials. *Biomaterials,* 2000, 21, 667-681.
[2]   Seaborn, C., Neilson, F., Dietary silicon affects acid and alkaline phosphatase and calcium uptake in bone of rats. *J. Elem. Exp. Med.,* 1994, 7, 11-18.
[3]   Reffit, D., Ogston, N., Jugdaohsingh, R., Cheung, H., Evans, B., Thompson, R., Powell, J. J., Hampson, G. N., Orthosilicic acid stimulates collagen type 1 synthesis and osteoblast differentiation in human osteoblast-like cells *in vitro. Bone,* 2003, 32, 127-135.
[4]   Shi, S., Kirk, M., Kahan, A., The role of type 1 collagen in the regulation of the osteoblast phenotype. *J. Bone miner. Res.,* 1996, 11, 1139-1145.
[5]   Chen, Q. Z., Thompson, J. D., Boccaccini, A. R., 45S5 Bioglass-derived glass-ceramic scaffolds for bone tissue engineering. *Biomaterials,* 2006, 27, 2414-2425.
[6]   Cho, Y. S., Hoelzer, D. T., Burdick, V. L., Amarakoon, V. R. W., Grain boundaries and growth kinetics of polycrystalline ferromagnetic oxides with chemical additives. *J. Appl. Phys.,* 1999, 85, 5220-5222.
[7]   Yang, B. C., *et al.,* Preparation of bioactive nanotitania ceramics with biomechanical compatibility. *J. Biomed. Mat. Res.,* 2006, 79 A, 210-215.
[8]   Mankani, M. H., *et al., In vivo* bone formation by human bone marrow stromal cells: Effect of carrier particle size and shape. *Biotech. and Bioeng.,* 2001, 72, 96-97.
[9]   Sepulveda, M., Jones, P., Jones, J. R., Hench, L. L., Bioactive sol-gel foams for tissue repair. *J. Biomed. Mater. Res.,* 2002, 59, 340-348.
[10]   Almirall, A., *et al.,* Fabrication of low temperature macroporous hydroxyapatite scaffolds by foaming and hydrolysis of an α-TCP paste. *Biomaterials,* 2004, 25, 3671-3680.
[11]   Saravanpavan, P., Hench, L. L., Low-temperature synthesis, structure and bioactivity of gel-derived glasses in the binary CaO-SiO_2 system. *J. Biomed. Mater. Res.,* 2001, 54, 608-618.
[12]   Sepulveda, P., Jones, J. R., Hench, L. L., *In vitro* dissolution of melt-derived 45S5 and sol-gel derived 58S bioactive glasses. *J. Biomed. Mater. Res. Part A,* 2002, 61, 310-311.

[13]   Joschek, S., Nies, B., Krotz, R., Göpferich, A., Chemical and physicochemical characterization of porous hydroxyapatite ceramics made of natural bone. *Biomaterials,* 2000, 21, 1645-1658.

[14]   Yuan, H., *et al.*, A preliminary study on osteoinduction of two kinds of calcium phosphate ceramics. *Biomaterials,* 1999, 20, 1799-1806.

[15]   Xia, W., Chang, J., Well-ordered mesoporous bioactive glasses (MBG): A promising bioactive drug delivery system. *J. Cont. Release,* 2006, 110, 522-530.

[16]   Yan, X., *et al.*, Highly ordered mesoporous bioactive glasses with superior *in vitro* bone-forming bioactivities. *Angew. Chem Int. Ed. Engl.,* 2004, 43, 5980-5984.

[17]   El-figi, A.; *et al.*, Capacity of mesoporous bioactive glass nanoparticles to deliver therapeutic molecules. *Nanoscale,* 2002, 4, 7475-7488.

[18]   Kalita, S. J., Bharadwaj, A., Bhatt, H. A., Nanocrystalline calcium phosphate ceramics in biomedical engineering. *Mat. Sci. & Eng. C.,* 2007, 27, 441-449.

[19]   Itälä, A., Nordstrom, E. G., Ylänen, H., Aro, H. T., Hupa, M., Creation of micro-rough surface on sintered bioactive glass microspheres. *J. Biomed. Mater. Res.,* 2001, 56, 282-285.

[20]   Deligianni, D. D., Katsala, N. D., Koutsoukos, P. G., Missirlis, Y. F., Effect of surface roughness of hydroxyapatite on human bone marrow cell adhesion, proliferation, differentiation and detachment strength. *Biomaterials,* 2000, 22, 87-96.

[21]   Xie, J., Blough, E. R., Wang, C. H., Sub micron bioactive glass tubes for bone tissue engineering. *Acta Biomater.,* 2012, 8, 811-819.

[22]   Juhasz, J. A., *et al.*, Mechanical properties of glass-ceramic A-W-Polyethylene composites: Effects of filler content and particle size. *Biomaterials,* 2004, 25, 949-955.

[23]   Zhang, Y., Lawn, B., Long term strength of ceramics for biomedical Applications. *J. Biomed. Mat. Res. Part B. Appl. Biomater.,* 2004, 6913, 166-172.

[24]   Silva, V. V., Domingues, R. Z., Microstructural and mechanical study of zirconia-hydroxyapatite (ZH) composite ceramic for biomedical applications. *Comp. Sci. and Technology,* 2001, 61, 301-310.

[25]   Deville, S., Saiz, E., Tomsia, A. P., Freeze casting of hydroxyapatite scaffolds for bone tissue engineering. *Biomaterials,* 2006, 27, 5480-5489.

[26]   Niu, Z. W., Li, L., Effect of whisker orientation on mechanical properties of hydroxyapatite-SiCw Composite. *Bioceramics key Engineering Material,* 2007, 334-335, 1165 in 'Advances in composite materials and structures', Edited by Kim, J. K., Wo, D. Z., Zhou, L. M, Huang, H. T., Lau, K. T and Wang, M.

[27]   Werener, J., Krcmar, B. L., Freiss, W., Greil, P., Mechanical properties and *in vitro* cell compatibility of hydroxyapatite ceramics with graded pore structure. *Biomaterials,* 2002, 23, 4285-4294.

[28]   Cao, W., Hench, L. L., Bioactive materials. *Ceramics International,* 1996, 22, 493-507.

[29]   Maquel, V., Boccaccini, A. R., Pravata, L., Notingher, I., Jérome, R., Porous poly (α-hydroxyacid)/Bioglass® composite scaffolds for bone tissue engineering. I: Preparation and *in vitro* characterization. *Biomaterials,* 2004, 25, 4185-4194.

[30]   Heuer, A. H., Ruthle, M., Marshall, D. B., On the Thermoelastic Martensitic Transformation in Tetragonal Zirconia. *J. Am. Ceram. Soc.,* 1990, 73, 1084-1093.

[31]   Porter, A. E., Patel, N., Skepper, J. N., Best, S. M., Bonfield, W., Comparison of *in vivo* dissolution processes in hydroxyapatite and silicon-substituted hydroxyapatite bioceramics. *Biomaterials,* 2003, 24, 4609-4620.

[32] Kalita, S. J., Bose, S., Hosick, H. L., Bandhyopadhyay, A., CaO-P_2O_5-Na_2O-based sintering additives for hydroxyapatite (HAP) ceramics. *Biomaterials,* 2004, 25, 2331-2339.

[33] Agathopoulos, S., *et al.*, A New model formulation of the SiO_2-Al_2O_3-B_2O_3-MgO-CaO-Na_2O-F glass ceramics. *Biomaterials,* 2005, 26, 2255-2264.

[34] Aza, P. N. D., Guitián, F., Aza, S. D., Bioeutectics: a new ceramic material for human bone replacement. *Biomaterials,* 1997, 18, 1285-1291.

[35] Park, J. H., Lee, Y. K., Kim, K. M., Bioactive calcium phosphate coating prepared on H_2O_2- treated titanium substrate by electrodeposition. *Surface and Coatings Technology,* 2002, 195, 252-257.

[36] Park, J. H., Lee, D. Y., Oh, K. T., Lee, Y. K., Kim, K-M., Kim, K. N., Bioactivity of calcium phosphate coatings prepared by electrodeposition in a modified simulated body fluid. *Mater. Letters,* 2006, 60, 2573- 2577.

[37] Rößler, S., *et al.*, Electrochemically assisted deposition of thin calcium phosphate coatings at near-physiological pH and temperature. *J. Biomed Mat. Res.,* 2002, 64 A, 655-663.

[38] Kim, H. W., *et al.*, Effect of CaF_2 on densification and properties of hydroxyapatite-zirconia composites for biomedical applications. *Biomaterials,* 2002, 23, 4113-4121.

[39] Lopes, M. A., Silva, R. F., Monteiro, F. J., Santos, J. D., Microstructural dependence of Young's and shear moduli of P_2O_5 glass reinforced hydroxyapatite for biomedical application. *Biomaterials,* 2000, 21, 749-754.

[40] Bellusi, D., Cannillo, V., Sola, A., A New Highly Bioactive Composite Scaffold Applications: A feasibility study. *Materials,* 2011, 4, 339-354.

[41] Adibnia, S., Nemati, A., Fathi, M. H., Baghshahi, S., Synthesis and characterization of sol-gel derived hydroxyapatite-Bioglass composite nanopowders for biomedical applications. *J. Biomimetics, Biomaterials & Tissue Engineering,* 2011, 12, 51-57.

[42] Lima, R. S, Maple, B. R., Thermal Spray Coatings Engineered from Nanostructured Ceramic Agglomerated Powders for Structural, Thermal Barrier and Biomedical Applications: A Review. *Journal of Thermal Spray Technology,* 2007, 16, 40-63.

[43] Park, Y. S. *et al.*, The effect of ion beam assisted deposition of hydroxyapatite on the grit-blasted surface of endosseous implants in rabbit tibiae. *Int. J. Oral Maxillofac Implants,* 2005, 20, 31-38.

[44] Cabañas, M. V., Regí, M. V., Calcium phosphate coatings deposited by aerosol chemical vapour deposition. *J. Mater. Chem.,* 2003, 13, 1104.

[45] Wolke, J. G. C., de Groot, K., Jansen, J. A., Subperiosteal implantation of various RF magnetron sputtered Ca-P coatings in goats. *J. Biomed. Mater. Res.,* 1998, 43, 270-276.

[46] Kannan, S., Balamurugan, A., Rajeswari, S., Development of calcium phosphate coatings on type 316L SS and their *in vitro* response. *Trends Biomater Artif. Organs,* 2002, 16, 8-11.

[47] Arias, J. L., *et al.*, Micro and nano-testing of calcium phosphate coatings produced by pulsed laser deposition. *Biomaterials,* 2003, 24, 3403-3408.

[48] Hashimoto, Y., *et al.*, Cytocompatibility of calciumphosphate coatings deposited by an ArF pulsed laser. *J. Mater. Sci. Mater. Med.,* 2008, 9, 327.

[49] Jansen, J. A., *et al.*, Application of magnetron sputtering for producing ceramic coatings on implant materials. *Clinical Oral Implants Reseacrh,* 1993, 4, 28-34.

[50] Regí, M. V., Hernández, E. H., Bioceramics: from bone regeneration to cancer nanomedicine. *Adv. Mater.,* 2011, 23, 5177-5218.

[51] Salinas, A. J., Merino, J. M., Hijón, N., Martín, A. I., Regí, M. V., Organic-inorganic hybrids based on CaO-SiO_2 sol-gel glasses. *Key Eng. Mater.,* 2001, 254, 481-484.

[52]   Sergey, V. D., Nanodimensional and Nanocrystalline Apatites and other calcium orthophosphates in Biomedical Engineering, Biology and Medicine. *Materials*, 2009, 2, 1975-2045.

[53]   Fang, L., Leng, Y., Gao, P., Processing of hydroxyapatite reinforced ultrahigh molecular weight polyethylene for biomedical applications. *Biomaterials*, 2005, 2, 3471-3478.

[54]   Sivakumar, M., Rao, K. P., Preparation, Characterization and *in vitro* release of gentamicin from coralline hydroxyapatite-gelatin composite microspheres. *Biomaterials*, 2002, 23, 3175-3181.

[55]   Verné, E., *et al.*, Surface functionalization of bioactive glasses. *J. Biomed. Mater. Res.*, 2009, 90A, 981-992.

[56]   Wu, C. *et al.*, Bioactive mesopore-glass microspheres with controllable protein-delivery properties by biomimetic surface modification. *J. Biomed Mater Res. Part A*, 2010, 95A, 476-485.

[57]   Hälä, A., Nordström, E. G., Ylänen, H., Aro, H. T., Hupa, M., Creation of micro rough surface on sintered bioactive glass microspheres. *J. Biomed. Mater. Res.*, 2001, 56, 282-288.

[58]   Eckert, K. L. *et al.*, Preparation and *in vitro* testing of porous alumina ceramics for cell culture applications. *Biomaterials*, 2000, 21, 63-69.

[59]   Li, Z. *et al.*, Effects of hydroxyapatite additive content on the bioactivity and biomechanical compatibility of bioactive nanotitania ceramics. *J. Biomed. Mater. Res. A*, 2008, 86, 333-338.

[60]   Bartold, P. M., Xiao, Y., Lyngstaadas, S. P., Paine, M. L., Snead, M. L., Principles and applications of cell delivery systems for periodontal regeneration. *Periodontology*, 2006, 41, 23-135.

[61]   Lowenstam, H. A., Weiner, S., On Biomineralization; Oxford University Press: New York, U. S. A. 1989, p. 324.

[62]   Hattar, S., *et al.*, Potential of biomietic surfaces to promote *in vitro* osteoblast-like cell differentiation. *Biomaterials*, 2005, 26, 839-848.

[63]   Zhang, Y., Cheng, N., Mion, R., Shi, B., Cheng, X., Delivery of PDGF-B and BMP-7 by mesoporous bioglass/silk fibrin scaffolds for the repair of osteoporotic defects. *Biomaterials*, 2012, 33, 6698-6708

[64]   Habraken, W. J. E. M., Wolke, J. G. C., Jansen, J. A., Ceramic composites as matrices and scaffolds for drug delivery in tissue engineering. *Adv. Drug Deliv. Reviews*, 2007, 59, 234-238.

[65]   Salinas, A. J., Román, J., Vallet-Regí, M., Oliveira, J. M., Correia, R. N., Fernandes, M. H., *In vitro* bioactivity of glass and glass-ceramics of the 3CaO. P_2O_5-CaO.SiO_2-CaO.MgO.2SiO_2 System. *Biomaterials*, 2000, 21, 251-257.

[66]   Arcos, D., Ibuprofen release from hydrophilic ceramic-polymer composites. *Biomaterials*, 1997, 18, 1235-1242.

[67]   Crouzier, T., *et al.*, The performance of BMP-2 loaded TCP/HAP porous ceramics with a poly electrolyte multilayer film coating. *Biomaterials*, 2011, 32, 7543-7554.

[68]   Andersson, J., Areva, S., Spliethoff, B., Linden, M., Sol-gel synthesis of a multi functional hierarchically porous silica/apatite composite. *Biomaterials*, 2005, 26, 6827-6835.

[69]   Zhang, X., *et al.*, Teicoplanin loaded borate bioactive glass implant for treating chronic bone infection in a rabbit tibia osteomyellitis model. *Biomaterials*, 2010, 31, 5865-5874.

[70] Popat, K. C., *et al.*, Titania Nanotubes: A Novel platform for Drug-Eluting coatings for Medical implant. *Small,* 2007, 3, 1878-1881.

[71] Otsuka, M., *et al.*, A novel skeletal drug delivery system using self-setting bioactive glass bone cement containing polymer-coated bulk powder. *Biomed. Mater. Eng.,* 1993, 3, 229-236.

[72] Soundarapandian, S., Datta, S., Kundu, B., Basu, D., Sa, B., Porous bioactive glass scaffolds for local delivery in osteomyelitis: Development and *in vitro* characterization. *AAPS Pharm. Sci. Tech.,* 2010, 11, 1675-1683.

[73] Dominguez, Z. R., *et al.*, Bioactive glass as a drug delivery system of tetracycline and tetracycline associated with beta-cyclodextrin. *Biomaterials,* 2004, 25, 327-333.

[74] Garnweitner, G., Zirconia nanomaterials:synthesis and biomedical Applications, Nanotechnologies for the Life Sciences, Published online 15 Oct 2010.

[75] Sareena, V., *et al.*, Zirconium nanoplatelets: a biocompatible nanomaterial for drug delivery to cancer. *Nanoscale,* 2003, 21, 2328-2336.

[76] Mukherjee, A., Mohammed, S. I., Prathna, T. C., Chandrasekharan, N., Antimicrobial activity of aluminium oxide nanoparticles for potential chemical applications-Science against microbial pathogens: communicating current research and technical advances. A. Méndez-Vilas (Ed.) 2011, *FORMATEX*

[77] Wu, C., Zreqiat, H., Porous bioactive diopside ($CaMgSi_2O_6$) ceramic microspheres for drug delivery. *Acta Biomaterialia,* 2010, 6, 820-829.

[78] Venkatasubbu, G. V., *et al.*, Nanocrystalline hydroxyapatite and zinc-doped hydroxyapatite as carrier material for controlled delivery of ciprofloxacin. *Biotech.,* 2011, 1, 173-186.

[79] Morcöl, T., Nagappan, P., Norenbaum, L., Mitchell, A., Bell, S. J., Calcium phosphate-PEG-insulin-casein (CAAPIC) particles as oral delivery systems for insulin. *Int. J. Pharm.,* 2004, 277, 91-97.

[80] Ramachandran, R., Paul, W., Sharma, C. P., Synthesis and characterization of PEGylated calcium phosphate nanoparticles for oral insulin delivery. *J. Biomed. Mater. ResB; Appl. Biomater.,* 2009, 88, 41-48.

[81] Arar, H., Bajpai, P. K., Insulin delivery by zinc calcium phosphate ceramics. *Biomed Sci Instrum.,* 1992, 28, 173-178.

[82] Wang, T. W., *et al.*, The development of magnetic degradable DP-Bioglass for hyperthermia cancer therapy. *J. Biomed. Mater. Res. A,* 2007, 3, 828-837.

[83] Hou, C. H., *et al.*, The *in vivo* performance of biomagnetic hydroxyapatite nanoparticles in cancer hyperthermia therapy. *Biomaterials,* 2009, 30, 3956-3960.

[84] Lii, G., *et al.*, Synthesis and characterization of magnetic bioactive glass-ceramics containing Mg ferrite for hyperthermia. *Mater. Sci. Eng. C,* 2010, 30, 148-53.

[85] Cheng, X., Kuhn, L., Chemotherapy drug delivery from calcium phosphate nanoparticles. *Int. J. Nanomedicine,* 2007, 2, 667-674.

[86] Singh, R. K., Srinivasan, A., Kothiyal, G. P., Evaluation of $CaO-SiO_2-P_2O_5-Na_2O-Fe_2O_3$ bioglass-ceramics for hyperthermia application. *J. Mater. Sci. Mater. Med.,* 2009, 20, S147-151

[87] Kawasita, M., *et al.*, Preparation of ceramic microspheres for *in situ* radiotherapy of deep-seated cancer. *Biomaterials,* 2003, 24, 2955-2963.

[88] Yamamuro, T. *et al.*, Intraoperative Radiotherapy and Ceramic prosthesis replacement for Osteosarcoma, in "New Developments for Limb salvage in musculoskeletal tumors". 1989, pp. 327-333. Springerlink.

[89]   Chen, F-M., Zhang, M., Wu, Z. F., Towards delivery of multiple growth factors in tissue engineering. *Biomaterials,* 2010, 31, 6279-6308.

[90]   Kumta, P. N., Sfeir, C., Lee, D-H., Olton, D., Choi, D., Nanostructured calciumphosphates for biomedical Applications: Novel synthesis and Characterization. *Acta Biomaterialia,* 2005, 1, 65-83.

[91]   Yuan, H., Yang, Z., Bruijn, J. D., de Groot, K., Zhang, X., Material-dependent bone induction by calciumphosphate ceramics: a 2.5 year study in dog. *Biomaterials,* 2001, 22, 2617-2623.

[92]   Jianqing, F., Huipin, Y., Xingdong, Z., Promotion of osteogenesis by a piezoelectric biologic ceramic. *Biomaterials,* 1997, 18, 1531-1534.

[93]   Wang, C. *et al.,* Phenotypic expression of bone-related genes in osteoblasts grown on calcium phosphate ceramics with different phase compositions. *Biomaterials,* 2004, 25, 2507-2514.

[94]   Nilles, J. L., Lapitsky, M., Biomechanical investigations of bone-porous carbon &porous metal interfaces, J. Biomed. Mater. Res., 1973, 7, 63-84.

[95]   Polonchuk, l., Elbel, J., Eckert, L., Blum, J., Wintermatel, E., Eppenberger, H. M., Titaniumdioxide ceramics control the differentiated phenotype of cardiac muscle cells in culture. *Biomaterials,* 2000, 21, 539-550.

[96]   Li, S. J., Niinomi, M., Aksahori, T., Kasuga, T., Yang, R., Hao, Y. L., Fatigue characteristics of bioactive glass-ceramic-coated Ti-29Nb-13Ta-4.6Zr for biomedical application. *Biomaterials,* 2004, 25, 3369-3378.

[97]   Oliviera, J. M., Correia, R. N., Fernandea, M. H., Surface modifications of a glass and a glass-ceramic of the MgO-3CaO.P_2O_5-SiO_2 system in a simulated body fluid. *Biomaterials,* 1995, 16, 849-854.

[98]   Kasuga, T. *et al.,* Bioactive calcium phosphate invert glass-ceramic coating on ß-type Ti-29Nb-13Ta-4.6Zr alloy. *Biomaterials,* 2003, 24, 283-290.

[99]   Agathopoulos, S., *et al.,* The fluorapatite-anorthite system in biomedicine. *Biomaterials,* 2003, 24, 1317-1331.

[100]   Xu, S., Lin, K., Wang, Z., Chang, J., Wang, L., Lu, J., Ning, C., Reconstruction of calvarial defect of rabbits using porous calcium silicate bioactive ceramics. *Biomaterials,* 2008, 29, 2588-2596.

[101]   Yao, J., *et al.,* The effect of bioactive glass content on synthesis and bioactivity of composite poly (lactic-co-glycolic acid)/bioactive glass substrate for tissue engineering. *Biomaterials,* 2005, 26, 1935-43.

[102]   Dalby, M. J., *et al.,* Increasing hydroxyapatite incorporation into poly (methylmethacrylate) cement increases osteoblast adhesion and response. *Biomaterials,* 2002, 23, 569-576.

[103]   Nevelos, J. E., Ingham, E., Doyle, C., Fisher, J., Nevelos, A. B., Analysis of retrieved alumina ceramic components from Mittelmeier total hip prostheses. Biomaterials, 1999, 20, 1833-1840.

[104]   Gauthier, O., Bouler, J. M., Aguado, E., Pilet, P., Daculsi, G., Macroporous biphasic calcium phosphate ceramics: influence of macropore diameter & macroporosity percentage on bone in growth. *Biomaterials,* 1998, 19, 133-139.

[105]   Wei, J., Chin, F., Shin, J-W., Hong, H., Dai, C., Su, J., Liu, C., Preparation and characterization of bioactive mesoporous wollastonite-polycaprolactone composite scaffold. *Biomaterials,* 2009, 30, 1080-1088.

[106] Couto, D. S., Hong, Z., Mano, J. F., Development of bioactive and biodegradable chitosan-based injectable systems containing bioactive glass nanoparticles. *Acta Biomaterialia,* 2009, 5, 115-123.

[107] http://www.accessdata.fda.gov/cdrh_docs/pdf4/k040278.pdf.

[108] Chevalier, J., What future for zirconia as a biomaterial. *Biomaterials,* 2006, 27, 535-543.

[109] Swaint, M. V., Shape memory behaviour in partially stabilized zirconia ceramics. Nature, 1986, 322, 234-236.

[110] Wei, Z. G., Sandström, R., Miyazaki, S., Review. Shape-memory materials and hybrid composites for smart systems. J. Mat. Sci., 1998, 33, 3743-3762.

Frontiers in Biomaterials, Vol. 1, 2014, 129-154 129

CHAPTER 5

Role of Scaffolds in Dentistry - From Conventional to Modern Innovative Biomaterials

M. Mozafari[*,1], M. Jafarkhani[2], A.M. Urbanska[3], H.H Caicedo[4,5] and S. Shahrabi Farahani[6]

[1]*Bioengineering Research Group, Nanotechnology and Advanced Materials Department, Materials and Energy Research Center (MERC), P.O. Box 14155-4777, Tehran, Iran;* [2]*School of Chemical Engineering, College of Engineering, University of Tehran, P.O. Box 11155-4563, Tehran, Iran;* [3]*Division of Digestive and Liver Diseases, Department of Medicine, Irving Cancer Research Center, Columbia University New York, NY 10032, USA;* [4]*Biologics Research, Biotechnology Center of Excellence, Janssen R&D, LLC, Pharmaceutical Companies of Johnson & Johnson, Spring House, PA 19477, USA;* [5]*National Biotechnology & Pharmaceutical Association, Chicago, IL 60606, USA; and* [6]*Division of Oral & Maxillofacial Pathology, Department of Diagnostic Sciences and Oral Medicine, College of Dentistry, University of Tennessee Health Science Center, Memphis, TN 38163, USA*

Abstract: Dental tissue injuries significantly affect the quality of life of hundreds of people worldwide. Although dental implants can be functionally effective in many cases, they are not able to completely satisfy all the aspects of regenerative dentistry. Tissue engineering using innovative biomaterial scaffolds that support cells for functional regenerative dental tissues offers new possibilities for clinical dentistry. There have been several attempts to examine different biomaterial scaffolds and cell sources to regenerate substitutes for natural extracellular matrix analogs. It is believed that regenerative dentistry involving scaffolds, stem cells, and growth factors will become common within the next twenty years. This chapter compiles a thorough review on the current developments and challenges in scaffolding techniques that are of particular significance for regenerative dentistry.

Keywords: Bioceramics, biopolymers, dentistry, fabrication, scaffolds, stem cells, tissue engineering.

*Corresponding Author M. Mozafari: Bioengineering Research Group, Nanotechnology and Advanced Materials Department, Materials and Energy Research Center (MERC), P.O. Box 14155-4777, Tehran, Iran; Tel: + 98 912 6490679; Fax: +98 263 6280034 (Ex. 477); E-mail: mozafari.masoud@gmail.com

INTRODUCTION

The tooth is an important organ that develops complex interactions between the epithelium, (a tissue composed of a layer of cells lining bodily organs and surfaces) and mesenchyme tissues, from which connective tissue, bone, cartilage, and the circulatory and lymphatic systems develop. A human tooth combines the roots, which affix to the central alveolar bone within the periodontal ligament and a crown facade for munching. Tooth roots are covered by a mineralized bone tissue (cementum) and are bonded to the adjacent alveolar bone *via* periodontal ligament tissue. This fibrous ligament permits the tooth to move and transfers the mechanical stimuli produced during mastication and orthodontic treatments to the primary and adjoining tissues [1].

Tooth damage or loss due to trauma, periodontal disease, post-cancer surgery, skeletal disease, congenital malformations, dental caries, or a variety of genetic disorders is common among old and young people alike. The task of restoring lost tooth tissue and the associated cost is still a challenge projected to remain for several years to come. In order to recuperate the lost masticatory function of the tooth, therapies such as artificial dentition, tooth transplantation, and dental implants are currently implemented [2].

In particular, the regeneration of the entire tooth and/or its root that can be integrated into the jaw bone is the main objective of regenerative dentistry. Therefore, with the recognition of the biological basis of teeth tissue, many efforts have been performed to design therapies promoting tooth tissue regeneration. Tooth engineering and regeneration is a very attractive solution as it offers unique opportunity to develop tissues, which is easily accessible and non-life-threatening [3].

Recently, in order to regenerate tooth-like structures, many different approaches have been applied such as the induction of a third dentition, chimeric tooth engineering, assembly of different bioengineered component parts, a novel three-dimensional pellet cultivation system for periodontal ligament stem cells (PDLSCs), gene-manipulated tooth regeneration, and scaffold-based tooth regeneration have been applied [4]. Among these approaches, implementing scaffold would be the most beneficial method for tooth regeneration since it is a well-established technology used routinely in many research and clinical laboratories which provides structural support for active biological components such progenitors cells, soluble factors, and extra cellular matrix proteins. The three key elements for dental tissue engineering are signals for morphogenesis, progenitor/stem cells, and scaffolds of extracellular matrix components, as shown in Fig. (**1**).

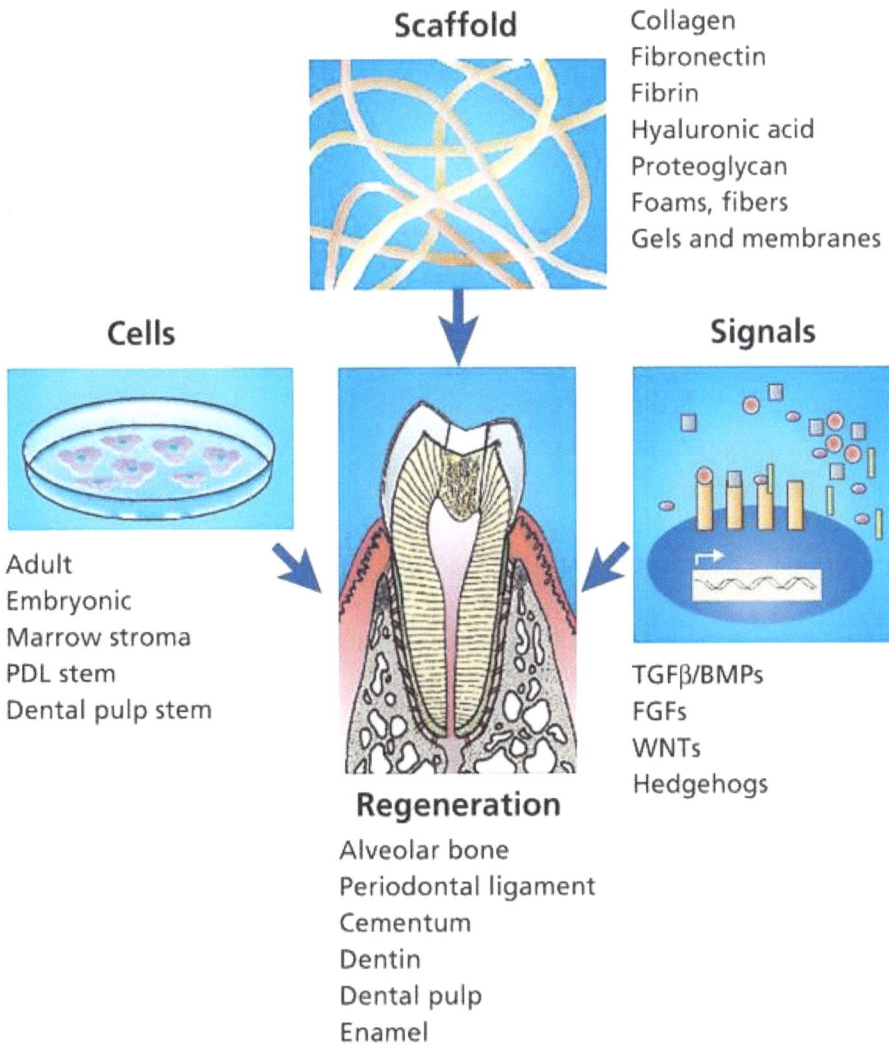

Fig. (1). Schematic illustration of three key elements for dental tissue engineering [5].

SCAFFOLDS FOR DENTAL TISSUE ENGINEERING

An ideal scaffold is surrounded by cells and provides structural support for the formation, maintenance and functionality of new tissues and eventually organs. The scaffolds, which are mainly composed of extracellular matrix proteins, provide cells with anchorage, sequestration of growth factors and signal cells to migrate, differentiate, proliferate and infiltrate integrin receptor-mediated signaling pathways [6]. Scaffolds play an important role in providing an environment that guides and assists the generation of a natural extracellular matrix. The scaffolds need to be designed and optimized to ensure mechanical integrity, stability, and functionality. Also, the surface of scaffolds should have the correct morphology for cell adhesion and differentiation. Another critical component to mimic the extracellular matrix of the replaced tissue is the selection of suitable scaffold materials. The tooth scaffold can be implemented with the suitable choice of cells and growth factors to initiate the forming of new tissues that can integrate with the surrounding tissues. In addition, scaffolds ought to be biocompatible and conductive as well as have the mechanical property and strength to restore the recipients' normal activities. In order to initiate the seeding of cells and growth factors and to support vascular ingrowth for oxygen and biomolecule transport, the scaffold should have a controllable interconnected porosity [7].

INNOVATIVE BIOMATERIALS FOR TEETH SCAFFOLDS

An organic scaffold is used to provide a construction on which cells may adhere, proliferate, grow, and spatially organize for regenerative strategies. Various classes of biomaterials are available to engineer such tissues. The biomaterials that are most commonly used in tissue engineering are synthetic polymers such as poly-L-lactide (PLLA), poly(glycolic) acid (PGA), poly(ε-caprolactone) (PCL), and matrices derived from biological sources such as collagen, chitosan, alginate, and finally bioceramics [8].

SYNTHETIC POLYMERS

PLLA is a synthetic, biodegradable polymer and chiral polyester usually found to be semicrystalline. It has suitable mechanical properties for biomedical applications and can be used in bioresorbable composites because of its biocompatibility and biodegradability [9]. Wang *et al.* [10] synthesized nanofibrous PLLA (NFPLLA) scaffolds to investigate the odontogenic differentiation of human dental pulp stem cells (hDPSCs) on these scaffolds *in vitro* and *in vivo*. They observed that the NFPLLA scaffold and the combination of bone morphogenetic protein (BMP) and dexamethasone (DXM) provides an excellent environment for DPSCs to regenerate dental pulp and dentin.

PGA is a biodegradable, thermoplastic polymer and the simplest linear, aliphatic polyester that was first used as a biodegradable suture. Young *et al.* [11] seeded the cells from tooth tissues onto biodegradable polyglycolate/poly-L-lactate (PGA/PLLA) polymers and reported that the bioengineering of tooth crowns was similar to that of naturally growing teeth [11-13]. After growing in rat hosts for thirty weeks, they found that some recognizable tooth structures containing dentin, odontoblasts, a well-defined pulp chamber, putative Hertwig's root sheath epithelia, putative cementoblasts, a fully formed enamel were formed. They established the first successful generation of tooth crowns from dissociated tooth tissue that contained both dentin and enamel. They also verified the presence of epithelial and mesenchymal dental stem cells in porcine third molar tissue. However, the disadvantages of PGA include, but are not limited to its insolubility in water, which leads to gycolic acid production, an ultimate generation of local acidosis, and potential tissue damage.

PCL is a slowly biodegrading polyester that has been tested as a scaffold material in many aspects of tissue engineering. Park *et al.* [14] have recently synthesized a new kind of PCL and PGA scaffold PCL and PGA for the specific cell implementation of genetically modified human cells so that a human tooth dentin-ligament-bone could be generated *in vivo*. Their results showed the interfacial production of parallel- and obliquely-oriented fibers and the creation of the tooth cementum-like tissue, ligament, as well as the bone assembly [14]. In addition, Goh *et al.* [15] fabricated PCL-based scaffolds containing different amounts of tricalcium phosphate (TCP) in order to study peri-implant bone regeneration and implant stability after its immediate implant placement into tooth sockets with facial wall defects. They reported the use of a PCL-TCP scaffold and showed better maintenance of the alveolar contour than the autogenous particulate bone at 6 months.

Polyether ester amide-based constructs containing self-assembling peptides are gaining popularity in tissue engineering applications, including bone, cartilage and dentin. Galler *et al.* [16] have recently combined two dental stem cell lines with peptide-amphiphile hydrogel scaffolds that showed differences in morphology, proliferation, and differentiation behaviors. The findings indicated that combining the cells with the scaffolds could simplify the process [16]. They demonstrated that due to the ease of handling and introducing into small defects, this novel system could be suitable for engineering both soft and mineralized matrices for dental tissue regeneration. In another study, Kiekham *et al.* [17] designed three-dimensional fibrillar scaffolds of peptides and suggested that self-assembling peptides may be useful in the modulation of mineral behavior during *in situ* dental tissue engineering.

NATURAL POLYMERS

As one of the most promising natural polymers, collagen has been frequently used in tissue engineering applications since it is the main protein of sinew, cartilage, bone, and skin. Collagen sponges possess many advantages due to their resemblance in structure to the extracellular matrix, their low immunogenicity and cytotoxicity, as well as efficiency and feasibility to form various shapes [18]. In a recent study, Sumita *et al.* [19] compared the performance of collagen sponge with polyglycolic acid fiber mesh as a scaffold material for tooth-tissue engineering. They showed that after 24 hrs, there was a significantly higher number of cells attached to the collagen sponge scaffold than to the polyglycolic acid fiber mesh scaffold. Similarly, the Alkaline Phosphatase (ALP) activity was significantly higher in the collagen sponge scaffold after 7 days of culture. Their results from *in vivo* experiments showed that the collagen sponge scaffold allowed tooth production with a higher degree of success than polyglycolic acid fiber mesh. In conclusion, the investigated collagen scaffold for tooth regeneration indicated that these natural materials support cell proliferation and differentiation and significantly help formation of calcified tissues [19]. Kim *et al.* [20] studied the growth and differentiation properties of human dental pulp cells (HDPC) on a variety of natural scaffolds, including 2 types of collagen (type I and type III). They found that dental pulp cells attached and proliferated rapidly on collagen. The cells plated on collagen exhibited high ALP activity and the expression peak of osteocalcin (OCN) mRNA from cells grown on collagen was found early and was followed by dentin sialophosphoprotein (DSPP) and dentin matrix protein-1 (DMP-1) mRNA expression. Iibuchi *et al.* [21] have reported that a scaffold constructed of synthetic octacalcium phosphate (OCP) and porcine atelocollagen sponge (OCP/Col) enhanced bone regeneration more than sintered b-tricalcium phosphate collagen composite or sintered hydroxyapatite (HA) collagen composite in a rat calvarial defect model.

Chitosan is a linear, biocompatible, and biodegradable polysaccharide composed of randomly distributed deacetylated and acetylated units and is currently used with other polymers in a variety of tissue engineering applications [22, 23]. Ravindran *et al.* [24] developed three-dimensional multilayered co-culture system collagen/chitosan and seeded with mesenchymal-derived dental pulp stem cells (DPSCs) and dental epithelial cells (HAT-7) to determine epithelial-mesenchymal interactions. The HAT-7 cell line is an epithelial stem cell line that initiates from the cervical loop of the murine incisor. This technique facilitated the co-culture of epithelial and mesenchymal cells, and after 24 days of culture, a substantial calcium deposition was observed. This class of scaffolds provided a macro scale bio-mimetic structure with tunable mechanical characteristics that supported the movement of cells in all directions [24].

Alginate is a natural, anionic polysaccharide derived from marine kelp, mainly brown sea algae. It has a number of attractive biophysical properties, such as excellent biocompatibility, mildness of gelation conditions, and low immunogenicity. Fujiwara *et al.* [25] have recently developed alginate-based scaffolds that were functionalized with rat dental-pulp-derived cells and human dental pulp cells simultaneously. The scaffolds were finally implemented in the back of nude mice. They reported that the seeded cells differentiated into odontoblast-likecells and stimulated calcification in the tooth [25]. Srinivasan *et al.* [26] synthesized nano-bioactive glass ceramic (nBGC) particles that were then incorporated in alginate composite scaffold to study periodontal tissue regeneration. They assessed the human periodontal ligament fibroblast (hPDLF) and observed that osteosarcoma (MG-63) cells were attached, viable, and proliferating in both alginate/bioglass composite scaffolds and alginate scaffolds. They reported that the presence of nBGC enhanced these factors of the hPDLF cells cultured on composite scaffolds.

Silk protein polymers are biodegradable, biocompatible, have controllable degradation rates, are non-immunogenic, and have been approved by Food and Drug Administration (FDA) [27]. They are spun into fibers by lepidoptera larvae such as silkworms, spiders, scorpions, mites, and flies and can be coupled to peptides such as arginine-glycine-aspartic acid (RGD). Due their impressive mechanical properties, silk proteins provide an important set of material options in the fields of biomaterials and scaffolds for tissue engineering. It was reported that silk-based scaffold could be useful in bone tissue engineering [28-31]. Xu *et al.* manufactured four scaffolds from silk protein (with or without RGD) peptide with various degrees of pores diameters ranging from 250 and 550 mm diameter, respectively. Then, they seeded these scaffolds with tooth bud cells and implemented them for 4 days in a postnatal rat tooth. They reported that the harvested scaffolds showed a regeneration of mineralized tissue in all scaffolds after implementation in the rat momentum for 20 weeks with the most robust of formation of bioengineered mineralized tissue in 550 mm pore RGD-containing scaffolds and the least robust in the 250 mm pore sized scaffolds without RGD [32].

Hyaluronic acid is an anionic, non-sulfated, glycosaminoglycan distributed widely throughout connective, epithelial, and neural tissues and an unbranched polysaccharide of repeating disaccharides consisting of D-glucuronic acid and N-acetyl-D-glucosamine [33]. Hyaluronic acid and its derivatives have excellent potential for tissue engineering because of their ability in modifying chemically and structurally for various applications. It is unique among glycosaminoglycans in that it forms in the plasma membrane. It has the appropriate physical structure, biocompatibility, and biodegradation as an implant for dental pulp regeneration. Hyaluronan as one of the main components of the extracellular matrix contributes significantly to cell proliferation and migration. Therefore, combinations of different growth factors with hyaluronic acid sponge are needed for the development of restorative treatment of dental pulp with sound dentin [34].

BIOCERAMICS

Dentin is composed of a mineral phase of HA and a soft hydrogel reinforcing phase generated primarily from type I collagen. Bioceramics and metals have been widely used as implant materials for joint and tooth replacement [35, 36]. HA is a part of various hard tissues, such as bone, dentin, and enamel, that has attracted much attention and is often used in conjunction with TCP [37]. The conventional metallic implants do not bond or integrate with natural bone tissues [38]. Therefore, bioactive coatings are of interest to improve the bone bonding performance of metallic implants.

Calcium phosphates have been proposed to provide additional advantages in endodontic therapy (repair of the dental pulp). They are biocompatible, nontoxic, and chemically similar to the mineral component of natural dentin in mammals and have the ability to form mineralized tissues. In addition, HA scaffolds are effective for the regeneration of dentin or the dentin-pulp complex [39-42]. The subject of fabricating of nano- or micro-structured scaffolds to mimic structural and three-dimensional configurations of natural bone or teeth has been of much interest. Hayakawa *et al.* [39] reported a new technique for self-assembling one-dimensional HA nano rods with a chosen location that simulated bone or 'enamel-like' structure. In order to assemble the teeth, Yoshikawa *et al.* [40] implemented a porous cylindrical HA implant with a hollow center for tooth regeneration where seeded bone marrow mesenchymal cells in the pores of the HA scaffold were pretreated with laminin to prepare the cell/HA composite scaffold. Then, they implanted these scaffolds in the dorsal subcutis of rats for 4 weeks, and observed that the osteogenesis in the pores of the cell/HA composite scaffold was clearly promoted [40]. Moreover, Mastrangelo *et al.* [41] synthesized HA scaffolds and seeded them with human dental follicle stem cells (hDFSCs) that were harvested from human dental cells and grew *in vitro* in order to study the morphological structure and extracellular matrix production. They observed an intense attachment and colonization of polygonal-shaped cells to the HA scaffold after week 1, a 3D organization of the cells after week 6, and the presence of dense material around the cell clusters [41]. Furthermore, Ando *et al.* [42] fabricated beta-tricalcium phosphate (b-TCP) scaffolds and seeded porcine dental papilla cells on them. Then, the cell-scaffold was transplanted into the nude mice.

The results indicated that an adentin-pulp complex-like structure could be successfully constructed [42]. Consequently, Liao *et al.* [43] synthesized a porous scaffold constructed from b-TCP/chitosan and seeded HPLCs into them. The result showed not only that vascular tissue ingrowths are multiplied and encouraged but also that the composite scaffold supported the differentiation of HPLCs headed for osteoblasts and cementoblasts [39]. It was reported that the HA-chitosan construct seeded with mainly fibroblast growth factor (bFGF) supplied an appropriate 3D setting for cellular structure, differentiation, proliferation, and mineralization [43]. In addition, electrospun PLLA/HA/multi-walled carbon nanotubes (MWNTs) nanofibrous scaffolds with high porosity and well-controlled pore seeded with hDPSCs cell culture could be useful for tooth tissue engineering [44]. However, the long term effects of using MWNTs in tissue engineering have not been well defined yet, and more research is needed.

Touri *et al.* [45] have recently reported the preparation of MWNT/45S5 Bioglass composite scaffolds by means of a new freeze casting process. As can be seen in Fig. (**2a**), the system consisted of ice lamellae, ceramic walls, and liquid particle suspension. The growing ice lamellae pushed the ceramic particles into the interlamellar spaces, where they formed ceramic walls consisting of random close packed ceramic particles dispersed in ice. They reported that the lamellar microstructure of the scaffolds consisted of plates with flat interconnected macropores, aligned along the ice growth direction, as shown in Fig. (**2b**). The width of the open interconnected macropores was between 20 and 100 μm, as shown in Fig. (**2c**). The addition of 0.25 wt.% MWCNTs increases the compressive strength and elastic modulus of 45S5 Bioglass scaffolds from 2.08 to 4.56 MPa, and 111.50 to 266.59 MPa, respectively.

In another study, this group isolated hDPSCs from dental pulp and seeded them on prepared scaffolds in order to evaluate cell viability, attachment, and proliferation [46]. They further reported that seeded cells showed high osteogenic capacity *in vitro*. They suggested that the combination of MWCNTs with Bioglass scaffolds could effectively optimize the approaches to dentin-pulp complex regeneration.

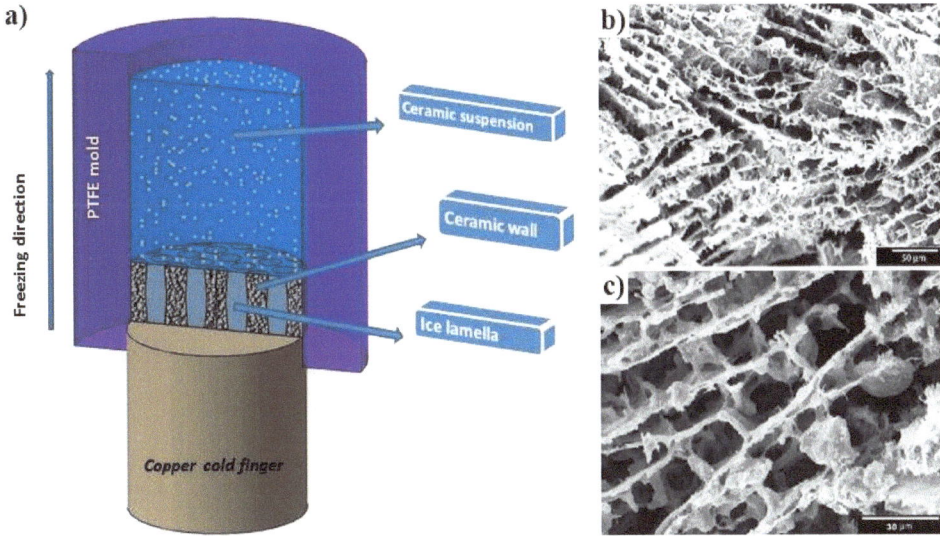

Fig. (2). (**a**) The schematic of freeze casting technique for the fabrication of the MWCNT/45S5 Bioglass scaffolds, (**b**) and (**c**) SEM micrograph of the cross sections parallel to the ice front, (**b**) with more details [45].

NEW TECHNOLOGIES IN SCAFFOLD PROCESSING

A number of conventional fabrication technologies have been applied to engineer biodegradable and bioresorbable materials into three-dimensional polymeric scaffolds of high porosity and surface area. For example, solvent casting/salt leaching allows for the preparation of porous structures with regular porosity, but with a limited thickness. In this method, a polymer is dissolved in an organic solvent and then particles, mainly salts, with specific dimensions are added to the solution. The mixture is shaped into its final geometry such as glass plate or in a three dimensional mold. Afterward, the solvent is evaporated to form a composite of the particles and polymer. The polymer remains and the particles are dissolved in a bath, leaving behind a porous structure [47].

Phase separation is a process which requires the use of a solvent with a low melting point to dissolve polymers. When a small quantity of water is added, phase separation is induced, and polymer-rich and polymer-poor phases are formed. Then, by cooling below the solvent melting point and evaporating the solvent, a porous scaffold is obtained. This method does not provide interconnectivity of pores in the porous structure [48].

In the emulsion freeze-drying technique, a synthetic polymer is dissolved into a suitable solvent first, and then water is added to the polymeric solution to obtain an emulsion. Subsequently, the emulsion is cast into a mold and frozen quickly before the two phases can separate. Finally, in order to remove the dispersed water and the solvent, the frozen emulsion is freeze-dried, thus leaving a solidified, porous polymeric structure. However, the problem with this method stems from that a relatively small pore size and often irregular porosity [49] of scaffolds produced with said technique.

Gas foaming is a technique that uses gas as a porogen to overcome the need to use organic solvents and solid porogens. In this method, initially disc-shaped structures made of the polymer are prepared, and, subsequently, the discs are placed in a chamber and exposed to high pressure carbon dioxide for several days. During this time carbon dioxide molecules escape the polymer, and pores are formed, resulting in a sponge-like structure. This method is fast and can fabricate micro-cellular configurations; however, its main drawback is that the pores do not form an interconnected structure [50].

In addition, the scaffolds produced by these techniques can be only constructed from one polymer and may produce inaccurate and uncontrollable porous morphology. Furthermore, almost all of these methods require organic solvent purification phases, which are time consuming and hence difficult for immediate implementation. Recently, tremendous amount of studies have been done aimed at exploring new techniques to custom-tailor scaffolds for teeth tissue engineering.

Electrospinning Technique

The electrospinning technique easily controls certain characteristics of scaffolds such as pore interconnectivity as well as internal and external scaffold geometry, to suit the structure and functionality of various tissue engineering applications. In this technique, a polymer in the liquid phase is pumped *via* a thin needle of specific diameter to assemble conductive object and so, the required high voltage is required. After the applied electric force over powers the surface tension forces of the polymer solutions, a jet of polymer fibers is developed. The main advantage of this method is the production of scaffolds, which are able to mimic the extracellular matrix in regard to a small pore size, density, and high surface area [51]. This technique can be used for many synthetic and natural polymers and can produce well-defined scaffolds. In regenerative dentistry, electrospinning has been successfully used to form membranes for periodontal tissue regeneration. This process also supports the fabrication of nanofibers from copolymers or polymer composites with biological molecules or minerals. Fig. (**3**) schematically indicates a diagram of fiber formation by electrospinning.

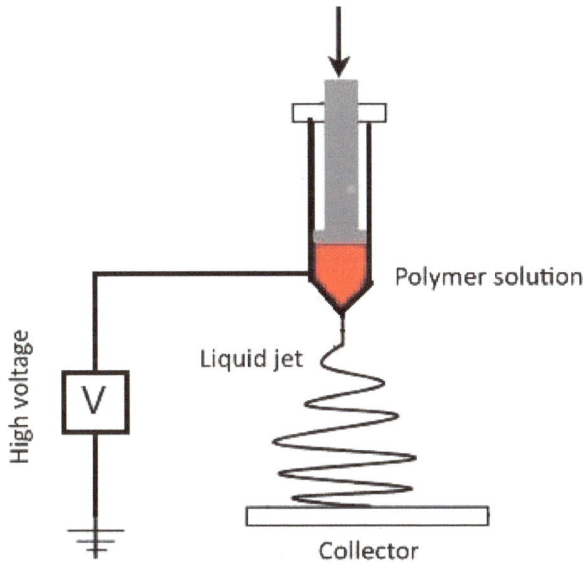

Fig. (3). Electro-spinning procedure [51].

Rapid Prototyping Technology

Rapid prototyping (RP) technologies have been widely applied in biomedical and tissue engineering applications. These techniques aim to design a computer controlled three-dimensional model and to construct a layer-by-layer cyclic deposition and the dispensation of material. Moreover, the detailed three-dimensional models can be potentially used as molds for manufacturing physical models of natural tissues or organs [52].

Hazeveld *et al.* [53], have recently investigated the accuracy and reproducibility of physical dental models reconstructed from digital data by using several RP techniques. They selected and served twelve mandibular and maxillary conventional plaster models from randomly chosen subjects as the gold standard. They then scanned the plaster models to form high-resolution three-dimensional models, and converted them into physical models using three rapid prototyping techniques: digital light processing, jetted photopolymer, and three-dimensional printing. The obtained results showed that the mean systematic differences for the measurements of the height of the clinical crowns were -0.02 mm for the jetted photopolymer models, 0.04 mm for the digital light processing models, and 0.25 mm for the three-dimensional printing models. For the width of the teeth, the mean systematic differences were -0.08 mm for the jetted photopolymer models, -0.05 mm for the digital light processing models, and -0.05 mm for the three-dimensional printing models (see Fig. **4**). They suggested that the dental models reconstructed by these techniques were considered clinically acceptable in terms of accuracy and reproducibility and could be appropriate for selected applications in orthodontics.

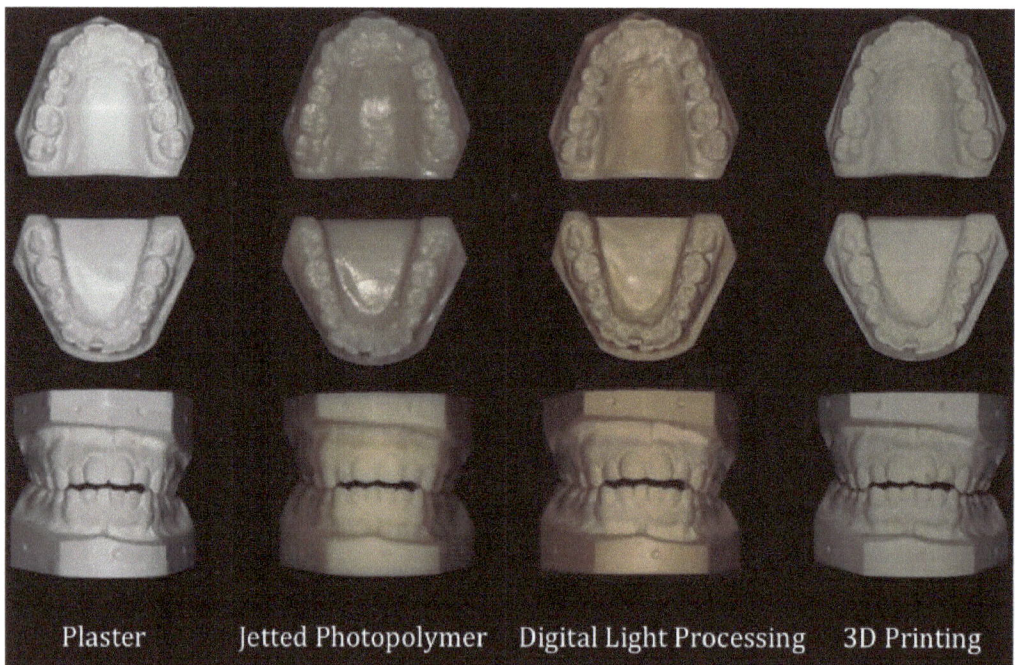

Plaster   Jetted Photopolymer   Digital Light Processing   3D Printing

Fig. (4). Typical illustrations of plaster model and corresponding replicas from the occlusal and frontal directions [53].

Supercritical Fluid-Gassing Process

A supercritical fluid-gassing approach can be used for creating suitable scaffolds for tissue engineering to address the main typical issue in the preparation of scaffolds, namely low connectivity between the pores. In a recent study, Maspero *et al.* [54] made a net-shaped porous scaffold in a few minutes by rapidly consolidating PLGA particles in a mold using sub-critical carbon dioxide and permitted the fast preparation of an exact porous copy of a tooth root without the use of any organic solvents. In this novel technique, a mold made from a sterile polyvinylsiloxane was constructed and copied the exact geometry of the tooth by placing the root of the tooth into the polyvinylsiloxane polymer. The aforementioned technique offers open porous scaffolds with desired shapes. Although this technique needs further optimization for clinical applications, the procedure offers a promising route in manufacturing open porous implants without the use of any organic solvent.

SELF-ASSEMBLING TECHNOLOGY

For the most part, current practice for treatment uses inert biomaterials as substitutes for soft and mineralized tissues. However, a tissue engineering technique using a hydrogel scaffold seeded with two dental stem cell lines together peptide-amphiphile (PA) has been used lately to establish a novel regenerative process to regenerate dental tissues. In addition, cell-matrix interactions can be guided by further inclusion of the tripeptide cell adhesion sequence, RGD, together with an enzyme-cleavable site. Galler *et al.* [16] cultured two types of stem cells from human exfoliated deciduous teeth (SHED) and DPSCs together with different osteogenic enhancements in PA hydrogels for 4 weeks. The results showed that the two types of cells differentiate and proliferate effectively with the hydrogel scaffolds. However, a certain degradation of the gels and extracellular matrix generation with clear disparities among both cell lines were observed by the histology data. The findings showed that SHED type cells had a spindle-shaped morphology, high proliferation rates, and collagen regeneration enabling soft tissue formation. DPSC cells had a drop in the rate of proliferation and produced an osteoblast-like phenotype with deposits of minerals. It was found that this technique established 3D PAs self-assembly configurations of nanofibers and tissues. In addition, due to the good biophysical properties of the hydrogels, they can be injected into small and irregular defects. Therefore, the developed process could be suitable for both soft and hard mineralized matrices for dental tissue engineering. Recently, a novel three-dimensional pellet cultivation technique was introduced to PDLSCs in order to produce a biological microenvironment similar to those of a regenerative milieu. The human PDLSCs were cultured with ascorbic acid and placed in media containing growing apical tooth germ cells. Correspondingly, the cells were assembled from the culture plate as an attaching cell piece that retains a substantial amount of extracellular matrix, and a single-cell pellet was produced from the detached cell-matrix. Furthermore, the PDLSCs implanted within this cell-matrix composite indicated many phenotypic characteristics of cementoblast lineages, as suggested by up regulation of alkaline phosphatase activity, the expression of bone sialoprotein, osteocalcin genes, and increased mineralization. However, it was reported that an aligned cementum/PDL-like composite was established when PDLSC pellets were implanted into immune-compromised mice. It was also found that the apical tooth germ cell-conditioned medium and endogenous extracellular matrix enriched the microstructure of the root/periodontal tissue regeneration. Moreover, the regeneration and enhancement of the physiological architecture of the cementum/PDL-like composite were found to be similar to that of the natural tissues. Therefore, the PDLSC pellet has the potential to deliver a good option to improve periodontal defect repair [55].

NOVEL SYNTHETIC POLYMERIC SCAFFOLDS

Synthetic polymers with a superior mechanical integrity, and machinability have been used extensively in dental repair [56]. For example, cells from tooth tissues were dissociated and seeded onto biodegradable PGA/PLLA, molecular evidence was obtained that the bioengineered tooth crowns similar to naturally growing teeth [57]. Moreover, the textile PGA fleece is a good candidate as the construct for human gingival fibroblasts and the structural factors of the fleece substantially influence the proliferation of cells [58]. In addition, it was reported that when stem cells from SHED were seeded into a synthetic open cell construct made from D, D-L, L-polylactic acid, the regeneration of the pulp tissue scaffolds was generated. After that, Gotlieb *et al.* [59] tested these constructs *in vivo* with a single cleaned and shaped root canal and reported that there was clear suggestion of cell adherence incorporated within all the pulp constructs investigated, according to ultra-structural assessment of SEM. Therefore, it was suggested that implanting tissue-engineered pulp constructs into teeth after cleaning and shaping is a justifiable technique [59]. Later, the use of multi-scale computational design and the fabrication of scaffolds consisting of PCL and PGA was studied for specific cell implementation of human cells so that a human tooth dentin-ligament-bone can be generated *in vivo*. The reports showed the interfacial creation of parallel- and obliquely-oriented fibers and the production of tooth cementum-like tissue [60]. Afterward, a new method of PLGA scaffold assembly using carbon dioxide as a solvent has been reported to make a net-shaped porous scaffold that had a high degree of porosity and interconnectivity [61]. Yang *et al.* [62] reported that the scaffolds made of PCL/gelatin/HA supported the proliferation and odontogenic differentiation of DPSCs, but the pore size of the scaffolds influenced tissue ingrowth. Lluch *et al.* [63] fabricated poly(ethyl methacrylate-co-hydroxyethyl acrylate) [P(EMA-co-HEA)] scaffolds with SiO_2 and aligned tubular pores which resembled natural dentin in regard to its structure and properties. Moreover, it induced the precipitation of apatite on dentin surfaces *in vitro*. Moreover, it is predicted that these scaffolds would expedite the amalgamation in the host mineralized tissue, encourage cell growth, and perform well *in vivo* dentin rejuvenation. Zhang *et al.* [64] combined tooth bud cell-seeded scaffolds with autologous iliac crest bone marrow stem cell-seeded scaffold to accelerate repair of mandibular defects in the Yucatan mini-pig. The generation of small tooth-like structures contained structured dentin, cementum, and periodontal was observed and enclosed by regenerated alveolar bone. These observations showed that the regeneration of teeth and associated alveolar bones in a single process can be achieved.

THE USE OF STEM CELLS, THEIR POTENTIAL AND THERAPEUTIC IMPLICATIONS IN DENTISTRY

Cell-based therapies are the most common approaches to tissue engineering and regenerative medicine [65]. Some of the most critical factors in using this approach clinically identifies the appropriate source of cells, finding methodologies to induce cell proliferation and differentiation, maintaining cell survival, and removing of any undesired cells. Stem cells not only possess an exceptional potential to proliferate and develop into many different cell types to form the desired organs but also hold great promise for regenerative therapies [66]. In addition, stem cell behavior closely correlates with cues that lie in their extracellular microenvironment [67, 68]. Embryonic stem cells, somatic or adult stem cells, and induced pluripotent stem cells are the most commonly investigated stem cells [69, 70]. The recent identification of adult mesenchymal stem cells in dental tissues also suggests that this cell population regrows into the tooth and regenerates the dentin-pulp complex [71, 72]. However, the exact mechanisms of the contribution of stem cells to clinical outcomes remain unclear.

Cell-Reprogramming Techniques

Embryonic stem cells have the capacity to multiply indefinitely, the ability to differentiate into any cell type under an appropriate microenvironment and are very useful in research and clinical applications in tissue engineering and regenerative medicine [73]. Somatic stem cells have limited applications; the derivation of human embryonic stem cells with matched immunogenotypes from fertilized human embryos also raises ethical issues. These cells can generate cell types of the tissue in which the cells reside but not cells of a very different origin. The new techniques for obtaining stem cells were developed due to the challenges stemming from working with human embryonic stem cells and somatic stem cells. Transdifferentiation and induced pluripotent stem cells are two such techniques.

Trans Differentiation

Transdifferentiation, or lineage reprogramming, converts a given cell type directly into another specialized cell type without bringing the cells back to a pluripotent state. This approach was successful for the conversion between two closely related cell types. For example, adult mesenchymal stem cells from teeth were shown to normally differentiate only into other mesenchymal cell types such as chondrocytes and adipocytes (see Fig. **5**) [74]. In addition, a combination of 3 neural transcription factors, achaete-scute complex homolog 1 (ASCL1), myelin transcription factor 1-like (MYT1L), and POU class 3 homeobox 2 (BRN2), was applied to convert mouse embryonic and postnatal fibroblasts into functional neurons *in vitro* [75]. The octamer-binding transcription factor 4 (OCT4) and cytokine treatment were used to convert human dermal fibroblasts into granulocytic, monocytic, megakaryocytic, and erythroid lineage cells [76].

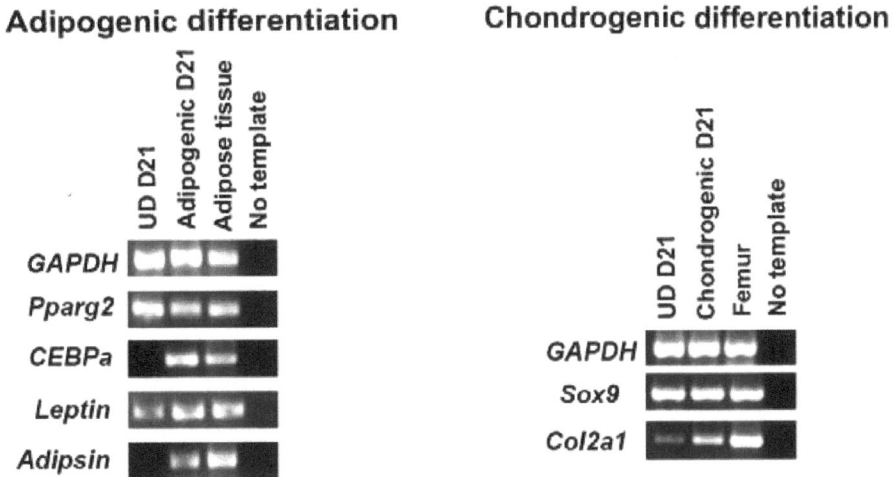

Fig. (5). Mesenchymal stem cells differentiate into chondrocytes and adipocytes [66].

Induced Pluripotent Stem Cells

This approach uses a quartet of transcription factors to reprogram somatic cells into pluripotent stem cells [77]. Yamanaka and Takahashi developed the first induced pluripotent stem (iPS) cells from adult mouse cells and from adult human cells [78, 79]. This technique offered a new way to dedifferentiate cells while maintaining donor-specific immune characteristics necessary to prevent rejection by the host's immune system. The iPS cells have almost identical properties to the ES cells in that they have the ability to multiply almost indefinitely without losing their potential to differentiate into any cells of the 3 germ layers: endoderm, mesoderm, and ectoderm. Instead of transdifferentiation, this approach is also applicable to the reprogramming of the adult stem cells to generate specialized cells of different origins [79].

CONCLUSION

Regenerative dentistry has a great potential to save millions of teeth each year and contribute to the overall improvement of human health. Synthetic and natural biodegradable bone regeneration materials, such as calcium phosphates, bioactive glasses, glass ceramics, calcium silicates, and *etc.*, are used to regenerate the bone defects of dental patients on regular basis. By taking advantage of stem cells, their intrinsic properties as well as growth factors and bioactive molecules, various characteristics of teeth can be repaired, and thus scaffolds can be used as a platform for the formation of engineered dental tissues. Molecular profiling of the genes that regulate dental stem cells to generate naturally formed dental tissues is of paramount importance. Moreover, establishing reliable and reproducible protocols to manipulate cell-scaffold interactions to bioengineer patient-specific dental tissues will allow for the field to generate more sound and robust solutions. This, in turn, would ultimately pave the way towards the tooth differentiation program, which could be fine-tuned to eventually lead to the formation of bioengineered dental tissues of even the whole tooth. There is a rising need for new and specialized scaffolds possessing surface properties and robustness of the natural extracellular matrix of bone and tooth. Future trends in this field are expected to revolutionize therapies for oral cavity regeneration and allow people to benefit from its use for years to come.

ACKNOWLEDGMENTS

None declared.

CONFLICT OF INTEREST

The authors confirm that this chapter contents have no conflict of interest.

ABBREVIATIONS

[P(EMA-co-HEA)]	=	Poly(ethyl methacrylate-co-hydroxyethyl acrylate)
3DP	=	Three-dimensional printing
ALP	=	Alkaline Phosphatase
ASCL1	=	Achaete-scute complex homolog 1
b-TCP	=	Beta-tricalcium phosphate

bFGF	= Fibroblast growth factor
BMP	= Bone morphogenetic protein
BRN2	= POU class 3 homeobox 2
DMP-1	= Dentin matrix protein-1
DPSCs	= Dental pulp stem cells
DSPP	= Dentin sialophosphoprotein
DXM	= Dexamethasone
FDA	= Food and Drug Administration
HA	= Hydroxyapatite
HAT-7	= Dental epithelial cells
hDFSCs	= Human dental follicle stem cells
HDPC	= Human dental pulp cells
hDPSCs	= Human dental pulp stem cells
hPDLF	= Human periodontal ligament fibroblast
iPS	= Induced pluripotent stem
MG-63	= Osteosarcoma
MWNTs	= Multi-walled carbon nanotubes
MYT1L	= Myelin transcription factor 1-like
nBGC	= Nano-bioactive glass ceramic
NFPLLA	= NanofibrousPLLA
OCN	= Osteocalcin
OCP	= Octacalcium phosphate
OCP/Col	= Porcine atelocollagen sponge

OCT4	= Octamer-binding transcription factor 4
PA	= Peptide-amphiphile
PCL	= Poly(ε-caprolactone)
PDLSCs	= Periodontal ligament stem cells
PGA	= Poly(glycolic) acid
PGA/PLLA	= Polyglycolate/poly-L-lactate
PLLA	= Poly-L-lactide
RGD	= Arginine-glycine-aspartic acid
RP	= Rapid prototyping
SHED	= Human exfoliated deciduous teeth
TCP	= Tricalcium phosphate

REFERENCE

[1] Alsberg E, Hill EE, Mooney DJ. Craniofacial tissue engineering. *Crit Rev Oral Biol Med* 2001; 12: 64-75.

[2] Honda M, Fong H, Iwatsuki S, Sumita Y, Sarikaya M. Tooth-forming potential in embryonic and postnatal tooth bud cells. *Med Mol Morphol* 2008; 41: 183-92.

[3] Anthony J, Paul T. Biological tooth replacement and repair. In: Robert P, Joseph V, editors. Principles of tissue engineering. *Academic Press*, 2007; 1067-77.

[4] Duailibi MT, Duailibi SE, Young CS, Bartlett JD, Vacanti JP, YelickPC. Bioengineered teeth from cultured rat tooth bud cells. *J Dent Res* 2004; 83: 523-8.

[5] Nakashima M, Reddi AH, The application of bone morphogenetic proteins to dental tissue engineering, *Nature Biotechnology*, 2003; 21: 1025-1032.

[6] Kim SH, Turnbull J, Guimond S. Extracellular matrix and cell signalling: thedynamic cooperation of integrin, proteoglycan and growth factor receptor. *J Endocrinol* 2011; 209: 139-51.

[7] Yen A, Sharpe P. Stem cells and tooth tissue engineering. *Cell Tissue Res* 2008; 331: 359-72.

[8] Murray PE, Constructs and Scaffolds Employed to Regenerate Dental Tissue, *Dent Clin N Am* 2012; 56: 577-588.

[9] Wan Y, Wu H, Yu A, Wen D, Biodegradable Polylactide/Chitosan Blend Membranes, *Biomacromolecules.* 2006; 7: 1362-1372

[10]   Wang J, Liu X, Jin X, Ma H, Hu J, Ni L. *et al.* The odontogenic differentiation of human dental pulp stem cells on nanofibrous poly(L-lactic acid) scaffolds *in vitro* and *in vivo*, *Acta Biomaterialia* 2010; 6: 3856-3863.

[11]   Young CS, Terada S, Vacanti JP, Honda M, Bartlett JD, Yelick PC. Tissue engineering of complex tooth structures on biodegradable polymer scaffolds. *J Dent Res* 2002; 81: 695-700.

[12]   Duailibi SE, Duailibi MT, Zhang W, Asrican R, Vacanti JP, Yelick PC. Bioengineered Dental Tissues Grown in the Rat Jaw, *J Dent Res* 2008; 87: 745-750.

[13]   Young C, Kimb S, Qinc C, Babac O, Butlerc W, Taylorb R, *et al.* Developmental analysis and computer modelling of bioengineered teeth. *Arch Oral Biol* 2005; 50: 259-65.

[14]   Park C, Rios H, Jin Q, Bland M, Flanagan C, Hollister S, *et al.* Biomimetic hybrid scaffolds for engineering human tooth—ligament interfaces. *Biomaterials* 2010; 31: 5945-52.

[15]   Goh BT, Chanchareonsook N, Tideman H, Teoh SH, Chow JK, Jansen JA. The use of a polycaprolactone-tricalcium phosphate scaffold for bone regeneration of tooth socket facial wall defects and simultaneous immediate dental implant placement in Macacafascicularis, *J Biomed Mater Res A.* 2014; 102(5): 1379-88

[16]   Galler K, Cavender A, Yuwono V, Dong H, Shi S, Schmalz G, *et al.* Self-assembling peptide amphiphile nanofibers as a scaffold fordental stem cells. *Tissue Eng* 2008; 14A: 2051-8.

[17]   Kirkham J, Firth A, Vernals D, Boden N, Robinson C, Shore RC, Brookes SJ, Aggeli A. Self-assembling peptide scaffolds promote enamel remineralization, *J Dent Res.* 2007; 86(5): 426-30.

[18]   Silver F, Pins G. Cell growth on collagen: a review of tissue engineering using scaffolds containing extracellular matrix. *J Long Term Eff Med Implants* 1992; 2: 67-80.

[19]   Sumita Y, Honda M, Ohara T, Tsuchiya S, Sagara H, Kagami H, *et al.* Performance of collagen sponge as a 3-D scaffold fortooth-tissue engineering. *Biomaterials* 2006; 27: 3238-48.

[20]   Kim NR, Lee DH, Chung PH, Yang HC, Distinct differentiation properties of human dental pulp cells on collagen, gelatin, and chitosan scaffolds, *Oral Surg Oral Med Oral Pathol Oral Radiol Endod.* 2009; 108: 94-100.

[21]   Iibuchi S, Matsui K, Kawai T, Sasaki K, Suzuki O, Kamakura S, Echigo S. Octacalcium phosphate (OCP) collagen composites enhance bone healing in a dog tooth extraction socket model. *Int. J. Oral Maxillofac. Surg.* 2010; 39: 161-168.

[22]   Madihally S, Matthew H. Porous chitosan scaffolds for tissueengineering. *Biomaterials* 1999; 20: 1133-42.

[23]   Suh J, Matthew H. Application of chitosan-based polysaccharidebiomaterials in cartilage tissue engineering: a review. *Biomaterials* 2000; 21: 2589-98.

[24]   Ravindran S, Song YQ, George A. Development of three-dimensionalbiomimetic scaffold to study epithelial—mesenchymalinteractions. *Tissue Eng Part A* 2010; 16: 327-42.

[25]   Fujiwara S, Kumabe S, Iwai Y. Isolated rat dental pulp cellculture and transplantation with an alginate scaffold. *Okajimas Folia Anat Jpn* 2006; 83: 15-24.

[26]   Srinivasan S, Jayasree R, Chennazhi KP, Nair SV, Jayakumar R, Biocompatible alginate/nano bioactive glass ceramic composite scaffolds for periodontal tissue regeneration, *Carbohydrate Polymers* 2012; 87: 274-283

[27]   Altman G, Diaz F, Jakuba C, Calabro T, Horan R, Chen J, *et al.* Silk-based biomaterials. *Biomaterials* 2003; 24: 401-16.

[28] Kim J, Kim U, Kim H, Li C, Wada M, Leisk G, *et al.* Bone tissue engineering with premineralized silk scaffolds. *Bone* 2008; 42: 1226-34.

[29] Uebersax L, Hagenmu"ller H, Hofmann S, Gruenblatt E, Muller R, Vunjaknovakovic G, *et al.* Effect of scaffold design on bone morphology *in vitro. Tissue Eng* 2006; 12: 3417-29.

[30] Hofmann S, Hagenmuller H, Koch AM, Muller R, Vunjak-Novakovic G, Kaplan DL, *et al.* Control of *in vitro* tissue-engineered bone-like structures using human mesenchymal stem cells and porous silk scaffolds. *Biomaterials* 2007; 28: 1152-62.

[31] Meinel L, Karageorgiou V, Hofmann S, Fajardo R, Snyder B, Li C, *et al.* Engineering bone-like tissue *in vitro* using human bone marrow stem cells and silk scaffolds. *J Biomed Mater Res* 2004; 71A: 25-34.

[32] Xu WP, Zhang W, Asrican R, Kim HJ, Kaplan DL, Yelick PC. Accurately shaped tooth bud cell-derived mineralized tissue formation on silk scaffolds. *Tissue Eng Part A* 2008; 14: 549-57.

[33] Morsi, YS. Tissue Engineering of the Aortic Heart Valve: Fundamentals and Developments (Paperback). *Gazelle Distribution* 2012; 30.

[34] Inuyama Y, Kitamura C, Nishihara T, Morotomi T, Nagayoshi M, Tabata Y, *et al.* Effects of hyaluronic acid sponge as a scaffold on odontoblastic cell line and amputated dental pulp. *J Biomed Mater Res* 2010; 92B: 120-8.

[35] HamlekhanA, MozafariM, NezafatiN, AzamiM, HadipourH, A proposedfabrication method of novel PCL-GEL-HApnanocomposite scaffolds for bone tissueengineering applications, *Adv Comp Lett* 2010; 19: 123-130.

[36] Azami M, Jalilifiroo zine zhadS, Mozafari M, Synthesis and solubility of calciumfluoride /hydroxyfluorapatitenanocrystals for dental applications, *Ceram Inter* 2011; 37: 2007-2014.

[37] Arinzeh TL, Tran T, McAlary J, *et al.* A comparative study of biphasic calciumphosphate ceramics for human mesenchymal stem-cell-induced bone formation. *Biomaterials* 2005; 26: 3631-8.

[38] Sepahvandi A, Moztarzadeh F, Mozafari M, Ghaffari M, Raee N, Photoluminescence in the characterization and early detection of biomimetic bone-likeapatite formation on the surface of alkaline-treated titanium implant: State of theart, *Colloids and Surfaces B: Biointerfaces*, 2011; 86: 390-396.

[39] Hayakawa S, Li Y, Tsuru K, Osaka A, Fujii E, Kawabata K. Preparation of nanometer-scale rod array of hydroxyapatite crystal. *Acta Biomater*2009; 5: 2152-60.

[40] Yoshikawa M, Tsuji N, Shimomura Y, Hayashi H, Ohgushi H. Effects of laminin for osteogenesis in porous hydroxyapatite. *Macromol Symp* 2007; 253: 172-8.

[41] Mastrangelo F, Nargi E, Carone L, Dolci M, Caciagli F, Ciccarelli R, *et al.* Tridimensional response of human dental follicularstem cells onto a synthetic hydroxyapatite scaffold. *J Heal Sci* 2008; 54: 154-61.

[42] Ando Y, Honda M, Ohshima H, Tonomura A, Ohara T, Itaya T, *et al.* The induction of dentin bridge-like structures by constructs of subcultured dental pulp-derived cells and porous HA/TCP in porcine teeth. *Nagoya J Med Sci* 2009; 71: 51-62.

[43] Liao F, Chen Y, Li Z, Wang Y, Shi B, Gong Z, *et al.* A novel bioactive three-dimensional beta-tricalcium phosphate/chitosanscaffold for periodontal tissue engineering. *J Mater Sci Mater Med* 2010; 21: 489-96.

[44] Akman A, Tigli R, Guemuesderelioglu M, Nohutcu R., bFGF loaded HA-chitosan: a promising scaffold for periodontal tissue engineering. *J Biomed Mater Res* 2010; 92A: 953-62.

[45] Touri R, Moztarzadeh F, Sadeghian Z, Bizari D, Mozafari M, The use of carbon nanotube to reinforce 45S5 bioglass-based scaffolds for bone tissue engineering and regenerative dentistry", *BioMed Research International* 2013; 2013: 1-8.

[46] Touri R, Moztarzadeh F, Sadeghian Z, Bizari D, Moztarzadeh S, Mozafari M, Carbon Nanotube-Reinforced Bioglass Scaffolds for Dental Pulp Tissue Engineering, *The First Iranian Annual Congress on Progress in Tissue Engineering and Regenerative Medicine, Artificial Organs* (John Wiley & Sons, Inc.) 2013, Vol. 37, No. 7: A3

[47] Mikos A, Thorsen A, Czerwonka L, Bao Y, Langer R, Winslow D. Preparation and characterization of poly(L-lactic acid) foams. *Polymer* 1994; 35: 1068-77.

[48] Nam Y, Park T. Biodegradable polymeric microcellular foams by modified thermally induced phase separation method. *Biomaterials* 1999; 20: 1783-90.

[49] Whang K, Thomas C, Healy K. A novel method to fabricate bioabsorbable scaffolds. *Polymer*1995; 36: 837-42.

[50] Harris L, Kim B, Mooney D. Open pore biodegradable matrices formed with gas foaming. *J Biomed Mater Res* 1998; 42: 396-402.

[51] Zhang L, MorsiY, WangY, Li Y, RamakrishnaS, Review scaffold design and stem cells for toothRegeneration, *Japanese Dental Science Review* 2013; 49: 14-26

[52] Lee J, Sachs E, Cima M. Layer position accuracy in powder-basedrapid prototyping. *Rapid Prototyping J* 1995; 1: 24-37.

[53] Hazeveld A, Huddleston Slater JJ, Ren Y, Accuracy and reproducibility of dental replica models reconstructed by different rapid prototyping techniques, *Am J Orthod Dentofacial Orthop* 2014; 145: 108-15.

[54] Maspero F, Ruffieux K, Muller B, Wintermantel E. Resorbable defect analog PLGA scaffolds using CO2 as solvent: structural characterization. *J Biomed Mater Res* 2002; 62: 89-98.

[55] Yang Z, Jin F, Zhang X, Ma D, Han C, Huo N, *et al.* Tissue engineering of cementum/periodontal-ligament complex using a novel three-dimensional pellet cultivation system for human periodontal ligament stem cells. *Tissue Eng C* 2009; 15: 571-81.

[56] Mozafari M, Functional nanomaterials for advanced tissue engineering, Editor: Aliofkhazraei M, Book Title: Handbook of Functional Nanomaterials (Volume 4 - Properties and Commercialization) [Hardcover] and [eBook]. NOVA Science Publishers Inc., New York, USA (2013).

[57] Sharma S, Srivastava D, Grover S, Sharma V. Biomaterials in Tooth Tissue Engineering: A Review, *J Clin Diagn Res* 2014; 8: 309-315.

[58] Baumchen F, Smeets R, Koch D, Graber H. The impact of defined polyglycolide scaffold structure on the proliferation of gingival fibroblasts *in vitro*: a pilot study. *Oral Surg Oral Med Oral Pathol Oral RadiolEndod* 2009; 108: 505-13.

[59] Gotlieb E, Murray P, Namerow K, Kuttler S, Garcia-godoy F. An ultrastructural investigation of tissue-engineered pulp constructs implanted within endodontically treated teeth. *J Am Dent Assoc* 2008; 139: 457-65.

[60] Horst OV, Chavez MG, Jheon AH, Desai T, Klein OD. Stem Cell and Biomaterials Research in Dental Tissue Engineering and Regeneration, *Dent Clin North Am* 2012; 56: 495-520.

[61] Young CS, Abukawa H, Asrican R, Ravens M, Troulis MJ, Kaban LB, Vacanti JP, Yelick PC. Tissue-engineered hybrid tooth and bone, *Tissue Eng.* 2005; 11(9-10): 1599-610.

[62] Yang X, Yang F, Walboomers X, Bian Z, Fan M, Jansen J. The performance of dental pulp stem cells on nanofibrous PCL/gelatin/nHA scaffolds. *J Biomed Mater Res* 2010; 93A: 247-57.

[63] Lluch AV, Fernandez AC, Ferrer GG, Pradas MM. Bioactive scaffolds mimicking natural dentin structure. *J Biomed Mater Res* 2009; 90B(1): 182-94.

[64] Zhang W, Walboomers X, van Kuppevelt T, Daamen W, Bian Z, Jansen J. The performance of human dental pulp stem cells on different three-dimensional scaffold materials. *Biomaterials* 2006; 27: 5658-68.

[65] Jaenisch R, Young R. Stem cells, the molecular circuitry of pluripotency and nuclear reprogramming. *Cell* 2008; 132(4): 567-82.

[66] Quante M, Wang TC. Stem cells in gastroenterology and hepatology. *Nat Rev Gastroentero lHepatol* 2009; 6(12): 724-37.

[67] Discher DE, Mooney DJ, Zandstra PW. Growth factors, matrices, and forces combine and control stem cells. *Science* 2009; 324(5935): 1673-7.

[68] Guilak F, Cohen DM, Estes BT, Gimble JM, Liedtke W, Chen CS. Control of stem cell fate by physical interactions with the extracellular matrix. *Cell Stem Cell* 2009; 5(1): 17-26.

[69] Jaenisch R. Stem cells, pluripotency and nuclear reprogramming. *J Thromb Haemost* 2009; 7: 21-3

[70] Han J, Sidhu KS. Current concepts in reprogramming somatic cells to pluripotent state. *Curr Stem Cell Res Ther* 2008; 3(1): 66-74.

[71] Li N, Liu N, Zhou J, Tang L, Ding B, Duan Y, Jin Y. Inflammatory environment induces gingival tissue-specific mesenchymal stem cells to differentiate towards a pro-fibrotic phenotype. *Biol Cell* 2013; 105(6): 261-75.

[72] Komada Y, Yamane T, Kadota D, Isono K, Takakura N, Hayashi S, Yamazaki H. Origins and properties of dental, thymic, and bone marrow mesenchymal cells and their stem cells. *PLoS One* 2012; 7(11): e46436.

[73] Arnhold S, Klein H, Semkova I, *et al.* Neurally selected embryonic stem cellsinduce tumor formation after long-term survival following engraftment into thesubretinal space. *Invest Ophthalmol Vis Sci* 2004; 45: 4251-5.

[74] Janebodin K, Horst OV, Ieronimakis N, *et al.* Isolation and characterization of neural crest-derived stem cells from dental pulp of neonatal mice. *PLoS One* 2011; 6: e27526.

[75] Vierbuchen T, Ostermeier A, Pang ZP, *et al.* Direct conversion of fibroblasts tofunctional neurons by defined factors. *Nature* 2010; 463: 1035-41.

[76] Szabo E, Rampalli S, Risueno RM, *et al.* Direct conversion of human fibroblaststo multilineage blood progenitors. *Nature* 2010; 468: 521-6.

[77] Yamanaka S, Takahashi K. Induction of pluripotent stem cells from mouse fibroblast cultures. *TanpakushitsuKakusanKoso* 2006; 51: 2346-51.

[78] Takahashi K, Yamanaka S. Induction of pluripotent stem cells from mouseembryonic and adult fibroblast cultures by defined factors. *Cell* 2006; 126: 663-76.

[79] Takahashi K, Tanabe K, Ohnuki M, *et al.* Induction of pluripotent stem cells fromadult human fibroblasts by defined factors. *Cell* 2007; 131: 861-72.

CHAPTER 6

Polyester Biomaterials for Regenerative Medicine

Diana-Elena Mogosanu[1,2], Elena-Diana Giol[1], Mieke Vandenhaute[1], Diana-Maria Dragusin[1], Sangram Keshari Samal[1] and Peter Dubruel[*,1]

[1]*Polymer Chemistry and Biomaterials Research Group, Ghent University, Krijgslaan 281 S4bis, Ghent 9000, Belgium; and* [2]*Center for Microsystems Technology (CMST), Ghent University - IMEC, Technologiepark - Building 914-A, Gent-Zwijnaarde 9052, Belgium*

Abstract: Polyesters represent a class of polymers comprised of backbone ester linkages offering opportunities to tune the macromolecular properties according to the needs of specific applications. The polyesters developed to date have generated an enormous interest because of their applicability in the biomedical field. Although these are flexible materials in the sense that they can be chemically tuned to obtain the desired properties, one of the important parameters that has to be considered when designing the material for biomedical applications represents the biocompatibility.

The present book chapter aims to review the recent advances for the most commonly studied polyester biomaterials. The first section of this chapter will focus on the synthesis strategies of polyesters as well as possible modification strategies. The second section of this chapter will highlight several polymer processing methods used to obtain scaffolds with different architectures for tissue engineering applications.

Keywords: Biodegradability, biomaterials, polyesters, poly(ethylene terephthalate), poly(glycerol sebacate), polyhydroxyalkanoates, poly(lactic-*co*-glycolic acid), poly(ε-caprolactone), prototyping techniques, scaffolds, tissue engineering.

INTRODUCTION

Polymers have generated an enormous interest because of their applicability in the biomedical field. The utility of polymers arises from a number of useful intrinsic properties, such as ease of processing, biocompatibility and low cost. However, a

***Corresponding Author Peter Dubruel:** Polymer Chemistry and Biomaterials Research Group, Ghent University, Krijgslaan 281 S4bis, Ghent 9000, Belgium; Tel: 003292644466; E-mail: Peter.Dubruel@ugent.be

noteworthy limitation in biological applications is given by their surface hydrophobicity and lack of natural cell recognition sites or functional groups along their backbones. Depending on the desired outcome, various polymer modification strategies such as plasma treatment, coating with bioactive components, blending with other polymers or copolymerization with functional monomers are often applied. These treatments introduce functionalities, improve hydrophilicity and enhance cell activity and tissue growth. In this chapter, we will focus on polyester scaffolds applied in regenerative medicine.

Scientists have focused their attention on providing novel synthesis strategies and complex scaffold designs suited for tissue engineering (TE) applications. In the 1990s, Langer *et al.* were the firsts to introduce the concept of delivering cells through polymeric scaffolds for regenerative purposes [1]. The main aim of a scaffold is to induce proper tissue development by guiding cells in a three-dimensional space (3D), allowing cell proliferation and extracellular matrix (ECM) deposition [2]. Whether the final scaffolds have to treat, support, regenerate or replace a certain tissue, optimal cell response, controllable biodegradation rate and minimum inflammatory response are vital. In this regard, researchers have introduced new functionalities to the existing synthetic material backbone [3], have performed surface modifications [4, 5], and elaborated new scaffold designs in order to mimic the ECM and therefore to attempt to reproduce living tissues [6].

Polyesters are considered attractive starting materials for scaffold production because they can be manufactured into various shapes with desired pore morphological features conductive to tissue in-growth. The most common classification of scaffolds architecture is in two-dimensional (2D) structures, defining mostly sheets or films, and three-dimensional (3D) structures such as porous solids, hydrogels, foams, or sponges [7]. Although electrospun membranes are sometimes reported as 2D structures [8], we will refer to all fiber-like structures (meshes and mats) as two-and-a-half dimensional (2.5D) structures. This extra category is justified by their apparent 2D structure (macroscopic scale), while in reality a 3D architecture is present (microscopic scale). To further support our statement, a high surface area-to-volume ratio is present in both 3D and electrospun scaffolds, the only difference being the size range (centi- or millimeter range for 3D and micro- or nanometer range for 2.5D scaffolds) [9].

This chapter reviews polyesters, focusing on their potential in regenerative medical applications. Biodegradable and non-biodegradable polyesters will be briefly discussed pointing out their synthesis strategies and properties. The use of polyesters as biomaterials in cardiovascular, neural, cartilage, bone and retinal tissue engineering will also be discussed in detail.

SYNTHESIS, MODIFICATION STRATEGIES AND PROPERTIES OF SYNTHETIC POLYESTERS

Biodegradable Polyesters

Poly (Glycerol-Sebacate) (PGS)

In the last decade, PGS has become one of the most studied elastomers for biomedical applications due to its biocompatibility and biodegradability. The polymer is synthesized *via* a polycondensation reaction between glycerol and sebacic acid, both being endogenous monomers found in the human metabolism [10]. The first reported synthesis involved mixing equimolar quantities of monomers, under inert atmosphere (120 °C, 24 hours) in order to form a pre-polymer. By applying subsequent curing treatments (*i.e.* vacuum), the pre-polymer undergoes crosslinking reactions that lead to an elastomer [11].

Intensive research has been performed on varying parameters such as molar ratio, type of reagents, and/or curing temperature [12, 13]. You *et al.* reported an epoxide ring opening polymerization of diglycidyl sebacate and sebacic acid, in the presence of tetrabutylammonium as a catalyst [14]. The replacement of the alcohol with an ester resulted in the synthesis of tougher elastomers with well-defined free hydroxyl groups. Nevertheless, the common limitations for the above mentioned synthesis strategies include high temperatures (used both for synthesis and curing), as well as long reaction times. The need of milder conditions was addressed by Nijst *et al.* [15] and Ifkovits *et al.* [16]. They reported the chemical modification of PGS with acrylate functions that allows rapid UV polymerization at room temperature in the presence of a photo-initiator. Liu *et al.* investigated the effect of blending PGS with citric acid and its effect in controlling the curing time [12]. The researchers blended the PGS pre-polymer with citric acid monohydrate in different molar ratios (glycerol/sebacic acid/citric acid) in order to render a higher mechanical strength and a shorter curing time. The next step was made by Wu *et al.* who reinforced poly(glycerol-sebacate-citrate) with nano-fumed silica [17]. It was reported that thus developed elastomers possessed improved mechanical properties due to the filler-polymer interaction. In addition, a lower cytotoxicity was observed, making these materials suitable for biomedical applications. Branched copolymers designed by blending the PGS elastomer with thermoplastic materials such as poly(L-lactide) or poly-ε-caprolactone also proved to possess good biocompatibility and diverse mechanical properties in comparison with the individual polymers [18, 19].

PGS Properties

PGS is a transparent, slightly yellowish polyester. Although it does not dissolve in water, it swells up to around 2% after 24 hours of incubation [11]. Mitsak *et al.* reported that the swelling degree decreases with the increase of curing time and temperature [20]. Thermal analyses of PGS revealed a totally amorphous polymer at 37 °C (similar to vulcanized rubber), as expected for a thermoset material. The initial study performed by Wang *et al.* [11] reported two melting temperatures (5.23 °C and 37.62 °C) and two crystallization temperatures (-52.14° and -18.50 °C). In another study, Cai *et al.* indicated a glass transition temperature at -37.02 °C and a broad melting transition ranging from -20 to 40 °C [21]. The authors stressed that the thermal stability of the polymer remains unaltered even after 50 cooling/heating cycles.

The mechanical properties of PGS can be tailored to exhibit a range of stiffnesses by modifying parameters such as molar ratio of monomers, and curing temperature and time. Mechanical properties provide an important insight into the possible applications of PGS. With an elongation of ~250%, this material can be classified as a soft, elastic material [11]. The Young's modulus of PGS classifies it between ligaments and myocardium, while its maximum elongation is similar to veins and arteries [22]. Therefore, PGS can be a suitable candidate for cardiovascular, cartilage and retinal tissue engineering.

The biocompatibility of PGS was studied both *in vivo* [23] and *in vitro* [24], the latter using different cell lines according to specific applications. In an initial study of its biocompatibility, Wang *et al.* seeded fibroblasts and reported PGS to be at least as biocompatible as the U.S. Food and Drug Administration (FDA) approved poly(lactic-*co*-glycolic acid) (PLGA). The *in vivo* response was also similar; the PGS subcutaneous implants were resorbed without granulation or scar tissue formation [11]. In later studies, different cell lines were used to successfully attest the *in vitro* compatibility of PGS. For cardiovascular tissue engineering applications, blood compatibility is a crucial factor. Motlagh *et al.* reported the hemocompatibility of this elastomer due to the reduced presence of inflammatory markers and long blood clotting times [25].

The *in vivo* studies suggest that PGS degrades *via* a surface erosion mechanism with a linear mass loss over time. While the *in vitro* degradation studies in buffer phosphate show that the polymer degrades only around 17% after 60 days, the *in vivo* experiments in rats attest a total resorption of PGS in the same time frame [11]. In an attempt to elucidate this phenomenon, Pomerantseva *et al.* studied the *in vivo* characteristics of PGS materials with different crosslinking densities [23]. They concluded that there is no significant correlation between the polymer mass loss and the crosslinking density (*i.e.* curing time). The authors suggest that the *in vivo* degradation mechanism is probably controlled by an enzymatic surface erosion process. Therefore, introducing new chemical functionalities in the PGS backbone might provide a solution for applications that require slower degradation rates.

Poly-ε-Caprolactone (PCL)

Poly(ε-caprolactone) (PCL) is one of the most important polyesters due to excellent mechanical properties, miscibility with a large range of other polymers, biodegradability and applications in multiple sectors, ranging from the biomedical field to the areas of microelectronics [26], adhesives [27] and packaging [28]. In addition, this material is appealing as it has the lowest unit price among all commonly available biodegradable polymers [29].

PCL can be prepared *via* two different methods: polycondensation [30] and ring opening polymerization (ROP) [28, 31]. PCL can be synthesized by polycondensation of the corresponding hydroxyl acid, 6-hydroxyhexanoic acid

[32, 33]. Mahapatro *et al.* described the mild, solvent-free bulk polyesterification of linear aliphatic hydroxyacids of variable chain length, including 6-hydroxyhexanoic acid, catalyzed by immobilized Candida Antarctica Lipase B (Novozyme-435) [34]. After 8 hours, the relatively slower progress of 6-hydroxyhexanoic acid polymerization was evident. After 48h, the average degree of polymerization (DP) was 80 and the product showed a polydispersity index of 1.5. Polycondensation synthesis of PCL has been less investigated because of the shortcomings inherent to the reaction: harsh reaction conditions, long reaction times and low molecular weight [32]. As a consequence, ROP is the preferred route as it renders a polymer with a higher molecular weight and a narrow polydispersity [28].

The production of PCL by ROP of the cyclic monomer ε-caprolactone was studied as early as the 1930s [35]. Various ROP mechanisms exist and depend on the applied initiator/catalyst system. An overview of the ROP mechanisms is presented in Fig. (**1**). Each method has a profound effect on the resulting molecular weight and the end group composition [36].

o   Anionic ROP involves the formation of anionic species (by ring opening of a first monomer molecule using an initiator) which attacks the carbonyl carbon of a second monomer molecule. The reaction proceeds by the scission of the acyl carbon-oxygen bond leading to alkoxide growing species [37]. Initiators typically used for this type of polymerization include alkali metals, alkali metal alkoxides and alkaline earth metal-based catalysts [32, 33, 36, 38]. Evans *et al.* showed that ε-caprolactone can be polymerized by divalent samarium bis(phosphido) complexes [39]. At ambient temperatures, the reaction can be completed in less than 1 hour to yield PCL with narrow polydispersity.

o   Cationic ROP involves the formation of a cationic species which is subsequently attacked by the carbonyl oxygen of the monomer through a bimolecular nucleophilic substitution reaction [37]. Initiators typically used for this type of polymerization include protic acids, Lewis acids, stabilized carbocations and acylating agents [32, 36, 40]. This type of polymerization has not been frequently applied for the production of PCL since the control of the molecular weight is difficult and low DPs are obtained.

The coordination-insertion ROP mechanism is most commonly used to obtain high molecular weight PCL with high conversions, under mild conditions. It is a pseudo-anionic ROP where the propagation step proceeds through monomer coordination to the catalytic active site and insertion of the monomer into a metal-oxygen bond of the catalyst [41]. Since low reactive species are present in this stage, side reactions are suppressed and the reaction has the character of a living ROP. Initiators include dibutyl zinc, alkoxides and halides of aluminum, magnesium and titanium, stannous chloride and stannous octoate [32]. The most commonly used initiator is tin(II) 2-ethylhexanoate (Sn(Oct)$_2$), which is effective, commercially available and soluble in most organic solvents and lactones [42, 43].

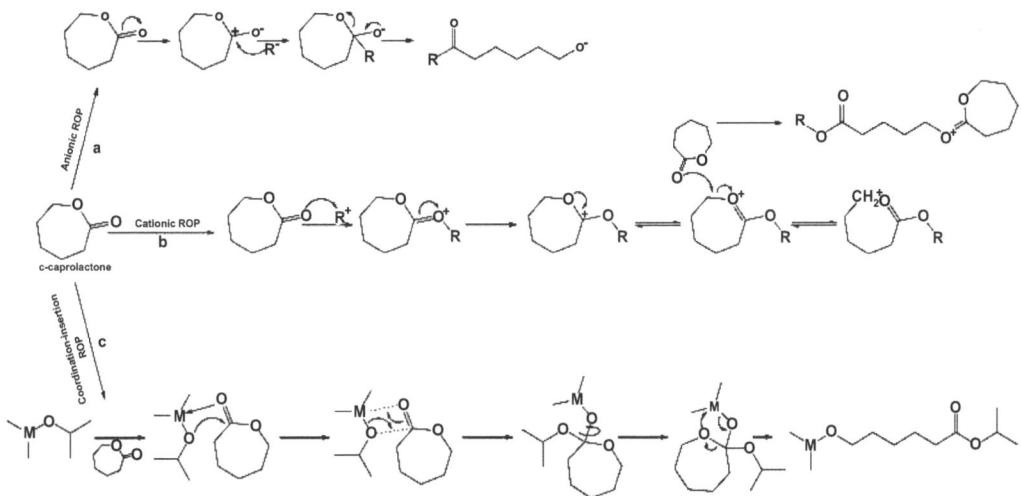

Fig. (1). Mechanism of the initiation step of the anionic (**a**), cationic (**b**) and coordination-insertion (**c**) ROP of ε-caprolactone.

PCL Properties

PCL is an aliphatic polyester composed of hexanoate repeat units [28]. It is a hydrophobic, semi-crystalline polymer [44]. The physical, thermal and mechanical properties of PCL depend mostly on its molecular weight and its degree of crystallinity. The number average molecular weight of PCL samples may vary from 530 to more than 100,000 g/mol. The degree of crystallinity increases as the molecular weight decreases, reaching up to 80% in case of a molecular weight of 5,000 g/mol. PCL exhibits several unusual properties not found among the other aliphatic polyesters. Most noteworthy are its exceptionally low glass transition temperature (-60 °C) [45] and low melting temperature (ranging between 56 °C-65 °C), both dictated by the crystalline nature of the polymer [32, 45-50]. PCL also shows a high thermal stability. Whereas most aliphatic polyesters have decomposition temperatures between 235° and 255°C, PCL displays a much higher value (350 °C) [51]. It has a low tensile strength, often below 20 MPa, but an extremely high elongation at break (up to 1 000%). At room temperature, PCL is highly soluble in chloroform, dichloromethane, carbon tetrachloride, benzene, toluene, cyclohexanone and 2-nitropentane; slightly soluble in acetone, dimethylformamide and acetonitrile; and insoluble in alcohols, diethyl ether and water [32, 46, 48]. The highly valuable property of PCL is that it is miscible with many other biodegradable and non-degradable polymers, such as starch, poly(lactic acid) (PLA), PLGA, poly(vinyl chloride), and poly(bisphenol-A) carbonates. Their blends present improved performances (*e.g.* improved stress crack resistance, dye-ability and adhesion), controllable degradation rate or the ability to serve as plasticizer [32, 46, 51]. Copolymers (block and random) of PCL can be formed using many monomers [46], such as ethyleneoxide [52, 53], styrene [54], diisocyanates (urethanes) [55], methyl methacrylate [56], glycolide [57] and lactide [58].

PCL can be enzymatically degraded by a number of organisms (bacteria and fungi), resulting in fast decomposition [32, 59-61]. In the human body, due to the lack of suitable enzymes, PCL undergoes a two-stage degradation process. Firstly, a non-enzymatic hydrolytic cleavage of labile aliphatic ester linkages takes place *via* surface and bulk degradation pathways. At this point the amorphous phase is degraded and free carboxylic acids autocatalyze the hydrolysis. Secondly, when the polymer is more crystalline and has a low molecular weight (less than 3,000 g/mol), it undergoes intracellular degradation due to uptake of macrophages and giant cells in phagosomes and fibroblasts [46, 48, 51]. Hydrolysis intermediates 6-hydroxyhexanoic acid and acetyl coenzyme A are formed and are eliminated from the body. The degradation of PCL is rather slow in comparison to polyglycolide (PGA), polylactide (PLA) and its copolymers [62]. Depending on the degradation conditions, molecular weight and degree of crystallinity, degradation can take from several months to several years [48]. This makes the material suitable for long term applications.

The good biocompatibility, biodegradability, structural stability and mechanical properties propelled PCL as an ideal candidate for TE applications. The main drawbacks are poor bioactivity (related to the absence of bioactive functional groups at the surface) and hydrophobicity that reduce cell affinity and cellular interactions, leading to low tissue regeneration rates [63]. This problem has been addressed by many researchers and led to the development of several surface modification strategies [64-69]. Among these techniques, the use of non-thermal plasma has proven to be of great potential, for 2D as well as 3D scaffolds [70, 71]. Jacobs *et al.* describe the use of medium pressure non-thermal plasma treatment in dry air, helium and argon atmosphere to enhance the surface properties of PCL [72]. The contact angle and XPS analyses showed that air and argon plasma treatments are able to enhance the surface wettability by incorporating oxygen-containing functionalities. In one of the most recent studies, Desmet *et al.* reported a multi-step modification protocol in which free amines were grafted on the PCL surface after plasma pre-treatment [4]. Subsequent coating with gelatin type B and fibronectin led to an enhanced osteosarcoma cell attachment and proliferation in comparison with the unmodified PCL surfaces.

Poly (Lactic-co-Glycolic Acid) (PLGA)

Some of the most versatile biodegradable polymers used in the medical field are those derived from poly lactic acid (PLA), poly glycolic acid (PGA) and their copolymers (PLGA). Although intensive research has been performed on both PLA and PGA, in the present book chapter we will focus on PLGA. PLGA is the most popular available biodegradable polymer and displays highly tunable properties. Moreover a lot of clinical experience with PLGA has been gained. Dating from the 1970s, the copolymers of PGA and PLA were the first commercialized biomaterials for surgical sutures, drug delivery systems and wound dressings [73].

PLGA can be obtained either *via* polycondensation or *via* ROP of lactide and glycolide [41, 74, 75]. The latter is the most widely used because of the higher control over the monomer sequence and over polymer chain ends. Similarly as with PCL production, different strategies are followed in order to obtain PLGA: anionic ROP, cationic ROP and coordination-insertion polymerization [74]. The use of a catalyst is critical, one of the most commonly used complexes for industrial preparation being $Sn(Oct)_2$, a FDA-approved food additive [74, 76]. Chain control agents (*i.e.* lauryl alcohol) are also used for better optimization of the polymerization [76, 77].

PLGA Properties

PLGA is a linear aliphatic polymer, soluble in common solvents such as chlorinated solvents, tetrahydrofuran, acetone or ethyl ether [78]. Its mechanical properties are dependent on the molecular weight, the polydispersity index and the crystallinity degree. Gilding *et al.* showed that PLGA is present in an amorphous state if the glycolic acid (GA) percentage is between 25% and 70% [76]. Generally, the monomer ratio influences the overall properties of the polymer. For instance, PLGA preparations with more lactide units are more hydrophobic and therefore degrade more slowly due to the methyl side groups in PLA [78, 79]. On the other hand, higher content of PGA leads to faster degradation, the exception being PLGA with a monomer ratio of 50/50 which exhibits the fastest degradation. In this regard, Middleton *et al.* stated that 50/50 PLGA degrades in approximately 1-2 months, the 75/25 copolymer in 4-5 months and the 85/15 copolymer in 5-6 months [80].

Although PLGA is a FDA approved polymer due to its optimal mechanical and degradation properties, its cell affinity is limited [81]. Additional coatings [82-84] or surface modification techniques [81, 83, 85-87] are required to improve biocompatibility. As for other materials, topography is a key factor for cell adhesion and proliferation [88, 89]. Recently, Zamani *et al.* found that aligned PLGA fibrous scaffolds can direct human nerve cell outgrowth without any post-processing modification [90]. A wide range of cell types were studied to assess the biocompatibility of this polymer and its application for regeneration of bone [84, 91-94], liver [95], nerve [96, 97], skin [98] and blood vessels [99, 100].

Polyhydroxyalkanoates (PHAs)

Polyhydroxyalkanoates (PHA) are a type of polyester produced by gram-negative and gram-positive bacteria and have been the subject of research since the 1920s, when the French bacteriologist Maurice Lemoigne discovered poly(3-hydroxybutyrate) (PHB). The polymer backbone is comprised of 3 carbon atoms with various alkyl groups in the β position, leading to more than 100 different polymers with properties ranging from stiff to elastomeric [101]. PHAs are considered "green" biomaterials and represent a solution to the pollution problem caused by synthetic plastic waste and dioxin emissions resulting from incineration disposal procedures [102].

Various bacteria have been reported [102-104] to produce PHAs under unfavorable growth conditions (excess of carbon source, limitation of oxygen, phosphorus, *etc.*), with a yield between 0.02-90 (w/v %) [102, 105, 106]. Some of the most used bacteria are *Alcaligeneseutrophus*, *Bacillus megaterium QMB1551*, *Klebsiellaaerogenes recombinants*, *Methylobacteriumrhodesianum*, *Pseudomonas (P.) aeruginosa*, *P. denitrificans*, *P. oleovorans*, *P. putida*, *Sphaerotilusnatans*, and *Escherichia coli* recombinants. When cells are subjected to unfavorable growth conditions they stimulate a survival mechanism through which accumulation of storage materials occurs. Phosphorus is stored in the form of polyphosphate and carbon in the form of PHA and/or glycogen [107]. PHAs are therefore accumulated as granules in the cytoplasmic membrane and cytoplasm of these bacteria [102].

The industrial production focuses mostly on batch and fed-batch fermentation procedures using carbon-rich substrates (sucrose, glucose, glycerol, *etc.*), followed by isolation and purification of PHA [108]. The most efficient method regarding the amount of obtained product is fed-batch fermentation due to the low quantity of used substrates. Despite the advantages they offer, PHAs have high production costs due to use of expensive substrates and long time lag between batch production.

PHAs Properties

PHAs are non-toxic, optically active, biocompatible and biodegradable thermoplastic materials. They are capable of having high crystallinity and a high number of repeating units, ranging from 100 to 30,000 [101]. Some of the most studied polymers of this class include PHB, poly(hydroxyvalerate) (PHV) and their copolymer, poly(3-hydroxybutyrate-*co*-3-hydroxyvalerate) (PHBV). PHB is a water insoluble, brittle material, with a melting temperature (179 °C) rather close to its degradation temperature (185 °C), making it a very challenging material for processing [109]. In order to tackle this problem, 3-hydroxyvalerate (HV) units have been incorporated as co-monomer of hydroxybutyrate (HB), leading to the development of a biomaterial with superior mechanical and thermal properties, PHBV. The addition of HV units provides more flexibility, an increased elongation at break and a decrease of the melting temperature [110].

Biodegradability is the key advantage of PHAs over synthetic plastics. The degradation rates depend on factors like exposure to microbes, pH, pressure, moisture, surface area and the physico-chemical properties of the polymers. PHAs degrade in anaerobic conditions into CO_2 and CH_4, while aerobic conditions render water and CO_2 as end products [109, 111]. Studies have shown that PHB copolymers with HV degrade faster than the polymer itself due to microorganisms that break down the polymer chain into hydroxyacids [102]. Other factors like low molecular weight and the low melting temperature favor enzymatic degradations. More specifically, PHBV were found to be compostable within 6, 75 and 350 weeks under anaerobic sewage, soil and sea water, respectively [109]. Due to the presence of low molecular weight PHB, PHAs and their monomers are considered non-toxic. This statement is supported by different patents [112, 113] that report the use of PHAs for therapeutical and nutritional applications.

NON-BIODEGRADABLE POLYESTERS

Polyethylene Terephthalate (PET)

Poly(ethylene terephthalate) (PET) or polyester (improperly called in the textile industry) has the IUPAC name "poly(oxyethyleneoxyterephthaloyl)". PET is a thermoplastic polymer obtained by a step-growth polycondensation reaction. The synthesis of PET implies a two-step process, where initially an oligomer (pre-polymer) is produced. The final polymer is obtained through further condensation reactions. At industrial scale, two main pathways for pre-polymer production are applied: the transesterification and the esterification reaction [114]. PET was initially produced on a large scale *via* the transesterification reaction between dimethyl terephthalate (DMT) and ethylene glycol (EG). The monomer mixture was treated at high temperatures (250 °C) in order to obtain the pre-polymer bis-hydroxy ethylene terephthalate and methanol. In the late 1960s, high purity terephthalic acid (TA) was introduced on the industrial market and the PET synthesis method switched towards the esterification reaction between diols and diacids. Nowadays, 70% of the industrial production of PET is based on the esterification reaction of EG and TA, in a temperature range of 235 °C-285 °C and under pressure (1-4 bars). The use of catalysts decreases the number of side reactions and the polymerization reaction time. The most commonly used catalysts include antimony compounds. Other compounds with catalytic activity, such as germanium, titanium oxide or zeolites are also applied for the production of PET [115-117]. By-products are formed regardless of the synthesis path (*i.e.* methanol for transesterification and water for esterification). Both transesterification and esterification reactions are equilibrium reactions; this implies that the rate of pre-polymer formation is highly dependent on the removal of these by-products. In order to achieve higher molecular weights of the polyester, a subsequent polycondensation can be applied. This late stage polycondensation is called solid state polycondensation and is performed at a temperature of 220 °C-235 °C, under vacuum and/or an inert gas atmosphere [114].

PET Properties

PET is a hard, stiff, dimensionally stable material that absorbs little water. It has good mechanical and thermal properties and it is considered an inert material. PET of different grades (either low or high grade) can be produced depending on the synthesis evolution. The low grade PET, also called fiber-grade PET, has an average molecular weight between 15,000 and 20,000 g/mol. Bottle-grade PET is typically obtained after the two-step polycondensation manufacturing procedure and, as the name indicates, it is mostly used for beverage packaging production. Through a subsequent step during the manufacturing process, the average molecular weight of the final product can be increased (between 24,000 and 36,000 g/mol) and high grade PET or bottle-grade PET can be obtained. The grade of PET is directly dependent on thermal degradation reactions, as the thermal properties of the product are reduced with the increased presence of carboxylic moieties in the PET structure.

In mild acidic and alkaline media, PET presents a good chemical resistance. Concentrated alkaline solutions lead to a hydrolysis reaction, nicely presented in the study of Chen *et al.* [118]. PET is insoluble in most common solvents. Only trifluoroacetic acid (TFA), solvent mixtures of TFA with dichloromethylene and aromatic and/or halogenated solvents (at increased temperatures) can dissolve this polymer. One parameter that determines PET solubility is crystallinity. Depending on the applied processing methods, PET exhibits a wide range of crystallinity degrees. Possible processing methods of PET include extrusion, spinning, electrospinning, and melt-blowing, through which films and fibers can be obtained. Commercially available PET films (biaxially oriented and thermal stabilized) are industrially produced under the trade names of Mylar®, Melinex® or Hostaphan® and PET fibers are known under the trade names of Dacron®, Trevira® and Terylene® [119].

To conclude this part of the chapter, we have presented in Fig. (**2**) the chemical structures of the polyesters discussed so far. Some of their most relevant properties are summarized in Table **1**.

APPLICATIONS OF POLYESTERS FOR BIOMEDICAL APPLICATIONS

Design of Scaffolds

At a time when medicine requires an increasing number of implantable materials and medical devices for tissue repair or regeneration, synthetic 3D scaffolds provide a solution for a wide range of medical problems. Scaffolds offer support for cells to proliferate and maintain their differentiated function, while providing mechanical and mass transport functions for tissue regeneration. These are facilitated by the internal architecture and physico-chemical properties of the polymer construct. Therefore, scaffolds must present navigational routes for cell

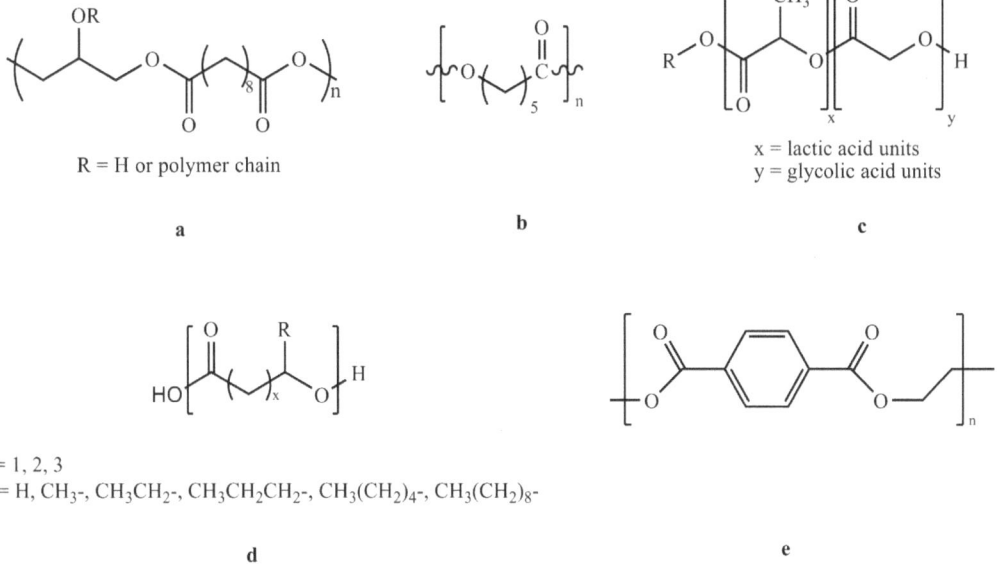

R = H or polymer chain

a

b

x = lactic acid units
y = glycolic acid units

c

x = 1, 2, 3
R = H, CH$_3$-, CH$_3$CH$_2$-, CH$_3$CH$_2$CH$_2$-, CH$_3$(CH$_2$)$_4$-, CH$_3$(CH$_2$)$_8$-

d

e

Fig. (2). Schematic representation of **a**: poly(glycerol sebacate), PGS; **b**: poly(e-caprolactone), PCL; **c**: poly(lactic-co-glycolic acid), PLGA; **d**: polyhydroxyalkanoates, PHA and **e**: poly(ethylene terephthalate), PET.

Table 1.   Summary of Relevant Polyester Properties

	T_m (°C)	T_g (°C)	Young's Modulus	Tensile Strength (MPa)	Elongation at Break (%)	Degradation Time	Refs.
PGS	5.23; 37.62	-37	0.282-2 MPa	0.5	250	60 days *in vivo*	[11, 22]
PCL	59-65	-60	343.9-364.3 MPa	10.5-16.1	1000	Slow degradation; Up to 4 years	[22, 62]
PLGA**	159.75	59.25	40.4-134.5 MPa	2.1-2.6	-	1-6 months	[22, 78, 79]
PHB	179	5	3.5 GPa	40 MPa	4	24-30 months *in vivo*	[22, 111]
PHBV*	137-170	-	0.7-2.9	30-38	20; 100	1-87 months	[109]
PET	245	76-80	2-4 GPa; 9-11 GPa (fibers)	80	60-165 (films); 36 (fibers)	-	[117, 119]

* Values depend on the HB:HV and LA:GA ratio, respectively; **PLGA fibers; T_m = melting temperature; T_g = glass transition temperature.

movement and migration *via* pores and channels. A wide range of scaffold fabrication methods enabling a controlled porosity (*i.e.* porosity degree, pore size or shape, interconnectivity) has been reported in the literature [120]. Some of the most frequently used methods include solvent casting, particulate leaching, membrane lamination, phase separation, emulsion freezing/drying or freeze drying procedures. Recently, other specialized methods such as electrospinning or rapid prototyping have evolved as novel scaffold manufacturing techniques [121]. These methods are often accompanied by imaging techniques (*i.e.* computed tomography (CT), magnetic resonance imaging) [48] and specialized computational topology design in order to produce a patient specific implants [1, 120, 121]. The main aforementioned techniques applied to date will be briefly discussed.

o *Particulate leaching* is one of the most straightforward scaffold fabrication techniques. Small particles (templates or porogens) are dispersed within a polymer or monomer solution that is fixed or gelled. Removal of the template results in desired porous scaffolds [46, 122].

o The *phase separation* technique involves the separation of a polymer solution into two phases, a polymer-rich (*i.e.* high concentration) phase and a polymer-lean (*i.e.* low concentration) phase. After the solvent is removed by extraction, evaporation or sublimation, the polymer-rich phase is solidified, generating porous membranes or scaffolds [46, 122, 123]. The main limitation of this technique is that detail limited structures are obtained.

o *Electrospinning* is a versatile technology that converts a polymer (either in solution or melt) into a fibrous structure by applying an electrical field. The resultant fibers are collected on a lower potential region (a grounded collector) under the form of fibers. Polymer properties (such as viscosity and concentration) and ambient parameters influence the morphology and characteristics of the obtained fibers. The main advantage of this method is its potential to produce materials with high porosity and high surface area-to-volume ratio [124].

o *Solid free-form fabrication* and *rapid prototyping techniques* [125] are used to build scaffolds through a selective deposition of the materials, in a layer-by-layer approach. These methods are based on computer software driven approach, where each layer is a cross-section of a computer-aided design

(CAD) model. This technology develops scaffolds with highly reproducible architectures and compositional variations across the entire matrix [46]. Stereolithography, selective laser sintering, 3D printing and systems based on extrusion (*i.e.* fused deposition modeling) are rapid prototyping techniques described in literature [46, 122, 126].

o In *stereolithograpy*, focused laser light [61] is used to scan the surface of a photo-sensitive material in order to produce 2D patterns of a polymerized material. A 3D construct is built-up using a layer-by-layer approach. Once a 2D layer is finished, the fabrication platform is moved stepwise in the Z-direction in order to add a new layer [46, 121, 122]. Although high accuracy structures and thin walls inside the scaffolds are obtained, photo-polymers are the only materials that can be processed *via* this method.

o *Selective laser sintering* is another technique that uses a focused laser beam to sinter or fuse areas of a loosely compacted powder. The powder is spread evenly onto a flat surface by a roller mechanism, and the powder particles irradiated by the laser beam are subsequently fused [46, 122, 127]. A variety of materials can be processed with this technique, but the mechanical properties are below those achieved with injection molding for the same material.

o *3D printing* is a cost efficient technology that is used to create a solid object by ink-jet printing of a binder (*i.e.* solvent) into selected areas of sequentially deposited layers of powder. The solvent drying rate is an important variable in the scaffolds production.

Fused deposition modeling involves the deposition of a thermoplastic filament material obtained through extrusion, using a layer-by-layer process. According to the specific CAD model, at the end of each finished layer, the collector platform is lowered and the next layer is deposited. The extruded filaments are fused together upon cooling [46, 122, 128]. Although this method has limited accuracy for small features, details and thin walls, the main advantage is that it is easy to manipulate (easy material changeover and office environment friendly).

TISSUE ENGINEERING

Tissue engineering (TE) has gained a spectacular interest due to its main goal: to **R**epair, **R**eplace or **R**egenerate an injured tissue [129]. The big three **R**s continue to raise questions regarding the nature of the materials. Natural materials present interesting properties, but also important limitations such as difficulty in controlling their mechanical properties and fast degradation rates. Synthetic biomaterials, on the other hand, are cheaper to fabricate (large scale production), have a long shelf life, and can be tailored to meet the stringent requirements imposed by different applications. Efforts have been made to surpass the limitations of the synthetic materials (*e.g.* limited material cell recognition) through different means such as manipulation of internal architecture and surface topography, and bio-functionalization. A schematic representation of what tissue engineering entails is presented in Fig. (**3**). An effect-cause relationship exists between polymer scaffolds and cells, and only an optimal co-existence results in formation of new tissue, neo-tissue. In this respect, polyesters are versatile polymeric materials and their usage extends in a broad suite of medical applications.

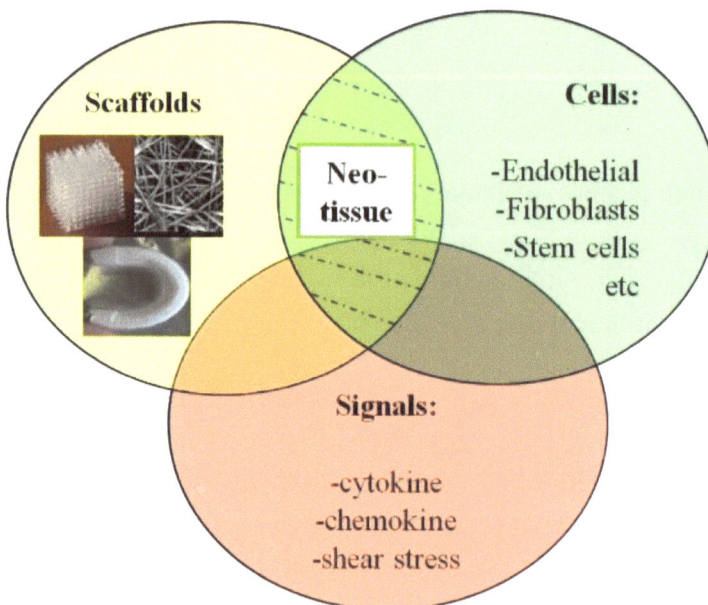

*bioplotted and electrospun (mesh and tubular) scaffolds

Fig. (3). Schematic concept of tissue engineering.

Cardiovascular Tissue Engineering

Heart failure is the result of a wide range of cardiovascular disorders such as coronary heart disease, cerebro-vascular disease, peripheral arterial disease, rheumatic heart disease, congenital heart disease, deep vein thrombosis and pulmonary embolism. Almost half of the adult population in Europe, the USA and Asia [130-133] suffer from one form of cardiovascular disease. At the current rate, 23.6 million people are estimated to die by 2030 either due to blood vessel disorders, or due to heart malfunctions [22]. Blood circulation is coordinated by contraction and expansion movements of the venous or aortic vessels performed in accordance with the heart pulses. The elastic nature of these highly organized structures is insufficient to ensure blood flow alone, and an anti-thrombogenic surface is also required to inhibit blood coagulation. Endothelial cells (the inner layer of blood vessels) offer this key feature of hemocompatibility. Both hemocompatibility and elasticity proved to be essential characteristics required in the blood vessel tissue engineering. Reduction of immunogenic reactions between implant and surrounding biological environment, and long term durability are essential complementary properties [134]. Examples of frequently used blood contact devices are catheters, guide-wires, stents, pacemakers, vascular grafts, stent-grafts, heart valve and patches. Out of these, the last four are mainly commercially available as polyester devices, with a worldwide reported consumption of 200,000 implantations per year [135].

In the case of PGS, Gao *et al.* reported the first covalently crosslinked cardiovascular scaffold with extensive micropores [136]. The scaffolds were developed by a fused-salt leaching technique and had an open structure with high porosity (89%). Muscle and endothelial progenitor cells were seeded on the scaffolds in order to mimic the *in vivo* blood vessel [137]. This co-culture of cells led to an increased deposition of collagen and elastin, similar to the ECM environment. Therefore, a highly compliant tissue engineered vessel was obtained. Porous tubular PGS scaffolds as possible grafts were also developed by Crapo *et al.*, who outlined the importance of the material stiffness in the *in vitro* tissue formation process [138]. An *in vitro* comparative study was conducted between PLGA and PGS scaffolds cultured with adult baboon arterial smooth muscle cells (SNCs) for 10 days. While SNCs culture increased the stiffness of both materials, the stiffness of PGS shifted towards that of the porcine carotid arteries. The authors explained that, in comparison with PLGA, PGS scaffolds promoted increased levels of elastin and decreased collagen deposition [139].

Dynamically cultured blood vessel substitutes were developed from PHB scaffolds seeded with enzymatically derived vascular smooth muscle cells. Significantly increased ECM deposition, DNA and protein content were noticed, showing that bioreactor cultured blood vessels based on PHAs can mimic the mechanical properties of the native aorta [140]. For the development of the complex anatomic structure of pulmonary and aortic grafts, rapid prototyping techniques are employed. Sodian *et al.* developed a human aortic root scaffold and a pulmonary heart valve scaffold from porous PHB and a polyhydroxyoctanoate [141]. In this study, a valve was scanned with a CT scanner and a stereolithograpy model was developed. This enabled the fabrication of a scaffold by thermal processing techniques [142]. In similar studies, tri-leaflet heart valve scaffolds were produced by a particulate leaching technique and seeded with cells harvested from ovine carotid artery. A confluent layer covered the pores of the scaffold, making PHAs viable for further *in vivo* studies. Implantation of these cell-seeded heart valve constructs in lambs confirmed that the scaffolds were covered by neo-tissue without thrombus formation [143].

PCL is also often used in vascular graft research due to its suitable mechanical strength and biocompatibility. It can be easily processed into fibers by electrospinning in order to form porous and cell-friendly scaffolds [144]. De Valence *et al.* evaluated the use of vascular grafts based on micro- and nano-PCL fibers in a rat abdominal aorta replacement model [144]. The scaffolds showed excellent structural integrity and patency, with no thrombosis and limited intimal hyperplasia. The 2.5D PCL grafts display ideal characteristics for wide-scale clinical use due to low cost production, ambient storage capability and ease of implantation.

Naito *et al.* synthesized a copolymer of lactic acid and ε-caprolactone (50:50 ratio) for the production of tubular scaffolds [145]. The intended application of these structures was as large caliber grafts in the venous and pulmonary circulation. The scaffolds had a diameter ranging from 12 to 24 mm, a length of 13 cm and a thickness of 0.6 to 0.7 mm. The fabrication was achieved by pouring the copolymer solution onto poly-L-Lactic acid (PLLA) or PGA woven sheets, used as reinforcement, followed by freeze-drying under vacuum. A number of 25 scaffolds have been implanted with follow-up throughout nine years. No evidence of graft related morbidity (*i.e.* aneurysm formation, graft rupture, graft infection, or ectopic calcification) was reported.

A non-biodegradable material worth mentioning for cardiovascular applications is PET, as it is the only polyester material commercialized as vascular graft. On an industrial scale, large caliber synthetic veins are manufactured from PET (trade name of Dacron®) [146]. PET based vascular grafts are commercially available as woven or knitted fibrous structures [147]. Industrially, fibers of micrometer range are obtained through drawing methods, while at the research level nano-scale fibers are achieved *via* electrospinning. Electrospun scaffolds are rapidly emerging as a viable processing technique to fabricate vascular grafts because of the preferential cell attachment to nanoscale fibreous structures. To the best of our knowledge, no electrospun PET graft is currently commercially available.

From the biological point of view, PET is an inert material that does not induce acute inflammation when implanted and presents adequate mechanical properties to sustain blood pressure. Even though PET presents excellent bulk properties, the main drawback is its hydrophobic surface [148]. In this context, many studies have focused on the surface modification of PET while preserving its excellent bulk properties. In order to improve its biocompatibility, different structural designs of the grafts (knitted or woven) and treatments such as preclotting with the patients' blood, or impregnation with different ECM derivatives (*i.e.* gelatin, collagen, heparin) are frequently reported in literature [149-155]. Feijen *et al.* studied the effect of heparin-albumin conjugates on endothelial cell seeding and platelet adhesion [152], as well as the mechanism of platelet compatibility on surface-treated 2.5D PET scaffolds [156]. Another study concluded that knitted structures are preferred as grafts, since woven structures tend to wrinkle, limiting PET ability to form tubular shapes [147]. The *in vivo* tests using endothelial cell cultures reported by Marois *et al.* support the previous study by presenting slightly improved results in the case of knitted PET grafts [149]. In the same report, grafts impregnated with various ECM derived proteins presented an enhanced biocompatibility than non-treated PET (woven or knitted). Criado *et al.* reported that soft straight Dacron® PET grafts, used for aortic aneurysm repairs, were completely endothelialized after three months of implantation [157]. The following step was patency improvement through biomolecule impregnation of the polyester graft (gelatin, collagen, fibronectin, heparin) [149, 158, 159]. Other surface modification approaches, such as irradiation based treatments (plasma [159-161], ion, γ-ray [162], electron beam or laser treatments [163]) were exploited both *in vitro* and *in vivo*. For PET, polymeric coatings were often reported as an initial step for subsequent covalent immobilization of biomolecules (*i.e.* gelatin) [159], biocompatible polymers (*i.e.* polyethylene glycol) [161] or anti-inflammatory agents [164, 165]. A detailed review on vinyl grafting of PET is nicely presented by Abdolahifard *et al.* [162]. An overwhelming number of research papers and patents, either on surface modification procedures or on scaffold processing techniques, have been reported for cardiovascular TE [166-169].

Another critical aspect of cardiovascular applications is the design of heart patches. Fig. (**4**) presents the general strategy of designing a patient-specific implant. For these specific applications, the fine design of the scaffold and the myocardium mechanical properties and architecture are of utmost importance. Various techniques including electrospinning [170], laser microablation, and film casting are used to render suitable geometries.

Electrospun mats of PGS blends with PLLA, PCL, PHBV were fabricated to match the properties of the heart muscle [19, 170, 171]. This approach comes as a solution to the fabrication of PGS-stand-alone fibers, which is rather difficult due to the low molecular weight and low viscosity of the pre-polymer. Kenar *et al.* described a thick myocardial patch created by stacking together layers of aligned microfiber mats. In this study, PHBV: PLLA: PGS blends were used to obtain fibers with diameters ranging from 1.16-1.37 μm [171, 172]. Other studies reported using gelatin [170, 173] and PLLA [19] as co-agents in obtaining core-shell PGS fibers for regeneration of myocardial infarction.

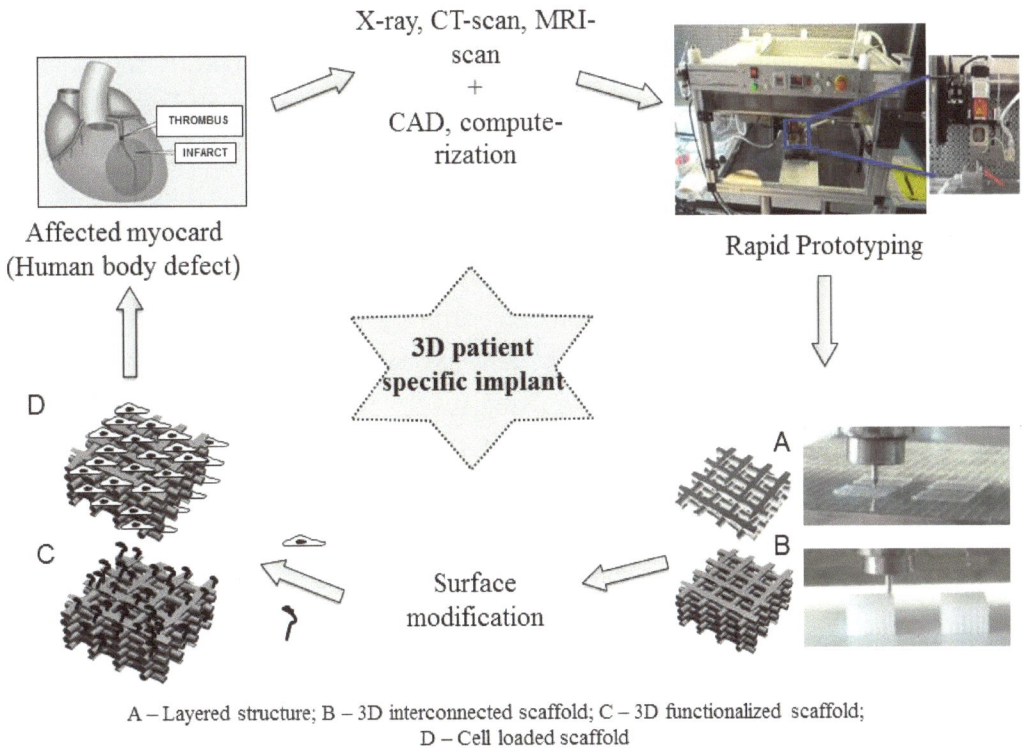

A – Layered structure; B – 3D interconnected scaffold; C – 3D functionalized scaffold;
D – Cell loaded scaffold

Fig. (4). Cardiovascular tissue engineering concept.

Neural Tissue Engineering

Nerve regeneration is a complex biological process and a challenge for scientists. While small nerve injuries can be remediated by self-regeneration, large injuries require grafts and surgical interventions. With an estimation of approximately 90,000 people per year affected by nervous system injuries, neural TE has emerged as an interesting field of study due to high associated disability levels and rehabilitation costs [174].

A variety of biomaterials have been evaluated for use in neural TE in order to provide a relevant matrix for cell adhesion and cell guidance. Poly(α-hydroxy esters) have received considerable attention, as they are bioresorbable and biocompatible with many cell types. Recent studies have focused on 2.5 and 3D scaffold fabrication. Nisbet *et al.* reported the effect of electrospun PCL scaffolds on the behavior of rat brain-derived neural stem cells [175]. The 2.5D PCL scaffolds were modified with ethylenediamine to determine the effect of amino functionalization and surface tension variation on cell proliferation and differentiation. The modified scaffolds were more hydrophilic and resulted in a significant increase of cells adhesion and spreading throughout the scaffold. Aligned PCL and collagen/PCL nanofibers were obtained by Schnell *et al. via* electrospinning as guidance structures for axonal nerve regeneration [176]. In their study, pure PCL (100%) fibers were compared with collagen/PCL blend fibers (25:75%) in terms of their biocompatibility (cell adhesion, survival and migration; effects on cell morphology; and axonal growth and guidance). Both electrospun fiber types presented promising results by sustaining oriented neurite outgrowth and glial migration from dorsal root ganglia explants. Different cell types (Schwann cells and fibroblasts) that play an important role in the pheripherical system were seeded on the scaffolds. The authors also studied olfactory ensheathing cells that support axon regeneration into the central nervous system. The data demonstrate that electrospun fibers composed of a collagen and PCL blend represent a suitable material for artificial nerve implants, as cell attachment, migration and axonal regeneration were enhanced.

Reconstruction of peripheral nerve defects was also pursued using PHB conduits, which were reported to provide a solution for spinal cord injuries [177]. An extensive study was performed on nerve regeneration using tubular scaffolds developed from copolymers of PCL, PGA and PHBV [178]. Herein, it was reported that 23 out of the 26 implanted nerve guides contained regenerated tissue. In addition, the inflammatory response due to polymer degradation did not influence the regeneration process [178]. Another study reported the use of PHB fibers coated with an alginate hydrogel and fibronectin as carrier scaffolds [179]. In this case, subsequent to Schwann cells seeding, regenerated axons entered the tubular construct from both ends and extended along its entire length.

PLGA scaffolds were used to generate *in vitro* artificial neuronal networks through distribution of genetically modified neuronal stem cells [180]. PLGA rods presenting longitudinal parallel-channels were fabricated by injection molding combined with thermally induced phase separation techniques. Li *et al.* have shown that artificial neuronal connections appear in PLGA scaffolds [97]. These constructs exhibited synaptic activities, as well as molecular signalling responding abilities to external stimuli.

Cartilage and Bone Tissue Engineering

The field of cartilage TE evolved as a solution to cartilage degenerative diseases that leads to little or no mobility (*i.e.* joint erosion due to osteoarthritis). Natural and synthetic scaffolds have been fabricated and investigated as potential graft substitutes. Amongst the natural polymers used for bone regeneration, chitosan, alginate and cellulose are worth mentioning [181]. Barbosa *et al.* have studied the biocompatibility [182-184] and mineralization [185-187] induced by these polymers. Although favorable biological results were obtained, natural polymers generally posses low mechanical, thermal and chemical stability. Alternatively, synthetic polymers can be tailored into materials with a broad range of properties. Further discussion entails some of the most used synthetic polymers in bone and cartilage TE, that include poly(α-hydroxy-esters) like PLA, PGA, PLGA, PHAs, PGS and PCL. These materials have shown to promote successfully chondrocyte growth and proliferation, as well as osteoblastic cell attachment.

Recently, Kemppainen *et al.* focused on scaffolds with mechanical properties similar to the native cartilage [188]. PGS and PCL porous 3D scaffolds were fabricated by a solid free form technique. *In vitro* studies showed higher levels of specific chondrocytes markers on PGS than on the PCL scaffolds. Izquierdo *et al.* described a particulate leaching technique to fabricate PCL scaffolds using poly(ethyl methacrylate) microspheres as templates [189]. Structures with high porosity (70%) and interconnected pores (< 200 μm) were produced and characterized. Human chondrocytes were seeded into the porous scaffolds and cell adhesion, viability and proliferation, and proteoglycan synthesis were tested. Promising results were obtained as cells maintained the same phenotype as chondrocytes within the native cartilage. Porous PCL/elastin composites were fabricated by Annabiet *et al. via* a rapid and solvent free process. High pressurized CO_2 was used as a foaming agent to create a PCL matrix with large pores (500 μm) and high porosity (91%) [190]. A subsequent impregnation in elastin of the 3D structure was performed. The fabrication of hybrid synthetic/natural scaffolds offered a suitable balance between biological and mechanical properties. In the same context, Declercq *et al.* demonstrated that different plotting and surface modification strategies of 3D PCL scaffolds have a synergistic effect on osteogenic cell colonization and differentiation [4]. Similar *in vitro* results were obtained with plotted PCL scaffolds of different architectures [191]. Honeycomb-like scaffolds were produced by fused deposition modeling. PCL-20% tricalcium phosphate constructs exhibited adequate mechanical properties for bone repair at medium load bearing sites [192]. *In vitro* tests with human mesenchymal stem cells over a 35-day culture period presented favorable results. Domingos *et al.* reported on how PCL scaffolds with controlled micro-architecture can be effectively produced *via* bioextrusion [63]. Low-pressure nitrogen-based coatings were employed to enhance cell adhesion and proliferation without altering the structural mechanical properties. The 3D PCL scaffolds were produced *via* a novel biomanufacturing device called BioCell Printing. The system enabled the fabrication of functional tissue engineering constructs through the integration and synchronization of the production, sterilization, cell seeding and dynamic *in vitro* culture stages. Extruded PCL scaffolds were plasma modified with a C_2H_4/N_2 deposition, followed by H_2 post-treatment. The purpose of the double process was to uniformly coat the internal and external surfaces of the 3D structures with a film rich in nitrogen-containing groups, in order to increase the hydrophilicity and cell affinity of the constructs. Shor *et al.* utilized a system called precision extrusion deposition consisting of a mini-extruder mounted on a high-precision positioning system to fabricate PCL and composite PCL/hydroxyapatite (PCL/HA) scaffolds [193]. Inclusion of HA significantly increased the compressive modulus independent of the scaffold porosity (59 to 84 MPa for 60% porous scaffolds; from 30 to 76 MPa for 70% porous scaffolds). *In vitro* cell-scaffold interaction studies were carried out using primary fetal bovine osteoblasts to assess the feasibility of scaffolds for bone tissue-engineering application and the results revealed that osteoblasts were able to migrate and proliferate during the culture time in both PCL and PCL/HA scaffolds.

Another polymer used for bone tissue applications is PLGA. Lee *et al.* obtained porous PLGA microspheres loaded with simvastatin (SIM, an FDA approved drug) for bone regeneration applications. Osteoblast cell line (MG-63) was cultivated up to 7 days upon it and important differences in gene expressions were observed between native PLGA and drug-loaded PLGA [194]. A positive correlation between SIM concentration and gene expressions (*i.e.* osteocalcin, osteonectin, collagen-1 and bone sialoprotein) was noticed for drug-loaded scaffolds. Besides bone tissue applications, PLGA scaffolds are designed for cartilage regenerative applications. Zhou *et al.* studied the impact of the scaffold orientation on *in vitro* cartilage regeneration [195]. In this regard, microtubular oriented scaffolds were obtained using PLGA, with a 50:50 monomer ratio. Oriented porous architectures were achieved through solid-liquid phase separation and lyophilization. Non-oriented porous structures with NaCl as porogen were manufactured for comparison purposes. The constructs with oriented morphology led to relatively homogeneous cell coverage; in this case, cartilage-like tissue was observed in both the outer and inner regions. Further *in vivo* implantation of these oriented scaffolds indicated a homogeneous and mature cartilage structure with abundant cartilage-specific ECM deposition.

Polymers from the PHA family are also considered for cartilage and bone tissue engineering. Although PHB shows good biocompatibility with osteoblasts, adrenocortical and epithelial cells [140, 196], its brittleness limits the application in cartilage TE. For this reason, blends of PHB and poly(3-hydroxybutyrate-*co*-3-hydroxyhexanoate) (PHBHHx), a more elastomeric member of the PHA family, were investigated. An initial *in vitro* study of the chondrocyte activity on blended scaffolds revealed that the cells proliferated and preserved their phenotype better than on PHB scaffolds [197]. Superior elongation at break was reported with the increase of the PHBHHx ratio in the blend, making these materials more suitable for cartilage TE applications [198]. Extensive biological and mineralization investigations are presented elsewhere, as complementary data [199, 200]. Furthermore, *in vivo* studies in rabbits demonstrated that the PHBHHx scaffolds seeded with allogeneic chondrocytes achieved cartilage repair in 16 weeks.

Retinal Tissue Engineering

Over 30 million people worldwide are affected by retinal degenerative diseases [22]. This type of diseases involves retina deterioration and possible loss of vision due to photoreceptor cell death. In the case of retinal tissue engineering, stem cells or retinal progenitor cells are cultured on scaffolds and transplanted to the subretinal space. In the last decades, scientists have devoted their time to deliver retinal progenitor cells (RPCs) to the retina using non-degradable solid implants, as well as biodegradable scaffolds [201, 202]. Mechanical and biological compatibility with the retina are essential characteristics and materials such as poly(hydroxyl ethyl methacrylate), PCL, PLGA, PLA, PGS and blends are suitable for retinal tissue engineering [203].

Due to its biodegradability, elasticity and good mechanical strength during transplantation procedures, PGS has proved to be suitable for RPC delivery, subretinal transplantation and retinal graft development [204-206]. Surface modification strategies for PGS were performed in order to promote graft-host integration. PGS membranes were coated with laminin/PCL electrospun electrospun fibers and modified with peptides containing an arginine-glycine-aspartic acid extracellular matrix ligand sequence [204]. These procedures promoted sufficient cell adhesion for simultaneous transplantation of isolated photoreceptor cells and PGS membranes.

Sodha *et al.* described the design, fabrication and evaluation of a complex 3D scaffold by stacking, aligning and bonding three uniquely designed PCL layers [203, 207]. The device elements were fabricated by photolithography, standard replica molding and soft lithography techniques. The 3D device was designed with a defined cage structure to encapsulate a large number of cells. The second layer allowed unidirectional cell migration into the subretinal space with the aid of contact guidance ridges, while the third layer allowed nutrient infiltration.

Tucker *et al.* published a study regarding retinal repopulation using PLGA polymeric constructs that contain MMP2, an active enzyme that degrade inhibitory ECM molecules responsible for poor cell integration following transplantation [208]. The MMP2-PLGA solid polymer fibers were obtained *via* electrospinning. Enzyme-polymer constructs seeded with RPCs were transplanted through an opening in the sclera into the subretinal space of mice. Delivery of active-MMP2 from the porous structure resulted in degradation/removal of inhibitory ECM deposited in the retina, priming the tissue for transplantation. The delivery of retinal progenitor cells loaded MMP2-polymer scaffolds resulted in an increase of the cellular integration, tissue-specific differentiation and retinal outer nuclear layer repopulation.

CONCLUSION AND OUTLOOK

From the present book chapter and from the vast amount of available (patent) literature, it is evident that polymers have been and will remain a very important class of biomaterials in the field of tissue engineering and regenerative medicine. The versatility of the building blocks that can be selected to develop a plethora of functional polymers with properties ranging from soft to hard, from biodegradable to biostable, from cell-interactive to cell-repelling is what makes polymers such an appealing materials class. This is supported by the large variety of applications in which polymers play a pivotal role. The most important ones including cardiovascular, ocular, orthopedic and neural have been dealt with in the second part of the chapter.

More recently, advanced rapid prototyping based polymer processing technologies have been applied to develop a next generation implant materials. Using earlier developed and novel polymers, patient specific porous perfectly interconnective scaffolds can now be produced. This technology thus opens up the possibility of developing more suitable scaffolds. Indeed, compared to previous generations, the newest generation of scaffolds enable a good control over internal geometry (dimension as well as geometry), perfusion capability (cell seeding purposes) and provide a perfect fit to the body defect. Looking at the pace at which new scaffold production technologies and new polymer(s) (coatings) are being developed, it can be anticipated that new breakthroughs will be achieved for various applications in which polymers play an important role. A continuous interaction with various disciplines including cell biologists, engineers, clinicians and regulatory authorities will be of the utmost importance in moving from the lab bench to commercialization.

ACKNOWLEDGEMENTS

The authors wish to thank Dr. Kenny Adesanya, Ms. Sheila Dunphy and Dr. Timothy Douglas for reading assistance.

CONFLICT OF INTEREST

The authors confirm that this chapter contents have no conflict of interest.

ABBREVIATIONS

3D	=	Three dimensional
2D	=	Two dimensional
2.5D	=	Two-and-a-half dimensional
CAD	=	Computer-aid design
CH4	=	Methane
CO2	=	Carbon dioxide
CT	=	Computed tomography
DMT	=	Dimethyl terephthalate
DNA	=	Deoxyribonucleic acid
DP	=	Degree of polymerization
ECM	=	Extra cellular matrix
EG	=	Ethylene glycol
FDA	=	Food and Drug Administration
HA	=	Hydroxyapatite
HB	=	Hydroxybutyrate
HV	=	3-hydroxyvalerate
IUPAC	=	International Union of Pure and Applied Chemistry
PCL	=	Poly(ε-caprolactone)
PET	=	Poly(ethylene terephthalate)
PGA	=	Poly(glycolic acid), poly(glicolide)
PGS	=	Poly(glycerol-sebacate)
PHA	=	Polyhydroxylalkanoates

PHB	=	Poly(3-hydroxy-butyrate)
PHV	=	Poly(hydroxyvalerate)
PHBHHx	=	Poly(3-hydroxybutyrate-co-3-hydroxyhexanoate)
PHBV	=	Poly (3-hydroxybutyrate-co-3-hydroxyvalerate)
PLA	=	Poly(lactic acid), poly(lactide)
PLGA	=	Poly(lactic-co-glycolic acid)
PLLA	=	Poly-L-lactic acid
ROP	=	Ring opening polymerization
RPCs	=	Retinal progenitor cells
SIM	=	Simvastatin
SNCs	=	Smooth muscle cells
Sn(Oct)2	=	Tin(II) 2-ethylhexanoate
TA	=	Terephthalic acid
TE	=	Tissue engineering
TFA	=	Trifluoroacetic acid
Tm	=	Melting temperature
Tg	=	Glass transition temperature
Td	=	Degradation temperature
UV	=	Ultra violet

REFERENCES

[1]   Hollister, S. J. Scaffold Design and Manufacturing: From Concept to Clinic. *Adv Mater.* 2009, 21, 3330-3342.

[2]   Dhandayuthapani, B., Yoshida, Y., Maekawa, T., Kumar, D. S. Polymeric Scaffolds in Tissue Engineering Application: A Review. *Int J Polym Sci.* 2011.

[3]   Amass, W., Amass, A., Tighe, B. A review of biodegradable polymers: Uses, current developments in the synthesis and characterization of biodegradable polyesters, blends of biodegradable polymers and recent advances in biodegradation studies. *Polym Int.* 1998, 47, 89-144.

[4]   Desmet, T., Billiet, T., Berneel, E., *et al.* Post-Plasma Grafting of AEMA as a Versatile Tool to Biofunctionalise Polyesters for Tissue Engineering. *Macromolecular Bioscience.* 2010, 10, 1484-1494.

[5]   Ma, Z., Mao, Z., Gao, C. Surface modification and property analysis of biomedical polymers used for tissue engineering. *Colloids Surf B Biointerfaces.* 2007, 60, 137-157.

[6]   Causa, F., Netti, P. A., Ambrosio, L. A multi-functional scaffold for tissue regeneration: the need to engineer a tissue analogue. *Biomaterials.* 2007, 28, 5093-5099.

[7]   Saha, K., Pollock, J. F., Schaffer, D. V., Healy, K. E. Designing synthetic materials to control stem cell phenotype. *Current Opinion in Chemical Biology.* 2007, 11, 381-387.

[8]   Goldberg, M., Langer, R., Jia, X. Q. Nanostructured materials for applications in drug delivery and tissue engineering. *J Biomat Sci-Polym E.* 2007, 18, 241-268.

[9]   Yang, S.-T., Robinson, C. Tissue Engineering, in Encyclopedia of Chemical Processing. *Taylor & Francis,* 2006, 3115-3124.

[10]   Barrett, D. G., Yousaf, M. N. Design and Applications of Biodegradable Polyester Tissue Scaffolds Based on Endogenous Monomers Found in Human Metabolism. *Molecules.* 2009, 14, 4022-4050.

[11]   Wang, Y. D., Ameer, G. A., Sheppard, B. J., Langer, R. A tough biodegradable elastomer. *Nat Biotechnol.* 2002, 20, 602-606.

[12]   Liu, Q. Y., Tan, T. W., Weng, J. Y., Zhang, L. Q. Study on the control of the compositions and properties of a biodegradable polyester elastomer. *Biomed Mater.* 2009, 4.

[13]   Liu, Q. Y., Tian, M., Ding, T., Shi, R., Zhang, L. Q. Preparation and characterization of a biodegradable polyester elastomer with thermal processing abilities. *J Appl Polym Sci.* 2005, 98, 2033-2041.

[14]   You, Z. W., Cao, H. P., Gao, J., *et al.* A functionalizable polyester with free hydroxyl groups and tunable physiochemical and biological properties. *Biomaterials.* 2010, 31, 3129-3138.

[15]   Nijst, C. L. E., Bruggeman, J. P., Karp, J. M., *et al.* Synthesis and characterization of photocurable elastomers from poly(glycerol-co-sebacate). *Biomacromolecules.* 2007, 8, 3067-3073.

[16]   Ifkovits, J. L., Padera, R. F., Burdick, J. A. Biodegradable and radically polymerized elastomers with enhanced processing capabilities. *Biomed Mater.* 2008, 3.

[17]   Wu, Y., Shi, R., Chen, D. F., Zhang, L. Q., Tian, W. Nanosilica Filled Poly(glycerol-sebacate-citrate) Elastomers with Improved Mechanical Properties, Adjustable Degradability, and Better Biocompatibility. *J Appl Polym Sci.* 2012, 123, 1612-1620.

[18]   Sant, S., Hwang, C. M., Lee, S. H., Khademhosseini, A. Hybrid PGS-PCL microfibrous scaffolds with improved mechanical and biological properties. *J Tissue Eng Regen M.* 2011, 5, 283-291.

[19]   Cheng, S. J., Yang, L. J., Gong, F. R. Novel branched poly(l-lactide) with poly(glycerol-co-sebacate) core. *Polym Bull.* 2010, 65, 643-655.

[20]   Mitsak, A. G., Dunn, A. M., Hollister, S. J. Mechanical characterization and non-linear elastic modeling of poly(glycerol sebacate) for soft tissue engineering. *J Mech Behav Biomed.* 2012, 11, 3-15.

[21]   Cai, W., Liu, L. L. Shape-memory effect of poly (glycerol-sebacate) elastomer. *Mater Lett.* 2008, 62, 2171-2173.

[22]   Rai, R., Tallawi, M., Grigore, A., Boccaccini, A. R. Synthesis, properties and biomedical applications of poly(glycerol sebacate) (PGS): A review. *Prog Polym Sci.* 2012, 37, 1051-1078.

[23]   Pomerantseva, I., Krebs, N., Hart, A., *et al.* Degradation behavior of poly(glycerol sebacate). *J Biomed Mater Res A.* 2009, 91A, 1038-1047.

[24]   Liang, S. L., Yang, X. Y., Fang, X. Y., *et al. In Vitro* enzymatic degradation of poly (glycerol sebacate)-based materials. *Biomaterials.* 2011, 32, 8486-8496.

[25]   Motlagh, D., Yang, J., Lui, K. Y., Webb, A. R., Ameer, G. A. Hemocompatibility evaluation of poly(glycerol-sebacate) *in vitro* for vascular tissue engineering. *Biomaterials.* 2006, 27, 4315-4324.

[26]   Hedrick, J. L., Magbitang, T., Connor, E. F., *et al.* Application of complex macromolecular architectures for advanced microelectronic materials. *Chem-Eur J.* 2002, 8, 3308-3319.

[27]   Joshi, P., Madras, G. Degradation of polycaprolactone in supercritical fluids. *Polym Degrad Stabil.* 2008, 93, 1901-1908.

[28]   Labet, M., Thielemans, W. Synthesis of polycaprolactone: a review. *Chem Soc Rev.* 2009, 38, 3484-3504.

[29]   Armani, D. K., Liu, C. Mircofabrication technology for polycaprolactone, a biodegradable polymer. *Journal of Micromechanics and Microengineering.* 2000, 10, 80-84.

[30]   Varma, I. K., Albertsson, A. C., Rajkhowa, R., Srivastava, R. K. Enzyme catalyzed synthesis of polyesters. *Prog Polym Sci.* 2005, 30, 949-981.

[31]   Albertsson, A. C., Srivastava, R. K. Recent developments in enzyme-catalyzed ring-opening polymerization. *Adv Drug Deliver Rev.* 2008, 60, 1077-1093.

[32]   Clark, J. H., Kraus, G. A., Osswald, T. A., Sharma, S. K., Mudhoo, A. A Handbook of Applied Biopolymer Technology: Synthesis, Degradation and Applications. *Royal Society of Chemistry*, 2011.

[33]   Persson, P. V., Schroder, J., Wickholm, K., Hedenstrom, E., Iversen, T. Selective organocatalytic ring-opening polymerization: A versatile route to carbohydrate-functionalized poly(ε-caprolactones). *Macromolecules.* 2004, 37, 5889-5893.

[34]   Mahapatro, A., Kumar, A., Gross, R. A. Mild, Solvent-Free ω-Hydroxy Acid Polycondensations Catalyzed by Candida a ntarctica Lipase B. *Biomacromolecules.* 2004, 5, 62-68.

[35]   Natta, F. J. v., Hill, J. W., Carothers, W. H. Studies of Polymerization and Ring Formation. XXIII. 1 ε-Caprolactone and its Polymers. *Journal of the American Chemical Society.* 1934, 56, 455-457.

[36]   Dubois, P., Coulembier, O., Raquez, J.-M. Handbook of ring-opening polymerization. *Wiley Online Library*, 2009.

[37]   Stridsberg, K. M., Ryner, M., Albertsson, A. C. Controlled ring-opening polymerization: Polymers with designed macromolecular architecture. *Degradable Aliphatic Polyesters.* 2002, 157, 41-65.

[38]   McLain, S., Drysdale, N. Living Ring-Opening Polymerization of epsilon-Caprolactone by Yttrium and Lanthanide Alkoxides. *Polymer Preprints(USA).* 1992, 33, 174-175.

[39]   Evans, W. J., Katsumata, H. Polymerization of epsilon-Caprolactone by Divalent Samarium Complexes. *Macromolecules.* 1994, 27, 2330-2332.

[40]   Okamoto, Y. Cationic ring - opening polymerization of lactones in the presence of alcohol. *Proccedings of Conference Cationic ring - opening polymerization of lactones in the presence of alcohol,* 1991, 42, 117-133.

[41]   Albertsson, A. C., Varma, I. K. Recent developments in ring opening polymerization of lactones for biomedical applications. *Biomacromolecules.* 2003, 4, 1466-1486.

[42]   Storey, R. F., Taylor, A. E. Effect of Stannous Octoate on the Composition, Molecular Weight, and Molecular Weight Distribution of Ethylene Glycol-Initiated Poly (ϵ-Caprolactone). *Journal of Macromolecular Science, Part A: Pure and Applied Chemistry.* 1998, 35, 723-750.

[43]   Okada, M. Chemical syntheses of biodegradable polymers. *Progress in polymer science.* 2002, 27, 87-133.

[44]   Iroh, J. O. Polymer Data Handbook, New York: *Oxford University Press,* 1999, 361-362.

[45]   Chandra, R., Rustgi, R. Biodegradable polymers. *Prog Polym Sci.* 1998, 23, 1273-1336.

[46]   Woodruff, M. A., Hutmacher, D. W. The return of a forgotten polymer—Polycaprolactone in the 21st century. *Progress in polymer science.* 2010, 35, 1217-1256.

[47]   Gross, R. A., Kalra, B. Biodegradable polymers for the environment. *Science.* 2002, 297, 803-807.

[48]   Sinha, V., Bansal, K., Kaushik, R., Kumria, R., Trehan, A. Poly-ϵ-caprolactone microspheres and nanospheres: an overview. *International journal of pharmaceutics.* 2004, 278, 1-23.

[49]   Ikada, Y., Tsuji, H. Biodegradable polyesters for medical and ecological applications. *Macromolecular rapid communications.* 2000, 21, 117-132.

[50]   Nair, L. S., Laurencin, C. T. Biodegradable polymers as biomaterials. *Progress in polymer science.* 2007, 32, 762-798.

[51]   Pachence, J. M., Kohn, J. Biodegradable polymers. *Principles of tissue engineering.* 2000, 3, 323-339.

[52]   Ge, H., Hu, Y., Jiang, X., *et al.* Preparation, characterization, and drug release behaviors of drug nimodipine - loaded poly (ϵ - caprolactone) - poly (ethylene oxide) - poly (ϵ - caprolactone) amphiphilic triblock copolymer micelles. *Journal of pharmaceutical sciences.* 2002, 91, 1463-1473.

[53]   Luo, L., Tam, J., Maysinger, D., Eisenberg, A. Cellular internalization of poly (ethylene oxide)-b-poly (ϵ-caprolactone) diblock copolymer micelles. *Bioconjugate chemistry.* 2002, 13, 1259-1265.

[54]   Nojima, S., Tanaka, H., Rohadi, A., Sasaki, S. The effect of glass transition temperature on the crystallization of ϵ-caprolactone-styrene diblock copolymers. *Polymer.* 1998, 39, 1727-1734.

[55]   Storey, R., Wiggins, J., Puckett, A. Hydrolyzable poly (ester - urethane) networks from L - lysine diisocyanate and D, L - lactide/ϵ - caprolactone homo - and copolyester triols. *Journal of Polymer Science Part A: Polymer Chemistry.* 2003, 32, 2345-2363.

[56]   Zhou, J., Villarroya, S., Wang, W., *et al.* One-Step Chemoenzymatic Synthesis of Poly (ϵ-caprolactone-b lock-methyl methacrylate) in Supercritical CO2. *Macromolecules.* 2006, 39, 5352-5358.

[57]   Bezwada, R. S., Hunter, A. W., Shalaby, S. W. Copolymers of. epsilon.-caprolactone, glycolide and glycolic acid for suture coatings.). *Google Patents,* 1991.

[58]   Cai, Q., Bei, J., Wang, S. Synthesis and degradation of a tri-component copolymer derived from glycolide, L-lactide, and ε-caprolactone. *Journal of Biomaterials Science, Polymer Edition*. 2000, 11, 273-288.

[59]   Tokiwa, Y., Suzuki, T. Hydrolysis of polyesters by lipases. *Nature*. 1977, 270, 76-78.

[60]   Chen, D., Bei, J., Wang, S. Polycaprolactone microparticles and their biodegradation. *Polymer degradation and stability*. 2000, 67, 455-459.

[61]   De Kesel, C., Wauven, C. V., David, C. Biodegradation of polycaprolactone and its blends with poly (vinylalcohol) by micro-organisms from a compost of house-hold refuse. *Polymer degradation and stability*. 1997, 55, 107-113.

[62]   Pachence, J. M., Bohrer, M. P., Kohn, J. Biodegradable polymers. *Academic Press: Burlington*, 2007, 1095-1109.

[63]   Domingos, M., Intranuovo, F., Gloria, A., *et al*. Improved osteoblast cell affinity on plasma-modified 3-D extruded PCL scaffolds. *Acta Biomaterialia*. 2013, 9, 5997-6005.

[64]   Amato, I., Ciapettia, G., Pagani, S., *et al*. Expression of cell adhesion receptors in human osteoblasts cultured on biofunctionalized poly-(epsilon-caprolactone) surfaces. *Biomaterials*. 2007, 28, 3668-3678.

[65]   Duan, Y., Wang, Z., Yan, W., *et al*. Preparation of collagen-coated electrospun nanofibers by remote plasma treatment and their biological properties. *J Biomat Sci-Polym E*. 2007, 18, 1153-1164.

[66]   Gabriel, M., Amerongen, G. P. V., Van Hinsbergh, V. W. M., Amerongen, A. V. V., Zentner, A. Direct grafting of RGD-motif-containing peptide on the surface of polycaprolactone films. *J Biomat Sci-Polym E*. 2006, 17, 567-577.

[67]   Marletta, G., Ciapetti, G., Satriano, C., Pagani, S., Baldini, N. The effect of irradiation modification and RGD sequence adsorption on the response of human osteoblasts to polycaprolactone. *Biomaterials*. 2005, 26, 4793-4804.

[68]   Zhang, H., Lin, C.-Y., Hollister, S. J. The interaction between bone marrow stromal cells and RGD-modified three-dimensional porous polycaprolactone scaffolds, *Biomaterials*. 2009, 30, 4063-4069.

[69]   Singh, S., Wu, B. M., Dunn, J. C. Y. The enhancement of VEGF-mediated angiogenesis by polycaprolactone scaffolds with surface cross-linked heparin. *Biomaterials*. 2011, 32, 2059-2069.

[70]   Kersemans, K., Desmet, T., Vanhove, C., Dubruel, P., De Vos, F. Radiolabeled gelatin type B analogues can be used for non-invasive visualisation and quantification of protein coatings on 3D porous implants. *J Mater Sci-Mater M*. 2012, 23, 1961-1969.

[71]   De Cooman, H., Desmet, T., Callens, F., Dubruel, P. Role of Radicals in UV-Initiated Postplasma Grafting of Poly-epsilon-caprolactone: An Electron Paramagnetic Resonance Study. *J Polym Sci Pol Chem*. 2012, 50, 2142-2149.

[72]   Jacobs, T., De Geyter, N., Morent, R., *et al*. Plasma treatment of polycaprolactone at medium pressure. *Surface and Coatings Technology*. 2011, 205, Supplement 2, S543-S547.

[73]   Samuel, J. H. Handbook of biodegradable polymers. *Rapra Technology Limited*, 2005, 287-302.

[74]   Dechy-Cabaret, O., Martin-Vaca, B., Bourissou, D. Controlled ring-opening polymerization of lactide and glycolide. *Chem Rev*. 2004, 104, 6147-6176.

[75]   Albertsson, A. C., Edlund, U., Stridsberg, K. Controlled ring-opening polymerization of lactones and lactides. *Macromol Symp*. 2000, 157, 39-46.

[76]   Gilding, D. K., Reed, A. M. Biodegradable Polymers for Use in Surgery - Polyglycolic-Poly(Actic Acid) Homopolymers and Copolymers.1. *Polymer*. 1979, 20, 1459-1464.

[77]   Kiremitci-Gumusderelioglu, M., Deniz, G. Synthesis, characterization and *in vitro* degradation of poly(dl-lactide)/poly(dl-lactide-co-glycolide) films. *Turk J Chem*. 1999, 23, 153-161.

[78]   Makadia, H. K., Siegel, S. J. Poly Lactic-co-Glycolic Acid (PLGA) as Biodegradable Controlled Drug Delivery Carrier. *Polymers-Basel*. 2011, 3, 1377-1397.

[79]   Nair, L. S., Laurencin, C. T. Polymers as biomaterials for tissue engineering and controlled drug delivery. *Adv Biochem Eng Biot*. 2006, 102, 47-90.

[80]   Middleton, J. C., Tipton, A. J. Synthetic biodegradable polymers as orthopedic devices. *Biomaterials*. 2000, 21, 2335-2346.

[81]   Croll, T. I., O'Connor, A. J., Stevens, G. W., Cooper-White, J. J. Controllable surface modification of poly(lactic-co-glycolic acid) (PLGA) by hydrolysis or aminolysis I: Physical, chemical, and theoretical aspects. *Biomacromolecules*. 2004, 5, 463-473.

[82]   Kim, T. G., Park, T. G. Biomimicking extracellular matrix: cell adhesive RGD peptide modified electrospun poly(D,L-lactic-co-glycolic acid) nanofiber mesh. *Tissue Eng*. 2006, 12, 221-233.

[83]   Dai, L. M., StJohn, H. A. W., Bi, J. J., *et al.* Biomedical coatings by the covalent immobilization of polysaccharides onto gas-plasma-activated polymer surfaces. *Surf Interface Anal*. 2000, 29, 46-55.

[84]   Ma, S. Q., Wang, K. Z., Dang, X. Q., *et al.* Osteogenic growth peptide incorporated into PLGA scaffolds accelerates healing of segmental long bone defects in rabbits. *J Plast Reconstr Aes*. 2008, 61, 1558-1560.

[85]   Khang, G., Lee, S. J., Jeon, J. H., Lee, J. H., Lee, H. B. Interaction of fibroblast cell onto physicochemically treated PLGA surfaces. *Polym-Korea*. 2000, 24, 869-876.

[86]   Nitschke, M., Schmack, G., Janke, A., *et al.* Low pressure plasma treatment of poly(3-hydroxybutyrate): Toward tailored polymer surfaces for tissue engineering scaffolds. *Journal of Biomedical Materials Research*. 2002, 59, 632-638.

[87]   Chu, P. K., Chen, J. Y., Wang, L. P., Huang, N. Plasma-surface modification of biomaterials. *Mat Sci Eng R*. 2002, 36, 143-206.

[88]   Flemming, R. G., Murphy, C. J., Abrams, G. A., Goodman, S. L., Nealey, P. F. Effects of synthetic micro- and nano-structured surfaces on cell behavior. *Biomaterials*. 1999, 20, 573-588.

[89]   Hollister, S. J., Murphy, W. L. Scaffold Translation: Barriers Between Concept and Clinic. *Tissue Eng Part B-Re*. 2011, 17, 459-474.

[90]   Zamani, F., Latifi, M., Amani-Tehran, M., Shokrgozar, M. A. Effects of PLGA nanofibrous scaffolds structure on nerve cell directional proliferation and morphology. *Fiber Polym*. 2013, 14, 698-702.

[91]   Huang, W., Shi, X. T., Ren, L., Du, C., Wang, Y. J. PHBV microspheres - PLGA matrix composite scaffold for bone tissue engineering. *Biomaterials*. 2010, 31, 4278-4285.

[92]   Ren, T. B., Ren, J., Jia, X. Z., Pan, K. F. The bone formation *in vitro* and mandibular defect repair using PLGA porous scaffolds. *J Biomed Mater Res A*. 2005, 74A, 562-569.

[93]   Yu, D., Li, Q., Mu, X., Chang, T., Xiong, Z. Bone regeneration of critical calvarial defect in goat model by PLGA/TCP/rhBMP-2 scaffolds prepared by low-temperature rapid-prototyping technology. *Int J Oral Max Surg*. 2008, 37, 929-934.

[94] Ge, Z. G., Tian, X. F., Heng, B. C., *et al*. Histological evaluation of osteogenesis of 3D-printed poly-lactic-co-glycolic acid (PLGA) scaffolds in a rabbit model. *Biomed Mater*. 2009, 4.

[95] Li, J., Tao, R., Wu, W., *et al*. 3D PLGA Scaffolds Improve Differentiation and Function of Bone Marrow Mesenchymal Stem Cell-Derived Hepatocytes. *Stem Cells Dev*. 2010, 19, 1427-1436.

[96] Xiong, Y., Zeng, Y. S., Zeng, C. G., *et al*. Synaptic transmission of neural stem cells seeded in 3-dimensional PLGA scaffolds. *Biomaterials*. 2009, 30, 3711-3722.

[97] Li, X. K., Cai, S. X., Liu, B., *et al*. Characteristics of PLGA-gelatin complex as potential artificial nerve scaffold. *Colloid Surface B*. 2007, 57, 198-203.

[98] Yang, J., Shi, G. X., Bei, J. Z., *et al*. Fabrication and surface modification of macroporous poly(L-lactic acid) and poly(L-lactic-co-glycolic acid) (70/30) cell scaffolds for human skin fibroblast cell culture. *Journal of Biomedical Materials Research*. 2002, 62, 438-446.

[99] Hu, X. X., Shen, H., Yang, F., Bei, J. Z., Wang, S. G. Preparation and cell affinity of microtubular orientation-structured PLGA(70/30) blood vessel scaffold. *Biomaterials*. 2008, 29, 3128-3136.

[100] Han, J. J., Lazarovici, P., Pomerantz, C., *et al*. Co-Electrospun Blends of PLGA, Gelatin, and Elastin as Potential Nonthrombogenic Scaffolds for Vascular Tissue Engineering. *Biomacromolecules*. 2011, 12, 399-408.

[101] Ojumu, T. V., Yu, J., Solomon, B. O. Production of Polyhydroxyalkanoates, a bacterial biodegradable polymer. *African Journal of Biotechnology*. 2004, 3, 18-24.

[102] Reddy, C. S. K., Ghai, R., Rashmi, Kalia, V. C. Polyhydroxyalkanoates: an overview. *Bioresource Technol*. 2003, 87, 137-146.

[103] Chen, G. Q., Wu, Q., Xi, J. Z., Yu, H. P. Microbial production of biopolyesters-polyhydroxyalkanoates. *Prog Nat Sci*. 2000, 10, 843-850.

[104] Jendrossek, D., Handrick, R. Microbial degradation of polyhydroxyalkanoates. *Annu Rev Microbiol*. 2002, 56, 403-432.

[105] Madison, L. L., Huisman, G. W. Metabolic engineering of poly(3-hydroxyalkanoates): From DNA to plastic. *Microbiol Mol Biol R*. 1999, 63, 21-+.

[106] Anderson, A. J., Dawes, E. A. Occurrence, Metabolism, Metabolic Role, and Industrial Uses of Bacterial Polyhydroxyalkanoates. *Microbiological Reviews*. 1990, 54, 450-472.

[107] Lee, S. Y., Choi, J. I. Production and degradation of polyhydroxyalkanoates in waste environment. *Waste Manage*. 1999, 19, 133-139.

[108] Rudnik, E. Compostable Polymer Materials. *Elsevier Science, ISBN 9780080453712*. 2007.

[109] Lee, S. Y. Bacterial polyhydroxyalkanoates. *Biotechnol Bioeng*. 1996, 49, 1-14.

[110] Holmes, P. A. Applications of Phb - a Microbially Produced Biodegradable Thermoplastic. *Phys Technol*. 1985, 16, 32-36.

[111] Wu, Q., Wang, Y., Chen, G. Q. Medical Application of Microbial Biopolyesters Polyhydroxyalkanoates. *Artif Cell Blood Sub*. 2009, 37, 1-12.

[112] Martin, D. P., Peoples, O. P., Williams, S. F., Zhong, L. *Nutritional and therapeutic uses of 3-hydroxyalkanoate oligomers*. Patent WO 00/04895 A2, 2000.

[113] Martin, D. P., Skraly F. A., Williams S. F. *Polyhydroxyalkanoate compositions having controlled degradation rates*. Patent WO 99/32536, 1999.

[114] Rieckmann, T., Volker, S. Poly(ethylene Terephthalate) Polymerization - Mechanism, Catalysis, Kinetics, Mass Transfer and Reactor Design. *John Wiley & sons*, 2003, 31-116.

[115] Ahmadnian, F., Velasquez, F., Reichert, K. H. Screening of Different Titanium(IV) Catalysts in the Synthesis of Poly(ethylene terephthalate). *Macromol React Eng.* 2008, 2, 513-521.

[116] Ahmadnian, F., Reichert, K. H. Kinetic studies of polyethylene terephthalate synthesis with titanium-based catalyst. *Macromol Symp.* 2007, 259, 188-196.

[117] Ravindranath, K., Mashelkar, R. A. Polyethylene Terephthalate. 1. Chemistry, Thermodynamics and Transport-Properties. *Chem Eng Sci.* 1986, 41, 2197-2214.

[118] Chen, W., McCarthy, T. J. Chemical surface modification of poly(ethylene terephthalate). *Macromolecules.* 1998, 31, 3648-3655.

[119] Goodfellow Cambridge Ltd. Available from http://www.goodfellow.com, Accessed 12 April 2013.

[120] Hollister, S. J. Porous scaffold design for tissue engineering. *Nat Mater.* 2005, 4, 518-524.

[121] Billiet, T., Vandenhaute, M., Schelfhout, J., Van Vlierberghe, S., Dubruel, P. A review of trends and limitations in hydrogel-rapid prototyping for tissue engineering. *Biomaterials.* 2012, 33, 6020-6041.

[122] Desmet, T., Schacht, E., Dubruel, P. Rapid Prototyping as an elegant Production Tool for Polymeric Tissue Engineering Scaffolds: a review. In: *Tissue Engineering: Roles, Materials and applications*). *Nova Science Publishers, Inc* 2008, Chapter 7, pp. 141-189.

[123] Ma, P. X. Scaffolds for tissue fabrication. *Materials Today.* 2004, 7, 30-40.

[124] Cipitria, A., Skelton, A., Dargaville, T., Dalton, P., Hutmacher, D. Design, fabrication and characterization of PCL electrospun scaffolds—a review. *Journal of Materials Chemistry.* 2011, 21, 9419-9453.

[125] Melchels, F. P. W., Feijen, J., Grijpma, D. W. A review on stereolithography and its applications in biomedical engineering. *Biomaterials.* 2010, 31, 6121-6130.

[126] Sachlos, E., Czernuszka, J. Making tissue engineering scaffolds work. Review: the application of solid freeform fabrication technology to the production of tissue engineering scaffolds. *Eur Cell Mater.* 2003, 5, 39-40.

[127] Peltola, S. M., Melchels, F. P., Grijpma, D. W., Kellomäki, M. A review of rapid prototyping techniques for tissue engineering purposes. *Annals of Medicine.* 2008, 40, 268-280.

[128] Zein, I., Hutmacher, D. W., Tan, K. C., Teoh, S. H. Fused deposition modeling of novel scaffold architectures for tissue engineering applications. *Biomaterials.* 2002, 23, 1169-1185.

[129] Theoret, C. Tissue Engineering in Wound Repair: The three "R"s-Repair, Replace, Regenerate. *Vet Surg.* 2009, 38, 905-913.

[130] European Cardiovascular Disease Statistics 2012. *European Heart Network and European Society of Cardiology,* 2012.

[131] Shurin, S. B. Morbidity and Mortality: 2012 Chart Book on Cardiovascular, Lung, and Blood Diseases.). *National Heart, Lung and Blood Institute,* 2012.

[132] Allender, S., Scarborough, P., Peto, V., *et al.* European Cardiovascular Disease Statistics. *Dept. of Public Health, University of Oxford,* 2008.

[133] (2012), O. W. Mortality from cardiovascular disease, in Health at a glance. Asia/Pacific: *OECD Publishing,* 2012.

[134] Venkatraman, S., Boey, F., Lao, L. L. Implanted cardiovascular polymers: Natural, synthetic and bio-inspired. *Prog Polym Sci.* 2008, 33, 853-874.

[135] Ratner, B. D. The catastrophe revisited: Blood compatibility in the 21st Century. *Biomaterials*. 2007, 28, 5144-5147.

[136] Gao, J., Crapo, P. M., Wang, Y. D. Macroporous elastomeric scaffolds with extensive micropores for soft tissue engineering. *Tissue Engineering*. 2006, 12, 917-925.

[137] Gao, J., Crapo, P., Nerem, R., Wang, Y. D. Co-expression of elastin and collagen leads to highly compliant engineered blood vessels. *J Biomed Mater Res A*. 2008, 85A, 1120-1128.

[138] Crapo, P. M., Gao, J., Wang, Y. D. Seamless tubular poly(glycerol sebacate) scaffolds: High-yield fabrication and potential applications. *Journal of Biomedical Materials Research Part A*. 2008, 86A, 354-363.

[139] Crapo, P. M., Wang, Y. Physiologic compliance in engineered small-diameter arterial constructs based on an elastomeric substrate. *Biomaterials*. 2010, 31, 1626-1635.

[140] Chen, G. Q., Wu, Q. The application of polyhydroxyalkanoates as tissue engineering materials. *Biomaterials*. 2005, 26, 6565-6578.

[141] Sodian, R., Sperling, J. S., Martin, D. P., *et al.* Fabrication of a trileaflet heart valve scaffold from a polyhydroxyalkanoate biopolyester for use in tissue engineering. *Tissue Engineering*. 2000, 6, 183-188.

[142] Sodian, R., Loebe, M., Hein, A., *et al.* Application of stereolithography for scaffold fabrication for tissue engineered heart valves. *ASAIO J*. 2002, 48, 12-16.

[143] Sodian, R., Hoerstrup, S. P., Sperling, J. S., *et al.* Early *in vivo* experience with tissue-engineered trileaflet heart valves. *Circulation*. 2000, 102, 22-29.

[144] de Valence, S., Tille, J.-C., Mugnai, D., *et al.* Long term performance of polycaprolactone vascular grafts in a rat abdominal aorta replacement model. *Biomaterials*. 2012, 33, 38-47.

[145] Naito, Y., Shinoka, T., Duncan, D., *et al.* Vascular tissue engineering: towards the next generation vascular grafts. *Advanced Drug Delivery Reviews*. 2011, 63, 312-323.

[146] Bos, G. W., Poot, A. A., Beugeling, T., van Aken, W. G., Feijen, J. Small-diameter vascular graft prostheses: Current status. *Arch Physiol Biochem*. 1998, 106, 100-115.

[147] Palmaz, J. C. Review of polymeric graft materials for endovascular applications. *J Vasc Interv Radiol*. 1998, 9, 7-13.

[148] Wang, X., Lin, P., Yao, Q., Chen, C. Development of Small-Diameter Vascular Grafts. *World Journal of Surgery*. 2007, 31, 682-689.

[149] Marois, Y., Sigot-Luizard, M. F., Guidoin, R. Endothelial cell behavior on vascular prosthetic grafts: Effect of polymer chemistry, surface structure, and surface treatment. *Asaio Journal*. 1999, 45, 272-280.

[150] Guidoin, R., Martin, L., Levaillant, P., *et al.* Endothelial Lesions Associated with Vascular Clamping - Surface Micro-Pathology by Scanning Electron-Microscopy. *Biomater Artif Cell*. 1978, 6, 179-197.

[151] Joseph, R., Shelma, R., Rajeev, A., Muraleedharan, C. V. Characterization of surface modified polyester fabric. *Journal of Materials Science-Materials in Medicine*. 2009, 20, 153-159.

[152] Bos, G. W., Scharenborg, N. M., Poot, A. A., *et al.* Blood compatibility of surfaces with immobilized albumin-heparin conjugate and effect of endothelial cell seeding on platelet adhesion. *Journal of Biomedical Materials Research*. 1999, 47, 279-291.

[153] Dekker, A., Reitsma, K., Beugeling, T., *et al.* Adhesion of Endothelial-Cells and Adsorption of Serum-Proteins on Gas Plasma-Treated Polytetrafluoroethylene. *Biomaterials*. 1991, 12, 130-138.

[154] Dekker, A., Beugeling, T., Wind, H., *et al.* Deposition of Cellular Fibronectin and Desorption of Human Serum-Albumin during Adhesion and Spreading of Human Endothelial-Cells on Polymers. *J Mater Sci-Mater M.* 1991, 2, 227-233.

[155] Dekker, A., Poot, A. A., Vanmourik, J. A., *et al.* Improved Adhesion and Proliferation of Human Endothelial-Cells on Polyethylene Precoated with Monoclonal-Antibodies Directed against Cell-Membrane Antigens and Extracellular-Matrix Proteins. *Thromb Haemostasis.* 1991, 66, 715-724.

[156] Klomp, A. J. A., Engbers, G. H. M., Mol, J., Terlingen, J. G. A., Feijen, J. Adsorption of proteins from plasma at polyester non-wovens. *Biomaterials.* 1999, 20, 1203-1211.

[157] Criado, E., Marston, W. A., Woosley, J. T., *et al.* An Aortic-aneurysm model for evaluation of endovascular exclusion protheses. *Journal of Vascular Surgery.* 1995, 22, 306-315.

[158] Gustafsson, Y., Haag, J., Jungebluth, P., *et al.* Viability and proliferation of rat MSCs on adhesion protein-modified PET and PU scaffolds. *Biomaterials.* 2012, 33, 8094-8103.

[159] Wilhelm, L., Zippel, R., von Woedtke, T., *et al.* Immune response against polyester implants is influenced by the coating substances. *Journal of Biomedical Materials Research Part A.* 2007, 83A, 104-113.

[160] Ramires, P. A., Mirenghi, L., Romano, A. R., Palumbo, F., Nicolardi, G. Plasma-treated PET surfaces improve the biocompatibility of human endothelial cells. *Journal of Biomedical Materials Research.* 2000, 51, 535-539.

[161] Wang, J., Pan, C. J., Huang, N., *et al.* Surface characterization and blood compatibility of poly(ethylene terephthalate) modified by plasma surface grafting. *Surface and Coatings Technology.* 2005, 196, 307-311.

[162] Abdolahifard M, Hajir Bahrami S., Malek R. M. A. Surface Modification of PET Fabric by Graft Copolymerization with Acrylic Acid and Its Antibacterial Properties. *International Scholarly Research Network (ISRN) Organic Chemistry.* 2011, 8.

[163] Bartnik, A., Fiedorowicz, H., Jarocki, R., *et al.* Physical and chemical modifications of PET surface using a laser-plasma EUV source. *Applied Physics a-Materials Science & Processing.* 2010, 99, 831-836.

[164] Karaszewska, A., Buchenska, J. Polyester Vascular Prostheses - Antibacterial and Athrombogenic Bio-Materials. Part I. Two-Stage Modification of Vascular Prostheses. *Polimery-W.* 2012, 57, 722-727.

[165] Bridges, A. Anti-Inflammatory Polymeric Coatings for Implantable Biomaterials and Devices. *Journal of Diabetes Science and Technology.* 2008, 2, 984-994.

[166] Mironov, V., Kasyanov, V., Markwald, R. R. Nanotechnology in vascular tissue engineering: from nanoscaffolding towards rapid vessel biofabrication. *Trends in Biotechnology.* 2008, 26, 338-344.

[167] Kumbar, S. Q., Nukavarapu, S. P., James, R., Hogan, M. V., Laurencin, C. T. Recent patents on electrospun biomedical nanostructures: an overview. *Recent Pat Biomed Eng.* 2008, 1, 68-7878.

[168] Sell, S. A., McClure, M. J., Garg, K., Wolfe, P. S., Bowlin, G. L. Electrospinning of collagen/biopolymers for regenerative medicine and cardiovascular tissue engineering. *Advanced Drug Delivery Reviews.* 2009, 61, 1007-1019.

[169] Ma, Z., Kotaki, M., Yong, T., He, W., Ramakrishna, S. Surface engineering of electrospun polyethylene terephthalate (PET) nanofibers towards development of a new material for blood vessel engineering. *Biomaterials.* 2005, 26, 2527-2536.

[170] Ravichandran, R., Venugopal, J. R., Sundarrajan, S., *et al*. Minimally invasive injectable short nanofibers of poly(glycerol sebacate) for cardiac tissue engineering. *Nanotechnology.* 2012, 23, 385102.

[171] Kenar, H., Kose, G. T., Hasirci, V. Design of a 3D aligned myocardial tissue construct from biodegradable polyesters. *J Mater Sci-Mater M.* 2010, 21, 989-997.

[172] Kenar, H., Kose, G. T., Toner, M., Kaplan, D. L., Hasirci, V. A 3D aligned microfibrous myocardial tissue construct cultured under transient perfusion. *Biomaterials.* 2011, 32, 5320-5329.

[173] Ravichandran, R., Venugopal, J. R., Sundarrajan, S., Mukherjee, S., Ramakrishna, S. Poly(Glycerol Sebacate)/Gelatin Core/Shell Fibrous Structure for Regeneration of Myocardial Infarction. *Tissue Eng Pt A.* 2011, 17, 1363-1373.

[174] Stabenfeldt, S. E., Garcia, A. J., LaPlaca, M. C. Thermoreversible laminin-functionalized hydrogel for neural tissue engineering. *J Biomed Mater Res A.* 2006, 718-725.

[175] Nisbet, D., Yu, L., Zahir, T., Forsythe, J., Shoichet, M. Characterization of neural stem cells on electrospun poly (ε-caprolactone) submicron scaffolds: evaluating their potential in neural tissue engineering. *Journal of Biomaterials Science, Polymer Edition.* 2008, 19, 623-634.

[176] Schnell, E., Klinkhammer, K., Balzer, S., *et al*. Guidance of glial cell migration and axonal growth on electrospun nanofibers of poly-ε-caprolactone and a collagen/poly-ε-caprolactone blend. *Biomaterials.* 2007, 28, 3012-3025.

[177] Novikova, L. N., Pettersson, J., Brohlin, M., Wiberg, M., Novikov, L. N. Biodegradable poly-beta-hydroxybutyrate scaffold seeded with Schwann cells to promote spinal cord repair. *Biomaterials.* 2008, 29, 1198-1206.

[178] Borkenhagen, M., Stoll, R. C., Neuenschwander, P., Suter, U. W., Aebischer, P. *In vivo* performance of a new biodegradable polyester urethane system used as a nerve guidance channel. *Biomaterials.* 1998, 19, 2155-2165.

[179] Mosahebi, A., Fuller, P., Wiberg, M., Terenghi, G. Effect of allogeneic Schwann cell transplantation on peripheral nerve regeneration. *Experimental Neurology.* 2002, 173, 213-223.

[180] Xiong, Y., Zeng, Y.-S., Zeng, C.-G., *et al*. Synaptic transmission of neural stem cells seeded in 3-dimensional PLGA scaffolds. *Biomaterials.* 2009, 30, 3711-3722.

[181] Barbosa, M. A., Granja, P. L., Barrias, C. C., Amaral, I. F. Polysaccharides as scaffolds for bone regeneration. *ITBM-RBM.* 2005, 26, 212-217.

[182] Granja, P. L., Pouysegu, L., Petraud, M., *et al*. Cellulose phosphates as biomaterials. I. Synthesis and characterization of highly phosphorylated cellulose gels. *J Appl Polym Sci.* 2001, 82, 3341-3353.

[183] Granja, P. L., Pouysegu, L., Deffieux, D., *et al*. Cellulose phosphates as biomaterials. II. Surface chemical modification of regenerated cellulose hydrogels. *J Appl Polym Sci.* 2001, 82, 3354-3365.

[184] Granja, P. L., De Jeso, B., Bareille, R., *et al*. Cellulose phosphates as biomaterials. *In vitro* biocompatibility studies. *React Funct Polym.* 2006, 66, 728-739.

[185] Granja, P. L., Ribeiro, C. C., De Jeso, B., Baquey, C., Barbosa, M. A. Mineralization of regenerated cellulose hydrogels. *J Mater Sci-Mater M.* 2001, 12, 785-791.

[186] Granja, P. L., Barbosa, M. A., Pouysegu, L., *et al*. Cellulose phosphates as biomaterials. Mineralization of chemically modified regenerated cellulose hydrogels. *J Mater Sci.* 2001, 36, 2163-2172.

[187] Healy, K., Guldberg, R. Bone tissue engineering. *Journal of Musculoskeleta and Neuronal Interactions*. 2007, 7, 328.

[188] Kemppainen, J. M., Hollister, S. J. Tailoring the mechanical properties of 3D-designed poly(glycerol sebacate) scaffolds for cartilage applications. *J Biomed Mater Res A*. 2010, 94A, 9-18.

[189] Izquierdo, R., Garcia - Giralt, N., Rodriguez, M., *et al*. Biodegradable PCL scaffolds with an interconnected spherical pore network for tissue engineering. *Journal of Biomedical Materials Research Part A*. 2008, 85, 25-35.

[190] Annabi, N., Fathi, A., Mithieux, S. M., Weiss, A. S., Dehghani, F. Fabrication of porous PCL/elastin composite scaffolds for tissue engineering applications. *The Journal of Supercritical Fluids*. 2011, 59, 157-167.

[191] Declercq, H. A., Desmet, T., Berneel, E. E., Dubruel, P., Cornelissen, M. J. Synergistic effect of surface modification and scaffold design of bioplotted 3-D poly-epsilon-caprolactone scaffolds in osteogenic tissue engineering. *Acta Biomater*. 2013, 9, 7699-7708.

[192] Rai, B., Lin, J. L., Lim, Z. X., *et al*. Differences between *in vitro* viability and differentiation and *in vivo* bone-forming efficacy of human mesenchymal stem cells cultured on PCL-TCP scaffolds. *Biomaterials*. 2010, 31, 7960-7970.

[193] Shor, L., Güçeri, S., Wen, X., Gandhi, M., Sun, W. Fabrication of three-dimensional polycaprolactone/hydroxyapatite tissue scaffolds and osteoblast-scaffold interactions *in vitro*. *Biomaterials*. 2007, 28, 5291-5297.

[194] Nath, S. D., Son, S., Sadiasa, A., Min, Y. K., Lee, B. T. Preparation and characterization of PLGA microspheres by the electrospraying method for delivering simvastatin for bone regeneration. *International Journal of Pharmaceutics*. 2013, 443, 87-94.

[195] Zhang, Y., Yang, F., Liu, K., *et al*. The impact of PLGA scaffold orientation on *in vitro* cartilage regeneration. *Biomaterials*. 2012, 33, 2926-2935.

[196] Wang, Y. W., Yang, F., Wu, Q., *et al*. Effect of composition of poly(3-hydroxybutyrate-co-3-hydroxyhexanoate) on growth of fibroblast and osteoblast. *Biomaterials*. 2005, 26, 755-761.

[197] Deng, Y., Zhao, K., Zhang, X. F., Hu, P., Chen, G. Q. Study on the three-dimensional proliferation of rabbit articular cartilage-derived chondrocytes on polyhydroxyalkanoate scaffolds. *Biomaterials*. 2002, 23, 4049-4056.

[198] Zhao, K., Deng, Y., Chen, J. C., Chen, G. Q. Polyhydroxyalkanoate (PHA) scaffolds with good mechanical properties and biocompatibility. *Biomaterials*. 2003, 24, 1041-1045.

[199] Ye, C., Hu, P., Ma, M. X., *et al*. PHB/PHBHHx scaffolds and human adipose-derived stem cells for cartilage tissue engineering. *Biomaterials*. 2009, 30, 4401-4406.

[200] Wang, Y., Bian, Y. Z., Wu, Q., Chen, G. Q. Evaluation of three-dimensional scaffolds prepared from poly(3-hydroxybutyrate-co-3-hydroxyhexanoate) for growth of allogeneic chondrocytes for cartilage repair in rabbits. *Biomaterials*. 2008, 29, 2858-2868.

[201] Colthurst, M. J., Williams, R. L., Hiscott, P. S., Grierson, I. Biomaterials used in the posterior segment of the eye. *Biomaterials*. 2000, 21, 649-665.

[202] Ward, M. A., Georgiou, T. K. Thermoresponsive Polymers for Biomedical Applications. *Polymers-Basel*. 2011, 3, 1215-1242.

[203] Sodha, S., Wall, K., Redenti, S., *et al*. Microfabrication of a three-dimensional polycaprolactone thin-film scaffold for retinal progenitor cell encapsulation. *Journal of Biomaterials Science, Polymer Edition*. 2011, 22, 443-456.

[204] Pritchard, C. D., Arner, K. M., Neal, R. A., *et al.* The use of surface modified poly(glycerol-co-sebacic acid) in retinal transplantation. *Biomaterials.* 2010, 31, 2153-2162.

[205] Redenti, S., Neeley, W. L., Rompani, S., *et al.* Engineering retinal progenitor cell and scrollable poly(glycerol-sebacate) composites for expansion and subretinal transplantation. *Biomaterials.* 2009, 30, 3405-3414.

[206] Neeley, W. L., Redenti, S., Klassen, H., *et al.* A microfabricated scaffold for retinal progenitor cell grafting. *Biomaterials.* 2008, 29, 418-426.

[207] Sodha, S. A Microfabricated 3-D Stem Cell Delivery Scaffold for Retinal Regenerative Therapy, Thesis. *Massachusetts Institute of Technology,* 2009

[208] Tucker, B. A., Redenti, S. M., Jiang, C., *et al.* The use of progenitor cell/biodegradable MMP2-PLGA polymer constructs to enhance cellular integration and retinal repopulation. *Biomaterials.* 2010, 31, 9-19.

CHAPTER 7

Crosslinked Electrospun Mats Made of Natural Polymers: Potential Applications for Tissue Engineering

Silvia Baiguera[*,1], Costantino Del Gaudio[2], Alessandra Bianco[2] and Paolo Macchiarini[3]

[1]*BIOAIRlab, University Hospital Careggi, Florence, Italy;* [2]*University of Rome "Tor Vergata", Department of Enterprise Engineering, Intrauniversitary Consortium for Material Science and Technology (INSTM), Research Unit Tor Vergata, Rome, Italy; and* [3]*Advanced Center for Translational Regenerative Medicine (ACTREM), Karolinska Institutet, Stockholm, Sweden*

Abstract : Bioresorbable polymers represent a valuable choice for the fabrication of innovative scaffolds for tissue engineering applications. However, their actual ability to support the regenerative process needs to be carefully assessed. The extracellular matrix (ECM) is a complex functional structure providing specific cues and it should be replicated to promote an effective tissue regeneration after implantation. In this regard, electrospinning is a straightforward technique for the production of ECM-like scaffolds. Natural polymers might be promising candidates due to cellular affinity, even if affected by fast degradation and low mechanical stability. This limitation can be overcome by means of a cross-linking process, giving a hydrogel-like behavior to the final structure that can be usefully considered for the long-term release of drugs and growth factors.

This chapter is aimed firstly to review the potential of cross-linked electrospun natural polymers. Experimental results of the evaluation of cross-linked electrospun gelatin scaffolds, as suitable substrates to be loaded with vascular endothelial growth factor, are also herein presented.

Keywords: Cross-linking, electrospinning, growth factor release, natural polymers, tissue engineering.

INTRODUCTION

Tissue engineering is a promising alternative for the realization of novel devices able to recover or restore the integrity and the functionality of tissues and/or

---

*Corresponding Author Silvia Baiguera: BIOAIRlab, University Hospital Careggi, Florence, Italy; Tel: 0039 (0) 55/7946066; Fax: 0039 (0) 55/7949874; E-mail: sbaiguer@libero.it

organs. For this aim, the technical approach is based on the implementation of the typical tissue engineering paradigm involving three main key-factors: scaffolds, cells and signalling cues. Properly combining these elements, different strategies can be developed to obtain a targeted therapeutic option. The tissue engineering paradigm can be assumed as a whole (*e.g.*, cells seeded on a scaffold and *in vitro* cultured in a bioreactor, in order to deal with an already committed engineered construct before surgical implantation) or in its "incomplete" form (*e.g.*, (*i*) cell-seeded scaffolds implanted without a period of *in vitro* maturation or (*ii*) scaffolds properly prepared to directly attract *in vivo* endogenous cells in order to repopulate and regenerate novel tissue) [1].

Reasonably, the scaffold plays a pivotal role, mimicking the extracellular matrix (ECM) and allowing cell proliferation, migration and differentiation and thus promoting the regeneration of specific tissues [2]. In addition, bioresorbable polymers, with specific mechanical properties, can provide a temporary template for the regeneration of novel tissue that will replace the artificial support. This approach is believed (*i*) to enhance the functional deposition of autologous ECM, reproducing the anatomical architecture of the biological structure to be replaced, and (*ii*) to avoid possible complications generally associated with a typical foreign body response. However, this is only the starting point of a significant regenerative approach. A suitable and functional "artificial" substitute should be readily available to the surrounding tissue, in order to be promptly vascularized and to promote an effective integration with the host. To actually address this issue, it should be underlined that angiogenesis is a multifactor process, which is regulated by an interplay of a large number of factors. The vascular endothelial growth factor (VEGF), one of the most important biochemical inducers, stimulates cells to produce matrix metalloproteinases that degrade the basement membrane and surrounding ECM, allowing endothelial cell proliferation, migration and sprouting [3]. A possible approach to promote angiogenesis is to administer growth factors by injection or, preferably, by a slow-release system such as a bioresorbable scaffold. The fabrication of suitable scaffolds by means of electrospinning can be regarded as a valuable ECM-like system for the proposed target.

ELECTROSPINNING: GENERAL CONSIDERATIONS AND APPLICATIONS

Electrospinning is a cost-effective technique for the production of randomly arranged or aligned micro- and/or nanometric fibers [4-6]. Several polymers can be processed with this technique, in order to develop tissue engineered scaffolds that can effectively contribute to elicit a positive biological response either *in vitro* or, most importantly, *in vivo*. Synthetic and natural polymers are characterized by a number of pros and cons that should be accurately evaluated. To improve the final result, it is possible to finely tune several parameters, selecting, for instance, an appropriate blend of both types of polymers or including active agents or fillers in the starting polymeric solutions before to be electrospun. Moreover, post-processing treatments, *e.g.,* chemical adsorption or surface modification can be usefully considered as well, in order to deal with an easy and flexible fabrication process.

Technically, high voltage is applied to a polymeric solution flowing through a capillary to establish mutual charge repulsion. In the first phase of the process, a hemispherical drop is formed at the tip of the capillary, due to the surface tension of the solution. Then, by increasing the applied voltage, the shape of the pendant drop changes from hemispherical to conical (the Taylor cone) and, for a critical value of the imposed electric field, the electrostatic force, generated within the solution, overcomes the surface tension and a charged jet is ejected from the tip of the Taylor cone [7]. The polymeric jet experiences instability phenomena that stretch and reduce its diameter travelling from the tip of the capillary to the target, while solvents start to evaporate, concurring to further decrease the jet diameter [8]. Fibers are then collected onto a grounded target, the deposition (random or aligned) being dependent by its configuration (*e.g.,* fixed, rotating or *ad hoc* designed target to guide fiber deposition following a predefined pattern). Fluid properties (viscosity, conductivity, surface tension, and dielectric constant), operating parameters (applied voltage, capillary-to-target distance, flow rate), and environmental conditions deeply affect the resulting morphology of the electrospun scaffold [9, 10].

The peculiar characteristics imparted to the collected mats by electrospinnig can be regarded as an effective improvement toward the definition of suitable platforms for tissue engineering applications. For this aim, natural polymers, *e.g.,* gelatin, collagen, chitosan, and hyaluronic acid, can furnish a number of cues and favour a signalling cascade that can speed-up the formation of novel autologous tissue. Unfortunately, this kind of polymers do not show sufficient mechanical properties and promptly dissolve in aqueous environments, being a strong limitation to their extensive applications. As an example, gelatin might be a suitable material to fabricate specific electrospun platforms, being a well-known natural polymer resulting from collagen denaturation. Depending on the route selected for its production, it is possible to obtain gelatin type A (acidic treatment) or type B (alkaline treatment). The alkaline process converts glutamine and asparagine residues into glutamic and aspartic acid, which leads to higher carboxylic acid content for gelatin type B compared to gelatin type A [11]. However, being a water-soluble protein, gelatin needs to be properly treated in order to deal with a suitable scaffold. For this aim, cross-linking is an effective method that can improve its starting characteristics.

CROSS-LINKING ELECTROSPUN NATURAL POLYMERS

Cross-linking is an effective process that can ameliorate the temporal stability and the structural characteristics of several polymers. Different cross-linking approaches (chemical or physical) have been evaluated to find an ideal procedure to stabilize mechanical integrity and preserve original features of natural-based biomaterials [12-19]. Various synthetic cross-linking reagents, including formaldehyde, glutaraldehyde, dialdehyde and epoxy compound, have been used [20-22]. However, the clinical application was limited by their side-effects, such as high cytotoxicity, mismatched mechanical properties and post-implantation calcification, which impaired the biocompatibility of the engineered tissues [18, 19, 21-24]. Differently, genipin is a completely natural-derived (obtained from geniposide, isolated from the fruits of *Gardenia jasminoides* [25, 26]) cross-linking agent, which results to be as effective as glutaraldehyde at improving the stability of natural-based biomaterials, forming stable cross-linked products, with lower *in vitro* cytotoxic (about 10000 times less than glutaraldehyde) and *in vivo* inflammatory response [19, 27-35]. It has been used to fix tissues prior to implantation [36], modulate the release of growth factors [37], and increase structural properties of tissue engineered scaffolds [38-40]. Recently, genipin has been used to improve the mechanical and pro-angiogenic properties of decellularized rat airway matrices, demonstrating that genipin cross-linked matrices were *in vivo* well accepted and did not induce any cytotoxic effects [41].

Cross-linking can also give a hydrogel-like behavior to the substrate, allowing to load specific agents (*i.e.* drug and/or growth factors) within the structure, that can be subsequently released to stimulate and enhance peculiar biological processes. The resulting scaffolds, possessing a high water content, *ad hoc* mechanical properties and controllable degradation rates, could then represent a versatile strategy to deliver or present bioactive proteins.

Electrospun gelatin mats were cross-linked with genipin using different methods in order to select the most promising one [42]. Gelatin type A was dissolved in 60/40 vol% acetic acid/double distilled water at a concentration of 30 % (w/v), adding or not genipin. Electrospun mats were then collected and cross-linked by soaking in a genipin-ethanol solution, at different concentrations, and for different time periods at 37 °C. The addition of genipin to the starting polymeric solutions did not prevent scaffold solubilisation upon water exposure, but improved the results of the subsequent cross-linking reaction. Mechanical properties were, indeed, enhanced and the *in vitro* cytocompatibility was confirmed by seeding mesenchymal stem cells, isolated from human femoral arteries. Depending on the cross-linking process, morphological modifications can be obtained and it is possible to deal with resulting different fibrous microstructures. This occurrence was prevented adding a silane-coupling agent (γ-glycidoxypropyltrimethoxysilane) to a gelatin solution, obtained by dissolving the polymer (type A) in demineralised water at 50 °C, and electrospinning the final solution at the same temperature [43]. The cytocompatibility of the scaffolds was demonstrated by the *in vitro* adhesion, proliferation and survival of glial-like cells (neonatal olfactory bulb ensheating cells). No cytotoxic organic solvents were also considered for the electrospinning of gelatin type A, using ethanol/phosphate buffer saline solution [44]. The scaffolds were then cross-linked with vapour of 1.5% glutaraldehyde solution in ethanol at room temperature. The proposed approach resulted to be effective to stabilize gelatin nanofibers and the biological assays showed that 3T3 fibroblasts, seeded on the scaffolds, displayed a normal spindle-like morphology. However, the use of glutaraldehyde as cross-linking agent might be a potential limitation, considering the valuable effort not to use toxic solvents, as stated by the authors themselves. The same cross-linking procedure was considered to stabilize electrospun collagen-chitosan nanofibers for different blend ratios [45]. Infrared spectroscopy showed that the collagen-chitosan nanofibers did not change significantly, except for the enhanced stability after cross-linking by glutaraldehyde vapour. The cytocompatibility was evaluated culturing endothelial cells and smooth muscle cells for 14 days and the cellular proliferation, on or within the nanofiber architecture, confirmed the biocompatibility of the obtained scaffolds. Skotak *et al.* [46] evaluated the influence of the matrix stiffness of cross-linked electrospun gelatin fibers on chondrocytes response. For this aim, gelatin type B was dissolved in a 2,2,2,-trifluoroethanol/acetic acid solution to prevent clogging of the nozzle during electrospinning. Nanofibrous scaffolds were then cross-linked with glutaraldehyde for 1 hour at 30 °C. After 8 days of cell culture, it was observed that the matrix stiffness, correlated to the concentration of the cross-linker agent, affected chondrogenesis: the cell density was significantly higher when 1% of glutaraldehyde was used compared to the 0.1% case. Electrospun mats for cardiac tissue engineering, made up of natural polymers, were obtained by electrospinning haemoglobin, fibrinogen and gelatin [47]. The resulting fibers, consisting of 37.5% haemoglobin, 37.5% fibrinogen and 25% gelatin, were cross-linked using phytic acid, a natural agent. Human mesenchymal stem cells were cultured on the scaffolds for 21 days to assess cellular response. Cells exhibited the characteristic cardiomyocyte-like morphology, were positive for cardiac specific marker proteins, such as actin and troponin, and differentiated into functional cardiomyocytes with high oxygen binding ability. The results suggested that the combination of a functional nanofibrous scaffold, composed of natural polymers cross-linked by a natural agent, and stem cell may prove to be a novel therapeutic strategy for the treatment of myocardial infarction. The influence of different cross-linking agents (*i.e.*, genipin, hexamethylene-1,6-diaminocarboxysulphonate (HDACS) and epichlorohydrin (ECH)) was tested treating electrospun chitosan [48]. Chitosan was dissolved in trifluoroacetic acid (2.7 wt%) and cross-linkers were then added to the solution before electrospinning. Subsequently, collected mats underwent either heat or base activation. Covalent chemical interactions were evaluated by infrared spectroscopy and a large range of mechanical properties were revealed with a decreasing in both Young's modulus and tensile strength, in the case of genipin without post treatment [49]. Similarly, the effect of different cross-linking agents and cross-linking approaches was tested with electrospun collagen [50]. For this aim, collected nanofibers were (*i*) soaked either in N-[3-(dimethylamino)propyl]-N'-ethylcarbodiimide hydrochloride/N-hydroxysuccinimide or genipin solutions, (*ii*) UV-irradiated (253.7 nm, 30 W, 30 min), and (*iii*) cross-linked with an enzymatic approach by dissolving transglutaminase in a phosphate buffer (pH 6.0, 37 °C). UV-treated samples did not resist to the contact with water-based medium, while the other ones were tested by seeding MG-63 osteoblasts. An increased cell density was evaluated in all the investigated scaffolds, in particular the genipin case was characterized by retarded viability values. However, its use can still be attractive from a therapeutic viewpoint, considering the suppression of α-TN4 lens cell fibrogenic behaviors of the inflammatory reactions.

THE NEED TO VASCULARIZE A TISSUE ENGINEERED TISSUE

The vascularisation of a regenerating tissue allows cell and graft survival since blood vessels provide not only blood, but also endothelial progenitor cells to the implant. However, the identification of an effective vascularization strategy for an implanted scaffold is still a critical issue to be addressed in the tissue engineering field. *In vivo*, most cells are within a few hundred microns away from the nearest capillary or blood vessel. Beyond this distance, diffusion is not effective and tends to reduce cell survival and function [51]. In order to overcame this drawback different approaches have been explored [52]: (*i*) scaffolds with different pore size were investigated to identify the most suitable condition for cellular adhesion and migration [53], (*ii*) cells have been included into the scaffold to initiate angiogenesis *in vitro* [54], or (*iii*) growth factors have been added into the scaffold to promote angiogenesis *in vivo* [55]. CO_2 laser cutter was used to produce uniformly sized and evenly spaced pores on electrospun poly(ε-caprolactone) fiber mats without modifying the fiber structure [56]. These scaffolds, after being coated with collagen and wrapped around a catheter, to impart a cylindrical structure with a radius of 2.5 mm, were implanted into the omentum of Lewis rats. It was observed that scaffolds with 300 μm pores allowed

40% more cellular infiltration and significant vascular in-growth into the rolled scaffolds compared to controls. Computational models were also considered to simulate angiogenesis in porous scaffold, verifying that homogeneous scaffolds with large pore size (275-400 μm) and high interconnectivity (normalized pore connectivity > 0.65) supported extensive vascularisation and rapid in-growth [57]. Although a proper scaffold is a necessary requirement to promote an effective biological response, seeded cells actually contribute to promote vascularization of the tissue engineered construct. For instance, the combination of adipose-derived stem cells and outgrowth endothelial cells formed *in vitro* vascular structures in a matrix made of fibrin, a naturally occurring product in the blood coagulation [58]. Fibrin gels alone or in combination with synthetic poly(L-lactic acid)/polylactic-glycolic acid sponges were also evaluated to support *in vitro* construct vascularization and to enhance neovascularization upon implantation [59]. For this aim, two multicellular seeding assays were tested: (*i*) co-culture of endothelial cells and fibroblast, and (*ii*) a tri-culture combination of endothelial cells, fibroblasts and tissue specific skeletal myoblast cells. The acquired results proved that implanted endothelial cells formed 3D interconnected vascular-like networks *in vivo* which interacted with host neo-vessels penetrating the graft. In this context, specific growth factors (such as VEGF, the most potent growth factor to promote formation of new blood vessels) can further ameliorate the expected performance of the scaffold to induce angiogenesis. It should be pointed out that the addition of a growth factor within a scaffold is strictly dependent to the method adopted: encapsulation or covalent binding can be more robust approaches in achieving predictive drug release; however they expose the selected agent to harsher conditions that can compromise its bioactivity. Conversely, adsorption is a straightforward method that prevents this risk [60].

An effective strategy to develop sufficient vasculature is still lacking. Recently, specific growth (such as Granulocyte colony-stimulating factor) and boosting (such as Erythropoietin) factors have been used, both intraoperatively and post-operatively, to improve endothelial progenitor cell recruitment, activate endogenous stem cells and stimulate *in situ* vascularisation and, as a consequence, tissue regeneration [61, 62]. Despite the successful clinical results, new clinical strategies to drive and boost neo-angiogenesis are still lacking and require further studies to provide suitable tissue regeneration. It would be desirable to develop an approach providing controlled release of angiogenic factors to maintain high local therapeutic concentrations in tissue, while minimizing potential unwanted systemic effects. For this aim, a tailored platform resembling the natural ECM might represent a valuable option as several features can be combined together. The replication of a tissue-like microenvironment with structural and biochemical cues can improve the expected biological response for *in vivo* applications. In this respect, electrospinning could be a suitable technique to fabricate scaffolds to address this issue, allowing to properly manipulate a large number of processing variables to finally deal with an *ad hoc* device.

INVESTIGATING ELECTROSPUN GELATIN MATS AS GROWTH FACTOR RELEASING SYSTEMS

Gelatin is a valuable candidate for the fabrication of tailored scaffolds that can actively contribute to plan an opportune regenerative strategy. The natural origin, the ease of being processed by several techniques, and the possibility to be modified by blending with other polymers (to improve specific features), or incorporating drugs or growth factors (to be then released to speed-up the healing process), represent an interesting starting point for the development of a specific substrate with multiple biological cues. In this section, the potential of genipin cross-linked electrospun gelatin mats as bioresorbable platforms for the long-term release of VEGF is presented. *In vitro* and *in vivo* experiments were performed to actually assess the angiogenic properties of the obtained tissue engineered constructs.

THE EXPERIMENTAL PROCEDURE

In order to collect a suitable ECM-like scaffold, gelatin powder (type A, from porcine skin, Sigma-Aldrich) was firstly dissolved in a mixture of acetic acid/deionized water (9:1), the concentration was 14% w/v. The polymeric solution was then electrospun in the following conditions: 12 kV applied voltage, 0.4 ml/h feed rate, and 10 cm needle-to-target distance. All samples were vacuum dried for 48 hrs and stored in a desiccator.

Electrospun gelatin mats were stabilized against disintegration in an aqueous environment by means of a cross-linking process. For this aim, genipin (Wako) was dissolved in ethanol (0.5% w/v) and the collected substrates were then soaked into the alcoholic solution for 3 days at 37 °C.

The microstructure of as-spun and cross-linked gelatin samples was investigated by means of scanning electronic microscopy (SEM; Leo-Supra 35), after being sputter coated with gold. The average fiber diameter was determined from SEM micrographs by measuring about 50 fibers randomly selected (ImageJ, NIH).

Fourier transform infra-red (FTIR) analysis of as-spun and cross-linked gelatin mats was performed by using a Perkin Elmer Spectrum 100. The spectra were collected in the range 4000-400 cm^{-1} at a resolution of 4 cm^{-1}.

The VEGF, dissolved in Hank's Balanced Salt Solution (HBSS) + bovine serum albumin (BSA, 0.1%), was loaded on squared gelatin mats (50 ng/mg dry mat, 5 µl/mg of dry mat) (5 x 5 mm), previously sterilized in 100% v/v ethanol solution. The solution was then allowed to dry and the amount of VEGF released from samples was quantified, up to 28 days, using a human VEGF quantikine ELISA kit (R&D Systems, Minneapolis, MN). The bioactivity of VEGF loaded within gelatin cross-linked mats was assessed by seeding human bone marrow mesenchymal stromal cell (hMSC) cultures and determining (*i*) cell viability, (*ii*) cell migration, (*iii*) *in vitro* (Matrigel assay) and (*iv*) *in vivo* (CAM) angiogenic response, and (*v*) *in vitro* endothelial differentiation.

RESULTS

Electrospun gelatin mats were characterized by randomly arranged homogeneous fibers free of beads (Fig. **1**), the average fiber diameter being 0.22±0.04 µm. Cross-linked mat was still characterized by a fibrous structure, even if fiber diameters were larger than those of the as-spun case (*i.e.*, 0.55±0.14 µm). Moreover, fused regions were observed at the overlapping fiber sites. Resistance to aqueous environment was tested by soaking the electrospun mat in HBSS (+0.1% BSA) for 28 days at 37 °C. SEM analysis confirmed that the fibrous structure was preserved.

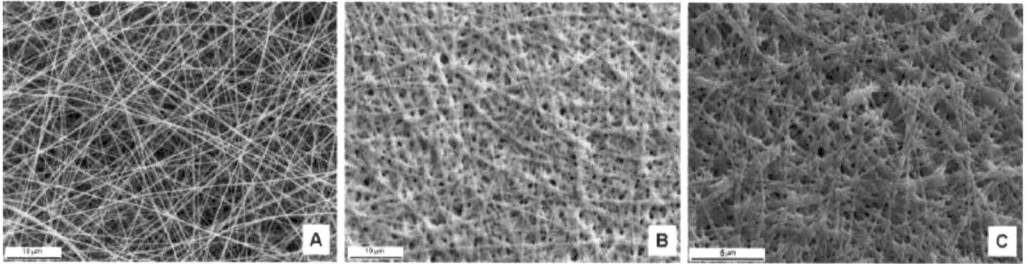

Fig. (1). SEM micrographs of as-spun gelatin (**A**), cross-linked gelatin (**B**), and after soaking in HBSS (+0.1% BSA) for 28 days (**C**).

In order to evaluate the influence of the cross-linker concentration on fiber stabilization to an aqueous environment, gelatin scaffolds were also chemically treated with a genipin solution at 0.1% w/v. Swelling assessment in PBS solution at 37 °C revealed that this type of scaffolds started to degrade after 4 days, suggesting that a mild cross-linking does not preserve the structure for a long period. However, this finding should be integrated by the type of the solution in which the sample was soaked in. Fig. (**2**) shows the macroscopic response of the same sample (*i.e.*, electrospun gelatin mat cross-linked with 0.1% w/v genipin) to three different media: Milli-Q water, PBS solution, and HBSS solution. It is evident that PBS solution turned to blue due to the dissolution of the mat just after 7 days; while the cross-linked mats remained stable in water and in HBSS solution up to 14 days. These results indicate that the definition of a suitable experimental protocol should be carried out in order (*i*) to univocally assess the properties of this kind of biomaterials and (*ii*) to perform a uniform comparison with literature data.

Infrared spectra of the investigated samples are shown in Fig. (**3**). Similar spectra were assessed for cross-linked and not cross-linked mats. Amide A peak (N-H stretching mode) was detected at 3300 cm^{-1} for the neat mat, while a little shift at 3320 cm^{-1} was observed for the cross-linked mat. Amide I (predominantly C=O stretching mode, with contributions from in-phase bending of the N-H bond and stretching of the C-N bond) and III (C-N stretching mode) were located at 1650 cm^{-1} and 1240 cm^{-1}, respectively, with no significant shifts for both samples. A little shift was also detected for amide II (N-H bending mode), from 1540 cm^{-1} for the as-spun sample to 1550 cm^{-1} for the cross-linked one [63, 64].

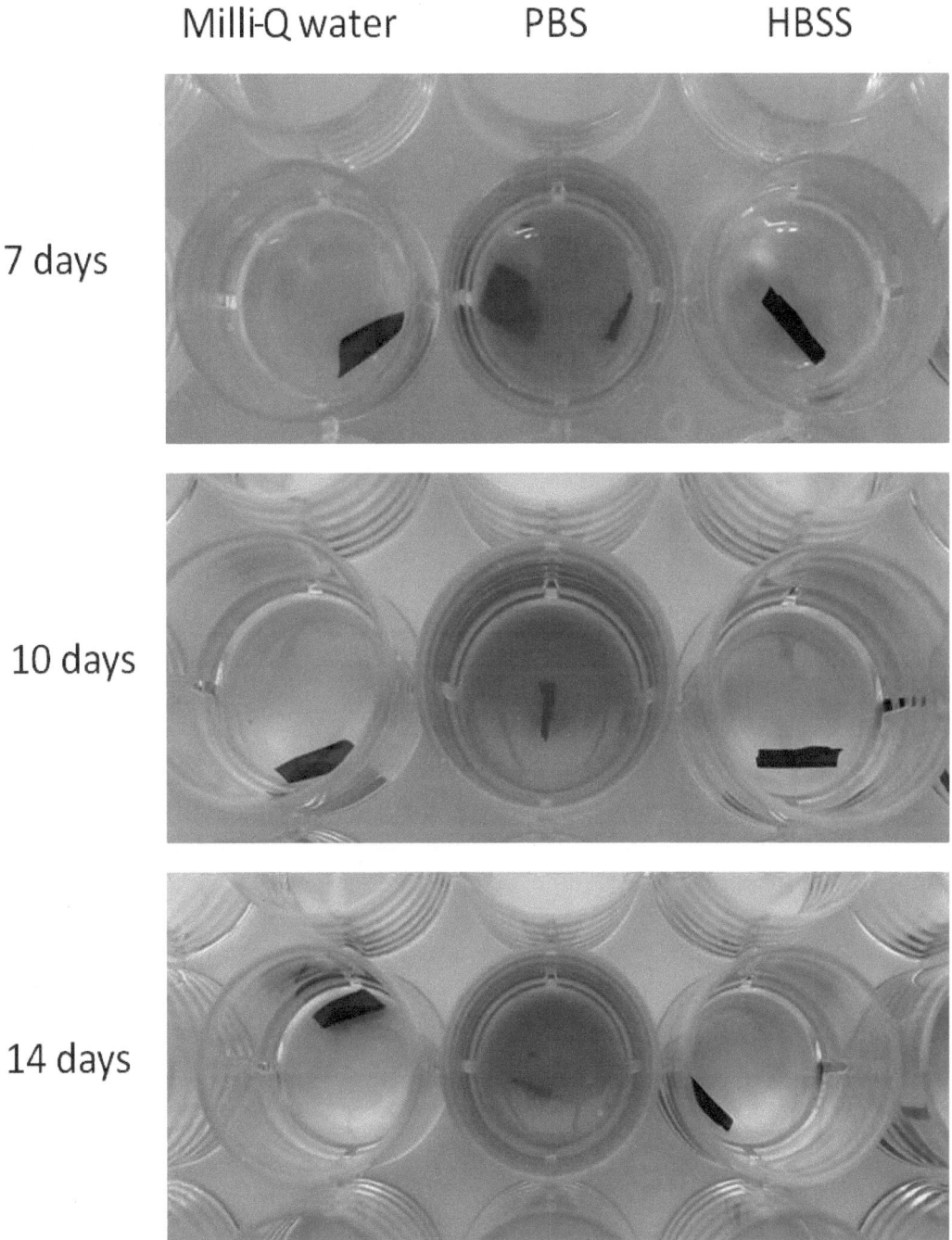

Fig. (2). Macroscopic evaluation of the temporal stability of the electrospun cross-linked (0.1% w/v genipin) gelatin mat to different media.

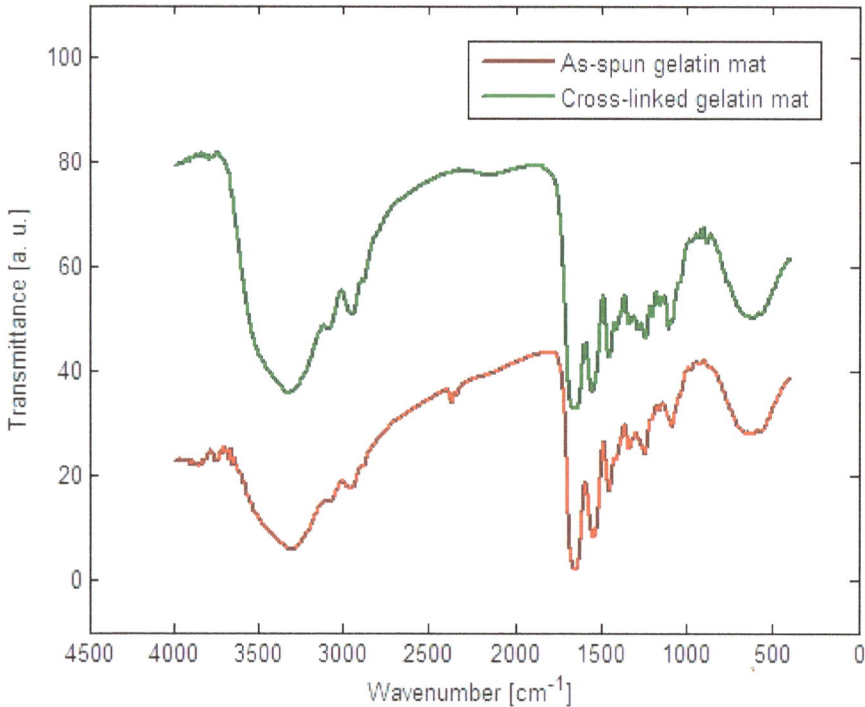

Fig. (3). FTIR spectra of electrospun gelatin mats before and after cross-linking.

The cumulative release trend of VEGF from the cross-linked mat was characterized by a burst release within the first day of incubation, followed by a prolonged sustained release. After 1 month the investigated scaffold released about 60% of the initial VEGF content (Fig. **4**).

In vitro studies demonstrated that VEGF loaded mat: (*i*) induced an increased cell viability with respect not only to negative control cultures (cells incubated only with culture medium), but also to positive ones (cells incubated with fresh VEGF (10 ng/ml) added directly into the culture medium); (*ii*) was characterized by *in vitro* chemoattractive properties, (*iii*) promoted hMSC spreading and alignment to form branching anastomotic tubes, which gave rise to a mesh of capillary-like structures (Fig. **5**), and (*iv*) induced the expression of KDR, the main mediator of VEGF-induced endothelial proliferation, survival, migration, tubular morpho-genesis and sprouting (% of expression of surface antigen anti KDR: negative cultures=6.63±1.07, positive culture=8.57±1.19, treated cultures=15.50±1.13,

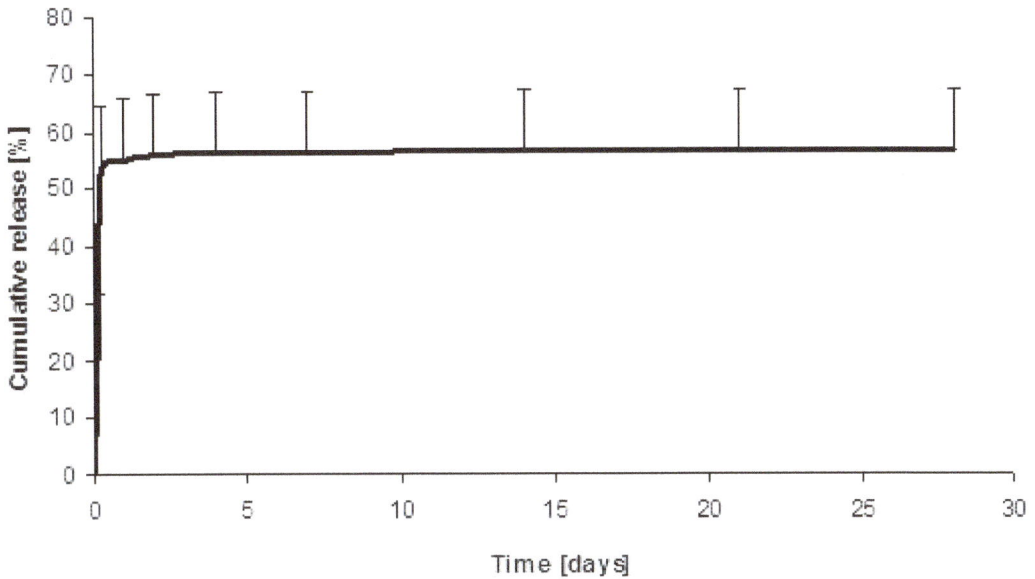

Fig. (4). VEGF cumulative release from the electrospun cross-linked gelatin mat.

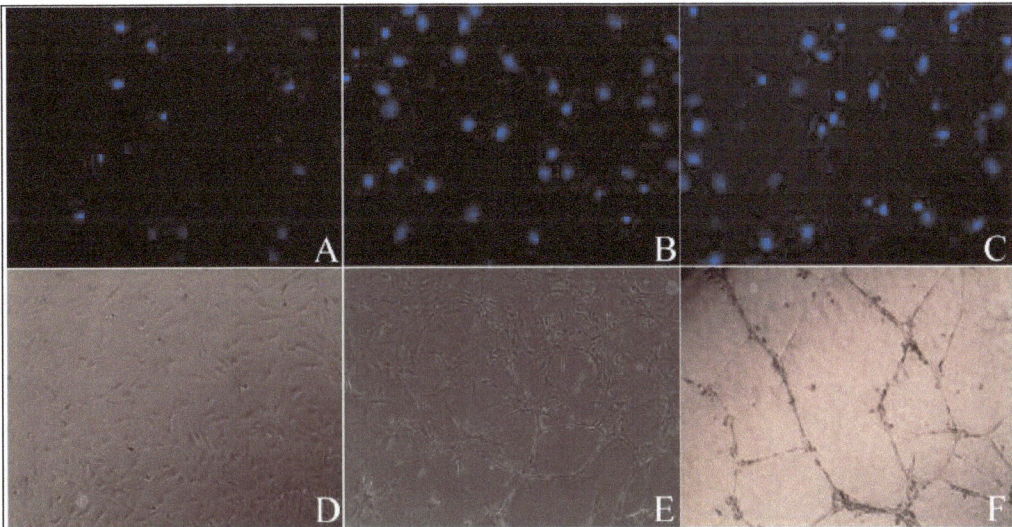

Fig. (5). Pro-angiogenic properties of VEGF loaded mats. (**A-C**) Representative images of hMSC migration in (**A**) culture medium only (negative control), (**B**) fresh VEGF (10 ng/ml; positive control), and (**C**) VEGF loaded cross-linked gelatin mat separate experiments. Nuclei were stained with DAPI. (**D-F**) Representative microscopic images of the capillary network observed in the presence of (**A**) culture medium only (negative control), (**B**) fresh VEGF (10 ng/ml; positive control), and (**C**) VEGF loaded cross-linked gelatin mat.

$p<0.05$). These results suggested that the VEGF loaded on mats has a positive cellular effect on hMSCs, retains its angiogenic potential and, most importantly, is able to induce cellular differentiation towards the endothelial pathway.

In vivo assessment of the potency of the VEGF-loaded mat, performed by chick chorioallantoic membrane (CAM) assay, showed that samples were surrounded by allantoic vessels that developed radially towards the implant in a spoke-wheel pattern, demonstrating that VEGF loaded on mats has *in vivo* angiogenic properties similar to fresh VEGF and is able to positively affect the growth and the organization of the network of CAM vessels.

CONCLUSION

Tissue engineering continuously shows its potential and versatility in the development of *ad hoc* strategies to treat a large number of pathologies, eliciting suitable tissue regeneration, positive host response and limiting the drawbacks associated to the conventional procedures. Moreover, in these last years, the route from bench to bedside has been started, and viable and functional substitutes have already been tested for human implantation with encouraging results [65-67]. However, even if positive, these have been isolated pioneering clinical therapies and the wide spectrum of the results presented in literature, clearly suggest that a suitable and safe approach is still to come, even for a single and specific clinical need. To move toward this goal, several requirements should be considered to produce a tissue-engineered construct that can effectively support a suitable and functional healing process. An active role for the scaffold should be therefore desirable because the nature of the material selected and the final microstructure are only preliminary requirements that could not assure the expected outcome. In this regard, natural polymers are a valuable alternative for biomedical applications, due to their origin and related intrinsic characteristics that can elicit a positive host response, but are also affected by several drawbacks, generally referred to the mechanical properties and degradation profile. Cross-linking represents a useful improvement that can aid to address this issue, but a critical review of the possible cross-linking agents and methods to chemically treat the polymers is needed. It is well known, in fact, that an appropriate selection of the agents and technical procedures to carry out the cross-linking procedure deeply affects the biological performance of the substrate that is in turn related to the scaffold properties. This implies to deal with a final scaffold with a preserved micro-architecture and cytotoxic degree, given by the nature of the cross-linker agent, as low as possible.

A major challenge in the field of tissue engineering is the integration of the implanted construct by the surrounding natural tissues and angiogenesis plays a fundamental role in this process. The addition of vascular growth factors represents an interesting strategy to promote angiogenesis within an tissue engineered scaffold.

In order to be compliant with these guidelines, genipin cross-linked electrospun gelatin mats were fabricated and investigated as a potential VEGF-release platform to induce angiogenesis. The morphological analysis confirmed the presence of uniform fibers randomly arranged that were still observed after being treated with genipin, even if a modification in terms of fiber dimensions was clearly revealed. A comparable result was previously reported when similar cross-linking conditions were considered [42, 47]. The VEGF release was assessed for 28 days: the investigated mat supported a prolonged factor release that can represent a relevant characteristic able to continuously induce the formation of blood vessels, as here demonstrated. Vascular endothelial or progenitor endothelial cells (predifferentiated stem cells with the potential to proliferate and differentiate into mature endothelial cells) are a common model to evaluate the efficacy of new strategies for revascularization [68]. However, their use in therapy is hampered by their limited expansion capacity and lack of autologous sources. Attracting and localizing mesenchymal stromal cells, which have been demonstrated to be promising source for obtaining endothelial cells able to create stable vascular networks [69, 70], could be a novel strategy for endothelialization. This was the rationale that led to the investigation of genipin cross-linked gelatin mats to act as a bioresorbable platform for the long-term release of VEGF on cultures of human bone marrow MSCs. Cell exposure to VEGF-loaded mats showed an increased viability, which resulted to be superior to that induced by fresh VEGF, and a positive chemoattractive and angiogenic activity, both *in vitro* and *in vivo*, was revealed, suggesting that cross-linked gelatin mats were able to release active VEGF. Moreover, this study demonstrates that hMSCs respond to absorbed VEGF not only by enhanced viability, migration and tube formation, but also by differentiating toward the endothelial pathway. As such, this approach could boost hMSCs to develop tissue vascularization.

ACKNOWLEDGEMENTS

This work was supported by European Project FP7-NMP-2011-SMALL-5: BIOtrachea, Biomaterials for Tracheal Replacement in Age-related Cancer *via* a Humanly Engineered Airway (No. 280584-2).

CONFLICT OF INTEREST

The authors confirm that this chapter contents have no conflict of interest.

ABBREVIATIONS

BSA   =   Bovine serum albumin

CAM   =   Chick chorioallantoic membrane

ECH   =   Epichlorohydrin

ECM   =   Extracellular matrix

FTIR   =   Fourier transform infra-red

HBSS   =   Hank's Balanced Salt Solution

HDACS   =   Hexamethylene-1,6-diaminocarboxysulphonate

hMSC   =   Human bone marrow mesenchymal stromal cell

KDR   =   Kinase insert domain receptor

PBS   =   Phosphate buffered solution

SEM   =   Scanning electron microscopy

VEGF   =   Vascular endothelial growth factor

REFERENCES

[1]   Rabkin, E; Schoen, FJ. Cardiovascular tissue engineering. *Cardiovasc. Pathol.*, 2002, 11, 305-317.

[2]   Murugan, R; Ramakrishna, S. Nano-featured scaffolds for tissue engineering: a review of spinning methodologies. *Tissue Eng.*, 2006, 12, 435-447.

[3]   Hoeben, A; Landuyt, B; Highley, MS; Wildiers, H; Van Oosterom, AT; De Bruijn, EA. Vascular endothelial growth factor and angiogenesis. *Pharmacol. Rev.*, 2004, 56, 549-580.

[4]   Yoshimoto, H; Shin, YM; Terai, H; Vacanti, JP. A biodegradable nanofiber scaffold by electrospinning and its potential for bone tissue engineering. *Biomaterials*, 2003, 24, 2077-2082.

[5]   Vaz, C; van Tuijl, S; Bouten, CVC; Baaijens, FPT. Design of scaffolds for blood vessel tissue engineering using a multi-layering electrospinning technique. *Acta Biomater.*, 2005, 1, 575-582.

[6]   Mo, XM; Xu, CY; Kotaki, M; Ramakrishna, S. Electrospun P(LLA-CL) nanofiber: a biomimetic extracellular matrix for smooth muscle cell and endothelial cell proliferation. *Biomaterials*, 2004, 25, 1883-1890.

[7]   Frenot, A; Chronakis, IS. Polymer nanofibers assembled by electrospinning. *Curr. Opinion Coll. Interface Sci.*, 2003, 8, 64-75.

[8]   Pham, QP; Sharma, U; Mikos, AG. Electrospinning of polymeric nanofibers for tissue engineering applications: a review. *Tissue Eng.*, 2006, 12, 1197-1211.

[9]   Lee, KH; Kim, HY; Khil, MS; Ra, YM; Lee, DR. Characterization of nano-strucutred poly(ε-caprolactone) nonwoven mats *via* electrospinning. *Polymer*, 2003, 44, 1287-1294.

[10]   Del Gaudio, C; Bianco, A; Folin, M; Baiguera, S; Grigioni, M. Structural characterization and cell response evaluation of electrospun PCL membranes: micrometric versus submicrometric fibers. *J. Biomed. Mater. Res. A*, 2009, 89, 1028-1039.

[11]   Zhang, Y; Ouyang, H; Lim, CT; Ramakrishna, S; Huang, ZM. Electrospinning of gelatin fibers and gelatin/PCL composite fibrous scaffolds. *J. Biomed. Mater. Res. B Appl. Biomater.*, 2005, 72, 156-165.

[12]   Nimni, ME; Cheung, D; Strates, B; Kodama, M; Sheikh, K. Chemically modified collagen: a natural biomaterial for tissue replacement. *J. Biomed. Mater. Res.*, 1987, 21, 741-771.

[13]   Cheung, DT; Tong, D; Perelman, N; Ertl, D; Nimni, ME. Mechanism of crosslinking of proteins by glutaraldehyde. IV: *in vitro* and *in vivo* stability of a crosslinked collagen matrix. *Connect. Tissue Res.*, 1990, 25, 27-34.

[14]   van Luyn, MJ; van Wachem, PB; Damink, LO; Dijkstra, PJ; Feijen, J; Nieuwenhuis, P. Relations between *in vitro* cytotoxicity and crosslinked dermal sheep collagens. *J. Biomed. Mater. Res.*, 1992, 26, 1091-1110.

[15]   van Wachem, PB; van Luyn, MJ; Olde Damink, LH; Dijkstra, PJ; Feijen, J; Nieuwenhuis, P. Biocompatibility and tissue regenerating capacity of crosslinked dermal sheep collagen. *J. Biomed. Mater. Res.*, 1994, 28, 353-363.

[16]   Schmidt, CE; Baier, JM. Acellular vascular tissues: natural biomaterials for tissue repair and tissue engineering. *Biomaterials*, 2000, 21, 2215-2231.

[17]   Courtman, DW; Errett, BF; Wilson, GJ. The role of crosslinking in modification of the immune response elicited against xenogenic vascular acellular matrices. *J. Biomed. Mater. Res.*, 2001, 55, 576-586.

[18]   Han, B; Jaurequi, J; Tang, BW; Nimni, ME. Proanthocyanidin: a natural crosslinking reagent for stabilizing collagen matrices. *J. Biomed. Mater. Res. A*, 2003, 65, 118-124.

[19]   Sung, HW; Chang, WH; Ma, CY; Lee, MH. Crosslinking of biological tissues using genipin and/or carbodiimide. *J. Biomed. Mater. Res. A*, 2003, 64, 427-438.

[20]   Schoen, FJ; Harasaki, H; Kim, KM; Anderson, HC; Levy, RJ. Biomaterial-associated calcification: pathology, mechanisms, and strategies for prevention. *J. Biomed. Mater. Res,.* 1988, 22(Suppl. A1), 11-36.

[21]   Nimni, ME; Cheung, D; Strates, B; Kodama, M; Sheikh, K. Bioprosthesis derived from crosslinked and chemically modified collagenous tissues. In: Nimni ME, editor. *Collagen*, Boca Raton, FL, CRC Press, 1988,. Volume-3. 1-38.

[22]   Yu, XX; Wan, C; Chen, HQ. Preparation and endothelialization of decellularized vascular scaffold for tissue engineered blood vessel. *J. Mater. Sci. Mater. Med.*, 2008, 19, 319-326.

[23]   Speer, DP; Chvapil, M; Eskelson, CD; Ulreich, J. Biological effects of residual glutaraldehyde in glutaraldehyde-tanned collagen biomaterials. *J. Biomed. Mater. Res.*, 1980, 14, 753-764.

[24]   Nishi, C; Nakajima, N; Ikada, Y. *In vitro* evaluation of cytotoxicity of diepoxy compounds used for biomaterial modification. *J. Biomed. Mater. Res.*, 1995, 29, 829-834.

[25]   Young S, Wong M, Tabata Y, Mikos AG. Gelatin as a delivery vehicle for the controlled release of bioactive molecules. J Control Release. 2005, 109, 256-274.

[26]   Tsm, TH; Westly, J; Lee, TF; Chen, CF. Identification and determination of geniposide, genipin, gardenoside, and geniposidic acid from herbs by HPLC/photodiode-array detection. *J. Liq. Chromatogr.*, 1994, 17, 2199-2205.

[27]   Schoen, FJ; Levy, RJ. Calcification of tissue heart valve substitutes: progress toward understanding and prevention. *Ann. Thorac. Surg.*, 2005, 79, 1072-1080.

[28]   Valente, M; Bortolotti, U; Thiene, G. Ultrastructure substrates of dystrophic calcification in porcine bioprosthetic valve failure. *Am. J. Pathol.*, 1985, 119, 12-21.

[29]   Chang, Y; Tsai, CC; Liang, HC; Sung, HW. *In vivo* evaluation of cellular and acellular bovine pericardia fixed with a naturally occurring crosslinking agent (genipin). *Biomaterials*, 2002, 23, 2447-2457.

[30]   Huang, LL; Sung, HW; Tsai, CC; Huang, DM. Biocompatibility study of a biological tissue fixed with a naturally occurring crosslinking reagent. *J. Biomed. Mater. Res.*, 1998, 42, 568-576.

[31]   Sung, HW; Huang, RN; Huang, LL; Tsai, CC; Chiu, CT. Feasibility study of a natural crosslinking reagent for biological tissue fixation. *J. Biomed. Mater. Res.*, 1998, 42, 560-567.

[32]   Sung, HW; Chang, Y; Chiu, CT; Chen, CN; Liang, HC. Crosslinking characteristics and mechanical properties of a bovine pericardium fixed with a naturally occurring crosslinking agent. *J. Biomed. Mater. Res.*, 1999, 47, 116-126.

[33]   Sung, HW; Liang, IL; Chen, CN; Huang, RN; Liang, HF. Stability of a biological tissue fixed with a naturally occurring crosslinking agent (genipin). *J. Biomed. Mater. Res.*, 2001, 55, 538-546.

[34]   Sung, HW; Huang, RN; Huang, LL; Tsai, CC. *In vitro* evaluation of cytotoxicity of a naturally occurring cross-linking reagent for biological tissue fixation. *J. Biomater. Sci. Polym. Ed.*, 1999, 10, 63-78.

[35]   Zhang, K; Qian, Y; Wang, H; Fan, L; Huang, C; Yin, A; Mo, X. Genipin-crosslinked silk fibroin/hydroxybutyl chitosan nanofibrous scaffolds for tissue-engineering application. *J. Biomed. Mater. Res. A*, 2010, 95, 870-881.

[36]   Englert, C; Blunk, T; Müller, R; von Glasser, SS; Baumer, J; Fierlbeck, J; Heid, IM; Nerlich, M; Hammer, J. Bonding of articular cartilage using a combination of biochemical degradation and surface cross-linking. *Arthritis. Res. Ther.*, 2007, 9, R47.

[37]   Liang, HC; Chang, WH; Lin, KJ; Sung, HW. Genipin-cross-linked gelatin microspheres as a drug carrier for intramuscular administration: *in vitro* and *in vivo* studies. J. Biomed. Mater. Res. A, 2003, 65, 271-282.

[38]   Somers, P; De Somer, F; Cornelissen, M; Bouchez, S; Gasthuys, F; Narine, K; Cox, E; Van Nooten, G. Genipin blues: an alternative non-toxic crosslinker for heart valves? *J. Heart. Valve Dis.*, 2008, 17, 682-688.

[39]   Avila, MY; Navia, JL. Effect of genipin collagen crosslinking on porcine corneas. *J. Cataract. Refract. Surg.*, 2010, 36, 659-664.

[40]   Bhrany, AD; Lien, CJ; Beckstead, BL; Futran, ND; Muni, NH; Giachelli, CM; Ratner, BD. Crosslinking of an oesophagus acellular matrix tissue scaffold. *J. Tissue Eng. Regen. Med.*, 2008, 2, 365-372.

[41]   Haag, J; Baiguera, S; Jungebluth, P; Barale, D; Del Gaudio, C; Castiglione, F; Bianco, A; Comin, CE; Ribatti, D; Macchiarini, P. Biomechanical and angiogenic properties of tissue-engineered rat trachea using genipin cross-linked decellularized tissue. *Biomaterials*, 2012, 33, 780-789.

[42]   Panzavolta, S; Gioffrè, M; Focarete, ML; Gualandi, C; Foroni, L; Bigi, A. Electrospun gelatin nanofibers: optimization of genipin cross-linking to preserve fiber morphology after exposure to water. *Acta Biomater.*, 2011, 7, 1702-1709.

[43]   Tonda-Turo, C; Cipriani, E; Gnavi, S; Chiono, V; Mattu, C; Gentile, P; Perroteau, I; Zanetti, M; Ciardelli, G. Crosslinked gelatin nanofibres: preparation, characterisation and *in vitro* studies using glial-like cells. *Mater. Sci. Eng. C*, 2013, 33, 2723-2735.

[44]   Zha, Z; Teng, W; Markle, V; Dai, Z; Wu, X. Fabrication of gelatin nanofibrous scaffolds using ethanol/phosphate buffer saline as a benign solvent. *Biopolymers*, 2012, 97, 1026-1036.

[45]   Chen, ZG; Wang, PW; Wie, B; Mo, XM; Cui, FZ. Electrospun collagen-chitosan nanofiber: a biomimetic extracellular matrix for endothelial cell and smooth muscle cell. *Acta Biomater.*, 2010, 6, 372-382.

[46]   Skotak, M; Noriega, S; Larsen, G; Subramanian, A. Electrospun cross-linked gelatin fibers with controlled diameter: the effect of matrix stiffness on proliferative and biosynthetic activity of chondrocytes cultured *in vitro*. *J. Biomed. Mater. Res. A*, 2010, 95, 828-836.

[47]   Ravichandran, R; Seitz, V; Reddy Venugopal, J; Sridhar, R; Sundarrajan, S; Mukherjee, S; Wintermantel, E; Ramakrishna, S. Mimicking native extracellular matrix with phytic Acid-crosslinked protein nanofibers for cardiac tissue engineering. *Macromol. Biosci.*, 2013, 13, 366-375.

[48]   Austero, MS; Donius, AE; Wegst, UGK; Schauer, CL. New crosslinkers for electrospun chitosan fibre mats. I. Chemical analysis. *J. R. Soc. Interface*, 2012, 9, 2551-2562.

[49]   Donius, AE; Kiechel, MA; Schauer, CL; Wegst, UGK. New crosslinkers for electrospun chitosan fibre mats. Part II: mechanical properties. *J. R. Soc. Interface*, 2013, 10, 20120946.

[50]   Torres-Giner, S; Gimeno-Alcañiz, JV; Ocio, MJ; Lagaron, JM. Comparative performance of electrospun collagen nanofibers cross-linked by means of different methods. *ACS Appl. Mater. Interfaces*, 2009, 1, 218-223.

[51]   Gauvin, R; Guillemette, M; Dokmeci, M; Khademhosseini, A. Application of microtechnologies for the vascularization of engineered tissues. *Vasc. Cell*, 2011, 3, 24.

[52]   Baiguera, S; Ribatti, D. Endothelialization approaches for viable engineered tissues. *Angiogenesis*, 2013, 16, 1-14.

[53]   O'Brien, FJ; Harley, BA; Yannas, IV; Gibson, LJ. The effect of pore size on cell adhesion in collagene-GAG scaffolds. *Biomaterials*, 2005, 26, 433-441.

[54]   Rickert, D; Moses, MA; Lendlein, A; Kelch, S; Franke, RP. The importance of angiogenesis in the interaction between polymeric biomaterials and surrounding tissue. *Clin. Hemorheol. Microcirc.*, 2003, 28, 175-181.

[55]   Pieper, JS; Hafmans, T; van Wachem, PB; van Luyn, MJ; Brouwer, LA; Veerkamp, JH; van Kuppevelt, TH. Loading of collageneheparan sulfate matrices with bFGF promotes angiogenesis and tissue generation in rats. *J. Biomed. Mater. Res.*, 2002, 62, 185-194.

[56]   Joshi, VS; Lei, NY; Walthers, CM; Wu, B; Dunn, JC. Macroporosity enhances vascularization of electrospun scaffolds. *J. Surg. Res.*, 2013, 183, 18-26.

[57]   Mehdizadeh, H; Sumo, S; Bayrak, ES; Brey, EM; Cinar, A. Three-dimensional modeling of angiogenesis in porous biomaterial scaffolds. *Biomaterials*, 2013, 34, 2875-2887.

[58]   Holnthoner, W; Hohenegger, K; Husa, AM; Muehleder, S; Meinl, A; Peterbauer-Scherb, A; Redl, H. Adipose-derived stem cells induce vascular tube formation of outgrowth endothelial cells in a fibrin matrix. *J. Tissue. Eng. Regen. Med.*, 2012. doi: 10.1002/term.1620.

[59]   Lesman, A; Koffler, J; Atlas, R; Blinder, YJ; Kam, Z; Levenberg, S. Engineering vessel-like networks within multicellular fibrin-based constructs. *Biomaterials*, 2011, 32, 7856-7869.

[60]   Singh, S; Wu, BM; Dunn, JC. Delivery of VEGF using collagen-coated polycaprolactone scaffolds stimulates angiogenesis. *J. Biomed. Mater. Res. A*, 2012, 100, 720-727.

[61]   Jungebluth, P; Moll, G; Baiguera, S; Macchiarini, P. Tissue-engineered airway: a regenerative solution. *Clin. Pharmacol. Ther.*, 2012, 91, 81-93.

[62]   Jungebluth, P; Bader, A; Baiguera, S; Möller, S; Jaus, M; Lim, ML; Fried, K; Kjartansdóttir, KR; Go, T; Nave, H; Harringer, W; Lundin, V; Teixeira, AI; Macchiarini, P. The concept of *in vivo* airway tissue engineering. *Biomaterials*, 2012, 33, 4319-4326.

[63]   Hashim, DM; Che Man, YB; Norakasha, R; Shuhaimi, M; Salmah, Y; Syahariza, ZA. Potential use of Fourier transform infrared spectroscopy for differentiation of bovine and porcine gelatins. *Food Chem.*, 2010, 118, 856-860.

[64]   Qian, YF; Zhang, KH; Chen, F; Ke, QF; Mo, XM. Cross-linking of gelatin and chitosan complex nanofibers for tissue-engineering scaffolds. *J. Biomater. Sci. Polym. Ed.*, 2011, 22, 1099-1113.

[65]   Jungebluth, P; Alici, E; Baiguera, S; Le Blanc, K; Blomberg, P; Bozóky, B; Crowley, C; Einarsson, O; Grinnemo, KH; Gudbjartsson, T; Le Guyader, S; Henriksson, G; Hermanson, O; Juto, JE; Leidner, B; Lilja, T; Liska, J; Luedde, T; Lundin, V; Moll, G; Nilsson, B; Roderburg, C; Strömblad, S; Sutlu, T; Teixeira, AI; Watz, E; Seifalian, A; Macchiarini, P. Tracheobronchial transplantation with a stem-cell-seeded bioartificial nanocomposite: a proof-of-concept study. *Lancet*, 2011, 378, 1997-2004.

[66]   Macchiarini, P; Jungebluth, P; Go, T; Asnaghi, MA; Rees, LE; Cogan, TA; Dodson, A; Martorell, J; Bellini, S; Parnigotto, PP; Dickinson, SC; Hollander, AP; Mantero, S; Conconi, MT; Birchall, MA. Clinical transplantation of a tissue-engineered airway. *Lancet*, 2008, 372, 2023-2030

[67]   Atala, A; Bauer, SB; Soker, S; Yoo, JJ; Retik, AB. Tissue-engineered autologous bladders for patients needing cystoplasty. *Lancet*, 2006, 367, 1241-1246.

[68]   Grieb, G; Groger, A; Piatkowski, A; Markowicz, M; Steffens, GC; Pallua, N. Tissue substitutes with improved angiogenic capabilities: an *in vitro* investigation with endothelial cells and endothelial progenitor cells. *Cells Tissues Organs*, 2010, 191, 96-104.

[69]   da Silva Meirelles, L; Caplan, AI; Nardi, NB. In search of the *in vivo* identity of mesenchymal stem cells. *Stem Cells*, 2008, 26, 2287-2299.

[70]   Janeczek Portalska, K; Leferink, A; Groen, N; Fernandes, H; Moroni, L; van Blitterswijk, C; de Boer, J. Endothelial differentiation of mesenchymal stromal cells. *PLoS One*, 2012, 7, e46842.

CHAPTER 8

Nanomaterials for Skin Regeneration

Huijun Zhu[*], Claudia Moia and Patrick Vilela

School of Applied Sciences, Cranfield University, Bedfordshire, MK43 0AL, UK

Abstract: Wound healing and its medical complications present a huge burden to health care worldwide. Current tissue engineering materials are far from satisfactory in meeting desirable safety and efficacy. Due to the intricate three-dimensional nanostructure, flexibility in shape design and multifunctional surface modification, advanced nanomaterials offer new hopes for revolutionising modern medicine. The potential of their applications in medical research and clinical practice include diagnosis, treatment, imaging and tissue regeneration. This chapter reviews the progress made in the application of nanomaterials in skin tissue engineering in the last decade. It mainly focuses on materials of biological origins that are biodegradable, non-toxic, and biocompatible with cells at target sites. The characteristics of novel biofunctional scaffolds, safety and future trend of nanomaterial application in tissue engineering are also discussed, aiming to promote continuous research effort in developing scaffold materials for optimisation of skin regeneration.

Keywords: Nanomaterial, scaffold, skin, tissue engineering, wound regeneration.

INTRODUCTION

Nanomaterials generally refer to materials with at least one dimension in the range of 1-100 nm [1, 2]. They offer a great potential for the revolution of almost all aspects of modern medicine, including diagnosis, treatment, imaging and tissue regeneration. This is due to their unique size, topology, and surface chemistry that allow them to interact with cells and cross physiological barriers, and subsequently to reach target site. The most desirable nanomaterials for biomedical applications are those that are biodegradable, biocompatible with healthy tissues/cells, and superior in biofunctionality over their conventional counterparts. Many types of nanomaterials, organic and inorganic origins, have been exploited for biomedical applications in the last two decades. Although the nanomaterials of

Corresponding Author Huijun Zhu: School of Applied Sciences, Cranfield University, Bedfordshire, MK43 0AL, UK; Tel: +44 (0)7766 923 186; Fax: +44 (0)1234 75 2971; E-mail: h.zhu@cranfield.ac.uk

various origins demonstrate great biological function individually, by combining these materials, their biological functions can be greatly enhanced.

The well characterized biological components such as lipids, proteins, sugars, peptides, surfactants and polymers have all been engineered into nanoformulations. Other most well-studied nanomaterials for medical applications include carbon nanotubes, titanium, silica, silver, magnetic iron oxide, and gold. The types of nanomaterials that are considered the most promising new generation of materials for medical applications have been reviewed previously and summarised in Tables **1** and **2**.

Table 1. **Inorganic Nanomaterials Applied in Medicine**

Nanomaterial	Application/Reference
Carbon Nanotubes	Optical biomedical sensors, drug delivery, neuronal tissue regeneration [3-5]
Fullerenes	Implantable sensors, therapeutics, drug delivery [6, 7]
Gold	Molecular imaging, theragnosis [8]
Gold	Drug delivery, therapeutics, and photothermal therapy [9-12]
Silica	Mesoporous: Drug/gene delivery, theranostic agent [13, 14]
Silica	Non-porous: Drug/Gene delivery, Molecular Imaging [15]
Ag, Au, Cu, Pt TiO_2, ZnO, CuO	As antimicrobial agent for treating infectious conditions [16, 17]
Iron oxide	Contrast agent for imaging, therapeutic agent, drug delivery, and cell tracking [18-20]
Quantum dots	Optical imaging [21]

This review mainly focuses on the progress made with these materials in the last decade in tissue engineering, an area of innovation initiated three decades ago by Burke *et al.*. Following their success in synthesis of a neodermis using a bovine collagen matrix-based bilayer and biocompatible dermal scaffold [36], the subsequent advances in tissue engineering have been largely fuelled by the advent of new materials

SKIN - THE LARGEST ORGAN OF HUMAN BODY

Skin is the largest organ in human body, contributing about 15% of the total body weight in adults. It is 2 m^2 in area and 2.5 mm in average thickness [37, 38], providing the greatest contact site with the exterior world. It functions as a first-line barrier, protecting the body against injuries due to physical damage, bacterial and virus infection, allergy attack and loss of water [39].

Table 2. **Organic Nanomaterials Applied in Medicine**

Nanomaterial/Origin	Chemical Composition/Bioactivity	Application/Reference
Lipids- hydrophobic or amphiphilic molecules from human, animals and vegetables	Categorised based on origins of ketoacyl and isoprene groups, main structure component of cell membranes.	Topical and systemic drug delivery [22, 23]
Collagen (Col)/gelatin	The most abundant protein in mammals, with a triple helix rigid structure; gelatin is derived from collagen by partial hydrolysis.	As scaffold for large-scale soft tissue regeneration [24]
Chitosan-the derivative of chitin.	Composed of repeating N-glucosamine units glucosamine and N-acetyl-glucosamine that are derived from partial deacetylation of chitin; anti-antibacterial activity and haemostatic.	Regenerative medicine, drug delivery [25-28]
Plant-derived nanofibrous materials	Indigoferaaspalathoides, Azadirachtaindica and Memecylonedule: anti-inflammatory and astringent properties.	All have been used traditionally as a medical plants; incorporated with Poly(Ɛ-caprolactone) PCL as scaffolds for wound dressing [29]
Synthetic polymers	PCL: high permeability to many drugs, slow degradation rate.	Drug delivery, wound healing [30, 31]
	Poly(l-lactide-co-glycolide) (PLGA): made of lactic acid and glycolic acid.	Drug/gene delivery, tissue regeneration [24, 32]
	Copoly(3-hydroxybutyrate-co-3-hydroxyvalerate) (PHBV): good mechanical property.	Used alone or in combination with collagen or gelatin to create wound dressing scaffolds [33, 34]
	Poly (vinyl alcohol) (PVA):	Often used as complex with natural molecules such as gelatine [35]

Normal human skin has a layered architecture, consisting of epidermis, dermis and subcutaneous tissue or subcutis. The epidermis, a non-vascularised epithelium representing the outermost layer of the skin, consists mainly of keratinocytes that are of different structural features. It also contains other cell types including melanocytes and epidermal stem cells that are located in the basal layer of the epidermis. The epidermal stem cells differentiate into keratinocytes that migrate to the surface of the skin to form a protective layer, the stratum corneum. Under the epidermis is the dermis, formed mainly by fibroblasts within connective tissue matrix that is comprised mostly of nano/microfibrous collagens, polysaccharides and water. It also houses other components including vascular, neural and lymphatic systems and its multiple accessories such as appendages. The two layers are separated by an intermediate acellularglycoproteinacous basement membrane layer, which is composed of protein microfilaments containing collagen, integrin, laminin, fibronectin, proteoglycans, and other complex nanometer sized fibrous topographies. The third layer of the skin, the sub-cutis or hypodermis, consists of fatty connective tissue, connecting the dermis to underlying skeletal components. The main cell types and components in different layers of human skin are illustrated in Fig. (**1**).

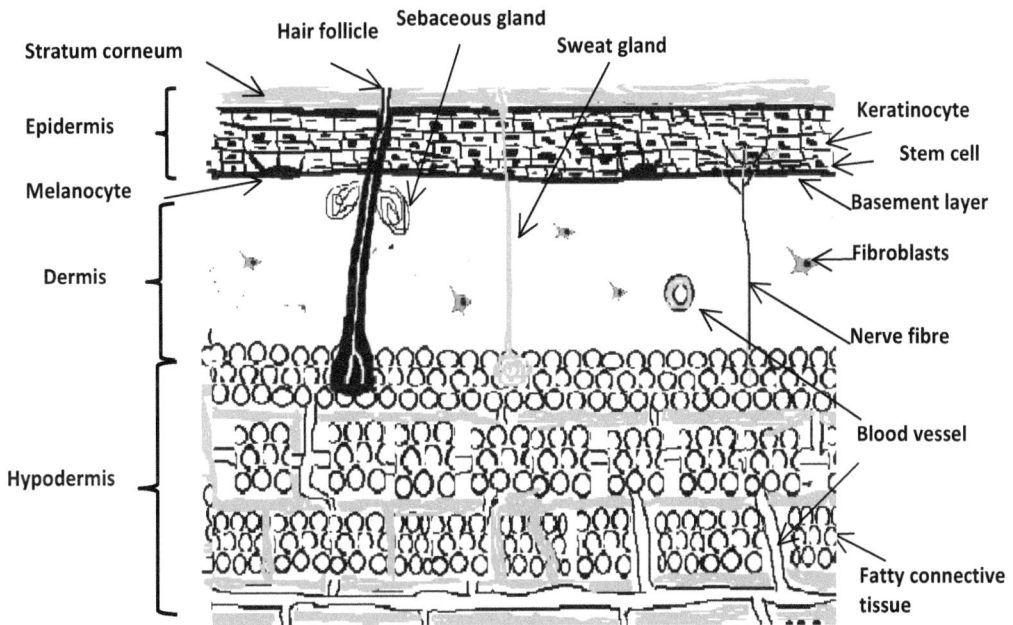

Fig. (1). Schematic illustration of human skin structure. The human skin consists of three layers, epidermis, dermis and subcutaneous tissue or subcutis. Each layer has its own distinct cell types and extracellular components, which provide different functionality.

The obvious function of the skin is to serve as a barrier between the inside of the body and the exterior world. This barrier is best known for its physical structure, consisting of the stratum corneum, cell-cell junctions, and extracellular matrix (ECM) that is a fibrillar network of self-assembled proteins and polysaccharides. The barrier function of the skin also constitutes biochemical components, including immune response mediators, proteins/ enzymes, and lipids [40]. Other functions of the skin include serving as a reservoir for soluble cell signalling molecules that contribute enormously to maintain skin morphogenesis and homeostasis, lipid and water storage, diffusion and absorption of certain compounds (oxygen, water, nitrogen, carbon dioxide, etc.), and thermoregulation through sweat. Therefore the skin is a highly dynamic organ rather than a mere structural barrier.

WOUND AND WOUND HEALING

Being permanently exposed to the external environment, the skin can suffer from different kinds of damages that result in the loss of variable volumes of extracellular matrix. The skin can be impaired not only by physical injuries and pathogen infections, but also as a secondary pathogenesis of some conditions such as diabetic ulcers. Wound healing and its medical complications present a huge burden to health care worldwide.

In normal skin wound healing, the fibroblasts and keratinocytes, at the edge of the wound, proliferate and migrate to restore intact epidermal barrier, and cellular and ECM function of the skin. In addition, the vascular endothelial cells also grow to form new blood vessels for supplying nutrients to the skin [41, 42]. Any factors that hinder the growth of any of these cells would lead to delayed skin regeneration. Fig. (**2**) depicts the normal process of wound healing.

A significant feature of biochemistry in skin wound is the presence of a high level of matrix metalloproteinase (MMP) secreted by fibroblasts, which are stimulated by activated inflammatory cells. MMP can denature the nonviable collagen in wound beds and also break down the viable collagen produced by fibroblasts for new tissue granulation and formation. In addition, fibroblasts in wound could not produce adequate levels of MMP inhibitors [43]. All these together result in the restriction of sufficient formation of matrix needed for cell migration and wound closure [44]. Moreover deep wounds do not heal autologously through regeneration due to lack of dermal tissue.

Wound coverage by autografts is the standard procedure for wound treatment, but its long term effect is controversial. Allografts and xenografts, on the other hand, carry the risk of pathogen transmission and immunological rejection. All these led to the development of skin substitutes. The characteristics of currently available skin substitutes have been reviewed recently by Yildirimer *et al.* [45]. Most synthetic materials currently used for tissue repair can elicit wound contraction, chronic inflammation, and do not integrate well into the host tissue, resulting in repeated tissue injury and eventual removal of implant [46, 47]. Synthetic materials are often resistant to degradation and consequently become encapsulated by a fibrous layer, which could not be replaced by healthy tissue. The toxicity of the chemicals utilized to crosslink the synthetic materials for strengthening their properties and improving their efficacy, is also of a concern.

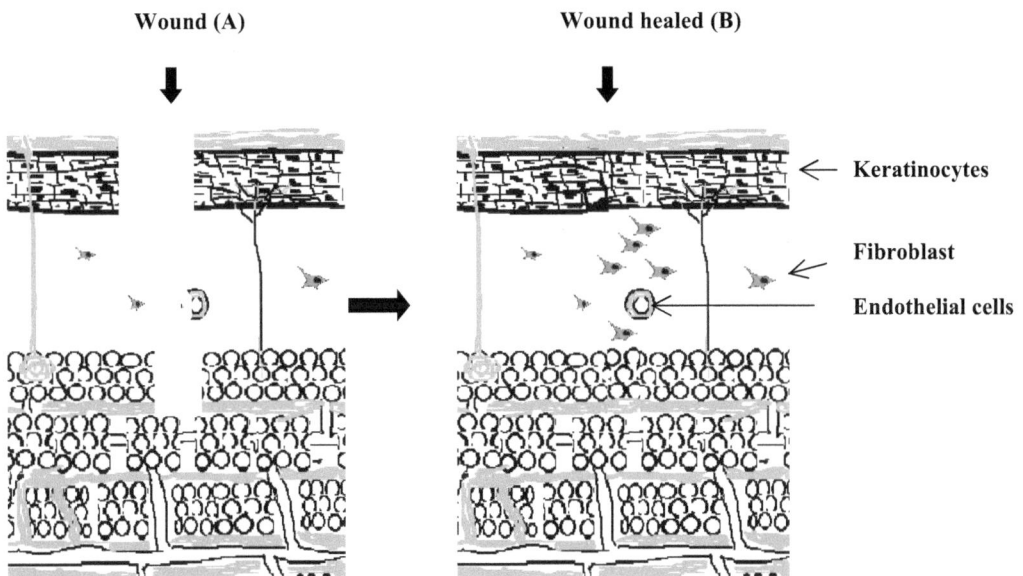

Fig. (2). Normal process of wound healing. In normal skin wound healing, the fibroblasts and keratinocytes at the edge of the wound proliferate and migrate to restore intact epidermal barrier, and cellular and ECM function of the skin. A. Wounded skin; B. Healed skin.

NANOMATERIALS FOR SKIN REGENERATION AND WOUND CARE

The main objective of tissue engineering is to create three-dimensional scaffolds as extracellular matrix (ECM) analogue that can, in combination with living cells and/or bioactive molecules, guide cell adhesion, growth, and differentiation to restore the function and structure of impaired skin. An ideal material for skin tissue regeneration and wound care should be biocompatible with all the cells in the skin, non-allergic, biodegradable at desirable rate, and allow proper nutrient and gas exchange. For incorporation of the bioadhesive character of ECMs, cell-recognizing domains such as integrin binding units Arg-Gly-Asp (RGD), Asp-Gly-Glu-Ala, and Tyr-Ile-Gly-Ser-Arg, or adhesive motif rich proteins, such as collagen, fibronectin, or vitronectin, can be directly grafted onto surface-active scaffold [48-51].

Biomaterials

Over the last few decades a class of materials commonly referred to as biomaterials, has emerged as an alternative to synthetic scaffold materials such as polypropylene. Natural biomaterials have the advantages of low toxicity and low chronic inflammatory response. Some even exhibit bioactivity that makes them readily integrate with the host tissue [27, 52]. These materials can be derived from different sources, such as extracellular matrices of human and animal tissues, plants and other organisms. They are profoundly used over synthetic materials in biomedical applications such as drug carrier, dermal grafts, neural implants, and burn dressings among others. For wound care, biomaterials including polypeptides, hydroxyl apatite, hyaluronic acid, fibronectin, collagen, chitosan and alginates have all been used, in the form of scaffolds, membranes, sponges, hydrogels, and some other alternatives.

The major limitations of the application of biomaterials as scaffold for tissue regeneration are the lack of strength, or enzymatic degradation of the materials before the recipient has fully healed, leading to early implant failure and reoperation. To overcome the shortcomings of synthetic and natural biomaterials as standalone tissue regeneration scaffolds, composites of organic-organic and inorganic-organic nanomaterials have been utilised. Table **3** lists some representative scaffolds developed from nanomaterials for skin regeneration.

Composite PLLA/PAA/Col I&III nanofibrous scaffolds, fabricated by electrospinning, were studied for their potential use as substrate for the differentiation of ADSCs in dermal regeneration [53]. The purpose for inclusion of a novel cell binding moiety PAA was to replace damaged extracellular matrix and to guide new cells directly into the wound bed with enhanced proliferation and overall organisation. The results showed that the cell proliferation was significantly increased in PLLA/PAA/Col I&III scaffolds compared to PLLA and PLLA/PAA nanofibrous scaffolds. The differentiation and morphology of ADSCs were also observed. This work suggested that combination of the epitome PLLA/PAA/Col I&III nanofibrous scaffold with stem cell therapy can induce paracrine signalling effect, therefore promoting faster regeneration of the damaged skin tissues [53].

Table 3.   Novel Organic/Inorganic Nanomaterial Scaffolds for Skin Tissue Engineering

Scaffold Components	Test Model/Reference
Nanofibrous Poly-l-lactic acid/poly(PLA) -(α,β)-dl-aspartic acid/collagen (PLLA/PAA/Col)	Adipose derived stem cells (ADSCs) [53]
Nano/microfibrous chitosan/collagen	3T3 fibroblasts and HaCaT keratinocytes; ex vivo human kin equivalent wound model [54]
Poly(ε-caprolactone) [PCL] and poly(ethyleneglycol) [PEG]	Mice diabetic with dorsal wound; human primary keratinocytes [55]
Nanofibrousindigoferaaspalathoides (IA), Azadirachta indica (AI), Memecylonedule (ME), Myristicaandamanica (MA)/PCL	Human dermal fibroblasts proliferation; adipose derived stem cells differentiation ME/PCL showed the highest effect on cell growth and differentiation [29]
Nanofibrous Chitosan/PVA	Rat burn with a hot brass cylinder in the dorsum skin [56]
Nanofibrous chitosan/PVA	Mouse 3T3 fibroblasts; *in vivo* with growth factor R-Spondin 1 [57]
Amine-functionalized gold nanoparticles and silicon carbide nanowires crosslinked to an acellular porcine tendon	L929 murine fibroblast cells [58]
PHBVNanofiber matrices	*In vitro* with dermal sheath cells and epithelial outer root sheath cells; *in vivo* in athymic nude mice with full thickness skin wound [33]
Gold colloid/chitosan film	Newborn mice keratinocytes [59]

Nano/microfibrous chitosan/collagen scaffold that approximates structural and functional attributes of native extracellular matrix has been developed and studied for applicability in skin tissue engineering [54]. 3T3 fibroblasts and HaCaT keratinocytes cultured on chitosan–collagen-based scaffolds showed superior cellular response in comparison to the ones without collagen. In an *ex vivo* human skin equivalent wound model keratinocyte migration and wound re-epithelization were demonstrated. Chitosan, a glycosaminoglycanlike biodegradable polymer, can promote would healing through hemostasis, antibacterial action, and accelerating collagen synthesis by fibroblasts [60, 61]. The type I collagen, on the other hand, is the major structural and functional protein of dermal matrix that interacts with keratinocytes to promote collagenase production; the collagenase in turn catalyses the disassociation of keratinocytes from collagen rich substrates which is required for keratinocytes migration [44]. However, the use of type I collagen in tissue engineering is restricted mainly due to the fast biodegradation, poor mechanical properties and issues related to contraction *in vivo* [60]. The incorporation of chitosan into collagen-based scaffolds was proposed to overcome these potential limitations, by providing mechanical stability to collagen scaffolds for efficient keratinocyte migration and wound closure [62].

Control infection is critical for chronic wound healing. In this respect nanofibers constructed from chitosan/PVA and chitosan/PLA-co-(D,L-lactide) [63] or chitosan/collagen [64] have all demonstrated a good antibacterial activity against the Gram-positive as well as Gram-negative bacteria. The wound covered with chitosan/PVA nanofibrous scaffolds recovered much rapid compared to untreated wounds as tested in rats that were burn with a hot brass cylinder in the dorsum skin. Moreover, the presence of stem cells on this scaffolds accelerated the wound healing process owing to their ability of collagen regeneration [56].

Amine-terminated block copolymers composed of biodegradable PCL and PEG were electrospun to form biocompatible nanofibers with functional amine groups on the surface *via* PEG linkers. Recombinant human epidermal growth factor (rhEGF) was immobilized on the electrospunnanofibers, which proved superior *in vivo* wound healing activities compared to control groups or EGF solutions as tested in diabetic mice with dorsal wounds. Furthermore, the rhEGF-nanofiber enhanced keratinocytic expression of human primary keratinocytes [55]. Nanofiber membranes composed from poly-N-acetyl-glucosamine (sNAG) and PHBV also proved beneficial for wound healing [33, 63, 65, 66].

In order to improve the mechanic property and durability of collagen matrices fabricated from purified forms of collagen, the extracellular matrix from many tissues of different origins including human dermis, porcine dermis, and porcine small intestine submucosa, are often utilized as scaffold in skin tissue engineering. Deeken *et al.* have looked into the suitability of the nanocomposite of amine-functionalised gold nanoparticles and silicon carbide nanowires crosslinked to an acellular porcine tendon as scaffold. Their work suggested that the crosslinking porcine diaphragm tissues with nanomaterials improved the resistance of the scaffold to enzymatic degradation and appropriate biocompatibility characteristics [58]. Compared with some commercially available scaffolds, utilisation of gold nanoparticles as "crosslinking" agents within biological scaffolds in pig skin wound model has shown some advantages including (1) increased cellular attachment; (2) delay in scaffold degradation; and (3) maintaining a more natural microstructure [67], although further studies are required to optimise the amount of crosslinking agents. It has also been demonstrated that gold colloid/chitosan film scaffold [59] can enhance cell attachment and accelerate proliferation of newborn mice keratinocytes [59].

Silver nanoparticles have antibacterial activity but can cause cell death when applied in wound dressing due to the influence of the surface chemistry. However, at optimal concentration or after coating with biomaterials, silver nanoparticles have been used in developing scaffold for tissue regeneration. Electrospun poly(L-lactic acid)-co-poly(ε-caprolactone) (PLLCL) nanofibres containing silver nanoparticles at 0.25 wt% has been demonstrated to have antibacterial activity with no effect on cell proliferation and morphology, suggesting that the PLLCL-silver scaffold is potentially suitable for skin tissue engineering [68]. Chitin/nanosilver composite scaffolds were found to have antibactericidal activities toward *S. aureus* and *E. coli*, and good blood clotting ability, which is important for wound healing. However, these scaffolds were cytotoxic to mouse fibroblasts under *in vitro* conditions. It is not sure whether this *in vitro* cytotoxicity will affect wound healing response *in vivo* [69].

Like in many other medical research and clinical practice areas, nanotechnology has brought huge opportunities for innovation in regenerative medicine. The last decade has witnessed an emergence of new generation of scaffolds, which are biocompatible, biodegradable and superior in physic-chemical material properties, being added to the pipeline as potential candidate materials for skin regeneration. Further studies of the characteristics that promote healthy wound healing are prominent.

CHARACTERISTICS OF NANOMATERIALS IN TISSUE ENGINEERING

The crucial requirements of scaffold materials in tissue engineering include biocompatibility, controlled porosity, permeability, and comparable physical-chemical properties to the targeted tissue. To promote cell adhesion and growth, the addition of nanotopographies, e.g. the surface roughness to the biomaterial surface improves its bioadhesive properties. The large surface area of nanostructured materials enhances the adsorption of adhesive proteins such as fibronectin and vitronectin, which mediate cell-surface interactions through integrin cell surface receptors [66, 70]. A recent trend in tissue engineering is to develop biomimetic scaffolds that can not only provide 3D structural support for cell to grow and differentiate in a spatially balanced manner, but also can deliver therapeutic agents, growth factors or cytokines required for cell function and tissue regeneration.

Nanofibers are currently one of the most intensively studied materials in biomedical applications, especially as scaffold in skin regeneration [71]. Their nanofibrous structure provides support for cell growth, which has proved attractive as an approach for treating various diseases [72]. In addition, their surface area, volume, and size of the pores all have considerable effect on cell adhesion, growth, and proliferation [71]. As compared with other methods such as phase separation and self-assembly for fiber material fabrication, the electrospinning method has received much attention primarily because it can produce nanofiber through a simple process without expensive or complex instruments [33, 55, 73, 74]. Nanofibres of polylactide, PCL, gelatin, polyamide and PLA/PAA/Col [71] have all been produced as candidate scaffolds for tissue regeneration.

It is worth mentioning that large-scale and highly efficient synthesis of micro- and nano-fiberspolyvinylpyrrolidone (PVP) and PLLA composite fibers with a novel centrifugal jet spinning process has been reported recently. This method allows better control of fiber morphology. Fibers with increased surface roughness and porosity showed a dramatic increase in hydrophilicity and a trend towards higher cell attachment and proliferation [75]. It is envisaged that continuous effort will be investigated in developing and improving methods for better controlled fabrication of different fiber materials for medical applications. Other different scaffold materials and fabrication techniques have been extensively reviewed elsewhere [76].

SAFETY CONCERNS OF SCAFFOLD MATERIALS

The safety of scaffold materials mainly depends on their degradability, compatibility to different types of skin cells and toxicity of molecules released from them. The ultimate goal of developing novel skin alternatives is to improve compatibility, allowing cells to homogenously attach and proliferate while secreting a high amount of natural ECM. After the restoration of skin structure and function the scaffolds have to be degraded. The scaffold should not release any harmful molecules due to degradation. As the use of nanomaterials in novel scaffolds has caused new concerns regarding the possible toxicity of these materials, it is a pressing requirement to address these concerns to allow optimally benefiting from nanotechnology while avoiding any adverse effects.

Toxicity Assessment of Nanomaterials

Chapter 10 in this book written by Dr Ferreira *et al.* focused on evaluating the evidence available so far regarding the compatibility and toxicity of nanomaterials. The nanomaterials used as skin scaffold are generally non-toxic, however the complexity of many formulations, which may contain chemicals used for material surface modification and as cross linking agents, presents a need for a broad spectrum of rigorous tests for toxicity.

Although an impressive number of new nanomaterials offer promises for improved skin regeneration, they have been tested mainly *in vitro* for effects on cell proliferation and differentiation and *in vivo* animal models for wound healing. Their toxicity, compatibility and long term effect in humans remain largely unknown. So far only few nanoengineered scaffolds reached clinical trial, including Silk Sericin Scaffold for wound dressing, Intgra (TM) Flowable Wound Matrix scaffold for cell invasion and capillary growth [77]. As in other areas of nanomedicine, the toxicity of nanomaterials has not been fully defined and more non-clinic and clinical studies are needed to translate nanoscience to the clinic.

The translation of nanoscience into clinic is a complex process. Due to the lack of studies over the long term effect of new scaffolds, it is envisaged that further work will focus on chronic toxicity of new scaffolds [76, 78] with emphasis on nanomaterials. As general consensus on critical parameters and harmonised protocols for assessing the possible adverse effects of nanomedicine have not yet established, it has been suggested that each novel nanoformulation should be tested on a case by case basis [79].

Regulation of Nanomaterials

The need for regulation of nanomaterials safety has been well recognized worldwide over the last decade, largely due to the concern about the nanosize specific effect. In the European Union, a framework involving different regulatory bodies was formed to develop approaches for managing safety issues related to nanomaterials [80]. The European Medicines Agency (EMEA) is actively engaged in assessing whether current regulatory framework and existing guidelines and requirements for medicine regulation are adequate for use in nanomedicine. The EMEA recently published a special report- Next-generation nanomedicines and nanosimilars: EU regulators' initiatives relating to the development and evaluation of nanomedicines. This report focused on the recent EMEA's activities relating to the development and evaluation of nanomedicine products while keeping patient and consumer safety at the forefront [81]. The United States Food and Drug Administration (USFDA) issued a draft guidance on considering whether a product contains nanomaterials (http://www.fda.gov/ScienceResearch/SpecialTopics/Nanotechnology/ucm257926.ht m, assessed on 28 August 2013). After creating an internal database of submitted and approved drugs containing nanoscale materials, the Nanotechnology Risk Assessment Working Group in the Center for Drug Evaluation and Research (CDER) within the USFDA assessed potential risks from administering nanomaterial active pharmaceutical ingredients (API) or nanomaterial excipients by various routes of administration. The group has also assessed the approaches used for Evaluation of Potential Risks from the Use of Nanomaterials in Drug Products [82].

Many other parts of the world are also involved in identifying potential areas where nanomaterials are used and potential risks need to be addressed. There are areas where improvements are needed in order to reach ultimate global consensus on assessment and management of nanotechnology related risk. These include: (1) instrumentation and training in nanomaterial characterisation; (2) modelling of particle size-product performance; (3) exposure monitoring and (4) nanotechnology-related education.

CONCLUSION AND OUTLOOK

The rapid progress of nanotechnology in recent years has led to the advancement in medicine. Tissue engineering scaffolds for skin regeneration is an area of ever-intensifying research due to the lack of products that meet the clinic requirements.

Natural wound healing is a complex process involving interactions between epidermal and dermal cells and ECM. It is desirable to create new scaffolds with properties that can promote the natural wound healing process, to replace damaged ECM and to direct cell migration into the wound area to form healthy organization with a desirable speed. Manipulating materials at the cellular; molecular and atomic levels can provide more controlled and effective approaches in treating sever skin conditions. Coupling engineering scaffolds with cells that has the potential to secrete growth signalling cytokines provides further avenue for seeking effective approach to skin regeneration.

Recent trends in skin regeneration include scaffold functionalisation that is to make the scaffold more bioactive by loading drugs or bioactive molecules; thereby the manifold cellular activities can be better orchestrated during the process of skin remodeling. The new engineering scaffolds are also expected to have tissue-mimicking structures of higher orders suitable for direct implantation into wounds. Moreover, the biocompatibility/toxicity and biodegradability are all important parts of future studies required for evaluation of new scaffolds.

ACKNOWLEDGEMENTS

The authors wish to acknowledge the European Commission for funding the FP7 project NANODRUG(grant number 289454) through the theme Marie Curie Actions-People Programme-Initial Training Network, which offers training opportunity for ambitious early career researchers to embark on the challenging area of advanced biomaterials. This chapter is devoted to the training on nanomaterials for treating skin disorders.

CONFLICT OF INTEREST

The authors confirm that this chapter contents have no conflict of interest.

ABBREVIATIONS

ADSCs = Adipose derived stem cells

AI   = Azadirachtaindica

API   = Active pharmaceuticalingredients

CDER   = Center for Drug Evaluation and Research

Col   = Collagen

ECM   = Extracellular matrix

EGF   = Epidermal growth factor

EMEA   = European Medicines Agency

EU   = EuropeanUnion

GT   = Gelatin

IA   = Indigoferaaspalathoides

MA   = Myristicaandamanica

ME   = Memecylonedulepcl: poly(ε-caprolactone)

MMP   = Matrixmetalloproteinase

PAA   = Poly-(α,β)-dl-aspartic acid

PEG   = Poly(ethylene glycol)

PCL   = Polycaprolactone

PHBV   = Copoly(3-hydroxybutyrate-co-3-hydroxyvalerate)

PLA   =   Poly[(L-lactide)

PLGA   =   Poly(l-lactide-co-glycolide)

PLLCL   =   Poly(L-lactic acid)-co-poly(ε-caprolactone)

PLLA   =   Poly(l-lactic acid

PVA   =   Poly(vinyl alcohol)

PVP   =   Polyvinylpyrrolidone

rhEGF   =   Recombinant human epidermal growth factor

sNAG   =   Poly-N-acetyl-glucosamine

USFDA   =   United States Food and Drug Administration

REFERENCES

[1]   Ansari A, Khan M, Alhoshan M, Aldwayyan A, Alsalhi M, Nanostructured materials: classification, properties, fabrication, characterization and their applications in biomedical sciences. *Nanoparticles: Properties, Classification, Characterization, and Fabrication*, Editors: Aiden E. Kestell and Gabriel T. DeLorey, Nova Science Publishers, Hauppauge, NY, USA, 2010, pp1-78.

[2]   Kreyling WG, Semmler-Behnke M, Chaudhry Q, A complementary definition of nanomaterial. *Nano Today,* 2010, 5, 165-8.

[3]   Jain KK, Advances in use of functionalized carbon nanotubes for drug design and discovery. *Expert Opinion on Drug Discovery,* 2012, 7, 1029-37.

[4]   Kruss S, Hilmer AJ, Zhang J, Reuel NF, Mu B, Strano MS, Carbon nanotubes as optical biomedical sensors. *Adv Drug Deliv Rev,* 2013, 65, 1933.

[5]   Nunes A, Al-Jamal K, Nakajima T, Hariz M, Kostarelos K, Application of carbon nanotubes in neurology: Clinical perspectives and toxicological risks. *Arch Toxicol,* 2012, 86, 1009-20.

[6]   Dellinger A, Zhou Z, Connor J, Madhankumar A, Pamujula S, Sayes CM *et al.,* Application of fullerenes in nanomedicine: An update. *Nanomedicine,* 2013, 8, 1191-208.

[7]   Wujcik EK, Monty CN, Nanotechnology for implantable sensors: Carbon nanotubes and graphene in medicine. *Wiley Interdisciplinary Reviews: Nanomedicine and Nanobiotechnology,* 2013, 5, 233-49.

[8]   Kim D, Jon S, Gold nanoparticles in image-guided cancer therapy. *InorgChimActa,* 2012, 393, 154-64.

[9]   Kumar A, Zhang X, Liang X-, Gold nanoparticles: Emerging paradigm for targeted drug delivery system. *BiotechnolAdv,* 2013, 31, 593-606.

[10]   Rana S, Bajaj A, Mout R, Rotello VM, Monolayer coated gold nanoparticles for delivery applications. *Adv Drug Deliv Rev,* 2012, 64, 200-16.

[11] Nguyen HT, Tran KK, Sun B, Shen H, Activation of inflammasomes by tumor cell death mediated by gold nanoshells. *Biomaterials,* 2012, 33, 2197-205.

[12] Choi WI, Sahu A, Kim YH, Tae G, Photothermal cancer therapy and imaging based on gold nanorods. *Ann Biomed Eng,* 2012, 40, 534-46.

[13] Slowing II, Trewyn BG, Giri S, Lin VS-, Mesoporous silica nanoparticles for drug delivery and biosensing applications. *Advanced Functional Materials,* 2007, 17, 1225-36.

[14] Mai WX, Meng H, Mesoporous silica nanoparticles: A multifunctional nano therapeutic system. *Integrative Biology (United Kingdom),* 2013, 5, 19-28.

[15] Tang L, Cheng J, Nonporous silica nanoparticles for nanomedicine application. *Nano Today,* 2013, 8, 290-312.

[16] Klasen HJ, A historical review of the use of silver in the treatment of burns. II. Renewed interest for silver. *Burns,* 2000, 26, 131-8.

[17] Moritz M, Geszke-Moritz M, The newest achievements in synthesis, immobilization and practical applications of antibacterial nanoparticles. *ChemEng J,* 2013, 228, 596-613.

[18] Laurent S, Forge D, Port M, Roch A, Robic C, Vander Elst L *et al.,* Magnetic iron oxide nanoparticles: Synthesis, stabilization, vectorization, physicochemical characterizations and biological applications. *Chem Rev,* 2008, 108, 2064-110.

[19] Ling D, Hyeon T, Chemical design of biocompatible iron oxide nanoparticles for medical applications. *Small,* 2013, 9, 1450-66.

[20] Sommer WH, Sourbron S, Huppertz A, Ingrisch M, Reiser MF, Zech CJ, Contrast agents as a biological marker in magnetic resonance imaging of the liver: Conventional and new approaches. *Abdom Imaging,* 2012, 37, 164-79.

[21] Na HB, Song IC, Hyeon T, Inorganic nanoparticles for MRI contrast agents. *Adv Mater,* 2009, 21, 2133-48.

[22] Kaur N, Puri R, Jain SK, Drug-cyclodextrin-vesicles dual carrier approach for skin targeting of anti-acne agent. *AAPS PharmSciTech,*2010, 11, 528-37.

[23] Wang G, Epand RF, Mishra B, Lushnikova T, Thomas VC, Bayles KW *et al.,* Decoding the functional roles of cationic side chains of the major antimicrobial region of human cathelicidin LL-37. *Antimicrob Agents Chemother,*2012, 56, 845-56.

[24] Alamein MA, Stephens S, Liu Q, Skabo S, Warnke PH, Mass production of nanofibrous extracellular matrix with controlled 3D morphology for large-scale soft tissue regeneration. *Tissue Engineering - Part C: Methods,*2013, 19, 458-72.

[25] Jayakumar R, Prabaharan M, Nair SV, Tamura H, Novel chitin and chitosan nanofibers in biomedical applications. *BiotechnolAdv,*2010, 28, 142-50.

[26] Muzzarelli RAA, Chitins and chitosans for the repair of wounded skin, nerve, cartilage and bone. *CarbohydrPolym,*2009, 76, 167-82.

[27] Anilkumar TV, Muhamed J, Jose A, Jyothi A, Mohanan PV, Krishnan LK, Advantages of hyaluronic acid as a component of fibrin sheet for care of acute wound. *Biologicals,*2011, 39, 81-8.

[28] Jayakumar R, Prabaharan M, Sudheesh Kumar PT, Nair SV, Tamura H, Biomaterials based on chitin and chitosan in wound dressing applications. *BiotechnolAdv,*2011, 29, 322-37.

[29] Jin G, Prabhakaran MP, Kai D, Annamalai SK, Arunachalam KD, Ramakrishna S, Tissue engineered plant extracts as nanofibrous wound dressing. *Biomaterials,*2013, 34, 724-34.

[30] Chawla JS, Amiji MM, Biodegradable poly(Îμ-caprolactone) nanoparticles for tumor-targeted delivery of tamoxifen. *Int J Pharm,*2002, 249, 127-38.

[31] Huber SC, Marcato PD, Barbosa RM, Duran N, Annichino-Bizzacchi JM, *In vivo* toxicity of enoxaparin encapsulated in mucoadhesive nanoparticles: Topical application in a wound healing model. *Journal of Physics: Conference Series,*2013, 429,.

[32] Jeon SY, Park JS, Yang HN, Woo DG, Park K-, Co-delivery of SOX9 genes and anti-Cbfa-1 siRNA coated onto PLGA nanoparticles for chondrogenesis of human MSCs. *Biomaterials,*2012, 33, 4413-23.

[33] Han I, Shim KJ, Kim JY, Im SU, Sung YK, Kim M *et al.*, Effect of poly(3-hydroxybutyrate-co-3-hydroxyvalerate) nanofiber matrices cocultured with hair follicular epithelial and dermal cells for biological wound dressing. *Artif Organs,*2007, 31, 801-8.

[34] Yuan J, Xing Z, Park S, Geng J, Kang I, Yuan J *et al.*, Fabrication of PHBV/keratin composite nanofibrous mats for biomedical applications. *Macromolecular Research,*2009, 17, 850-5.

[35] Choi SM, Singh D, Kumar A, Oh TH, Cho YW, Han SS, Porous three-dimensional PVA/gelatin sponge for skin tissue engineering. *International Journal of Polymeric Materials and Polymeric Biomaterials,*2013, 62, 384-9.

[36] Burke JF, Yannas OV, Quinby Jr. WC, Bondoc CC, Jung WK, Successful use of a physiologically acceptable artificial skin in the treatment of extensive burn injury. *Ann Surg,*1981, 194, 413-27.

[37] Tobin DJ, Biochemistry of human skin - Our brain on the outside. *ChemSoc Rev,*2006, 35, 52-67.

[38] Kanitakis J, Anatomy, histology and immunohistochemistry of normal human skin. *European Journal of Dermatology,*2002, 12, 390-401.

[39] Saraceno R, Chiricozzi A, Gabellini M, Chimenti S, Emerging applications of nanomedicine in dermatology. *Skin Research and Technology,*2013, 19, e13-9.

[40] Baroli B, Skin absorption and potential toxicity of nanoparticulatenanomaterials. *Journal of Biomedical Nanotechnology,*2010, 6, 485-96.

[41] Artlett CM, Inflammasomes in wound healing and fibrosis. *J Pathol,*2013, 229, 157-67.

[42] Barrientos S, Stojadinovic O, Golinko MS, Brem H, Tomic-Canic M, Growth factors and cytokines in wound healing. *Wound Repair and Regeneration,*2008, 16, 585-601.

[43] Cao Y, Croll TI, Rizzi SC, Shooter GK, Edwards H, Finlayson K *et al.*, A peptidomimetic inhibitor of matrix metalloproteinases containing a tetherable linker group. *Journal of Biomedical Materials Research - Part A,*2011, 96 A, 663-72.

[44] Brett D, A review of collagen and collagen-based wound dressings. *Wounds,*2008, 20, 347-56.

[45] Yildirimer L, Thanh NTK, Seifalian AM, Skin regeneration scaffolds: A multimodal bottom-up approach. *Trends Biotechnol,*2012, 30, 638-48.

[46] Rosch R, Lynen-Jansen P, Junge K, Knops M, Klosterhalfen B, Klinge U *et al.*, Biomaterial-dependent MMP-2 expression in fibroblasts from patients with recurrent incisional hernias. *Hernia,*2006, 10, 125-30.

[47]   Heniford BT, Park A, Ramshaw BJ, Voeller G, Hunter JG, Fitzgibbons Jr. RJ, Laparoscopic Repair of Ventral Hernias: Nine Years' Experience with 850 Consecutive Hernias. *Ann Surg,*2003, 238, 391-400.

[48]   Kim TG, Park TG, Biomimicking extracellular matrix: Cell adhesive RGD peptide modified electrospunpoly(D,L-lactic-co-glycolic acid) nanofiber mesh. *Tissue Eng,* 2006, 12, 221-33.

[49]   Shachar M, Tsur-Gang O, Dvir T, Leor J, Cohen S, The effect of immobilized RGD peptide in alginate scaffolds on cardiac tissue engineering. *ActaBiomaterialia,* 2011, 7, 152-62.

[50]   Ragetly G, Griffon DJ, Chung YS, The effect of type II collagen coating of chitosan fibrous scaffolds on mesenchymal stem cell adhesion and chondrogenesis. *ActaBiomaterialia,* 2010, 6, 3988-97.

[51]   Hansson A, Di Francesco T, Falson F, Rousselle P, Jordan O, Borchard G, Preparation and evaluation of nanoparticles for directed tissue engineering. *Int J Pharm,* 2012, 439, 73-80.

[52]   Nair LS, Laurencin CT, Biodegradable polymers as biomaterials. *Progress in Polymer Science (Oxford),* 2007, 32, 762-98.

[53]   Ravichandran R, Venugopal JR, Sundarrajan S, Mukherjee S, Sridhar R, Ramakrishna S, Composite poly-l-lactic acid/poly-(a,ß)-dl-aspartic acid/collagen nanofibrous scaffolds for dermal tissue regeneration. *Materials Science and Engineering C,* 2012, 32, 1443-51.

[54]   Sarkar SD, Farrugia BL, Dargaville TR, Dhara S, Chitosan-collagen scaffolds with nano/microfibrous architecture for skin tissue engineering. *Journal of Biomedical Materials Research - Part A,* 2013,.

[55]   Choi JS, Leong KW, Yoo HS, *In vivo* wound healing of diabetic ulcers using electrospunnanofibers immobilized with human epidermal growth factor (EGF). *Biomaterials,*2008, 29, 587-96.

[56]   Gholipour-Kanani A, Bahrami SH, Samadi-Kochaksaraie A, Ahmadi-Tafti H, Rabbani S, Kororian A *et al.,* Effect of tissue-engineered chitosan-poly(vinyl alcohol) nanofibrous scaffolds on healing of burn wounds of rat skin. *IET Nanobiotechnology,*2012, 6, 129-35.

[57]   Sundaramurthi D, Vasanthan KS, Kuppan P, Krishnan UM, Sethuraman S, Electrospun nanostructured chitosan-poly(vinyl alcohol) scaffolds: A biomimetic extracellular matrix as dermal substitute. *Biomedical Materials,* 2012, 7.

[58]   Deeken CR, Fox DB, Bachman SL, Ramshaw BJ, Grant SA. Characterization of bionanocomposite scaffolds comprised of amine-functionalized gold nanoparticles and silicon carbide nanowires crosslinked to an acellular porcine tendon. *Journal of Biomedical Materials Research - Part B Applied Biomaterials,*2011, 97 B :334-44.

[59]   Zhang Y, He H, Gao W-, Lu S-, Liu Y, Gu H-, Rapid adhesion and proliferation of keratinocytes on the gold colloid/chitosan film scaffold. *Materials Science and Engineering C,* 2009, 29, 908-12.

[60]   Ma L, Gao C, Mao Z, Zhou J, Shen J, Hu X *et al.,* Collagen/chitosan porous scaffolds with improved biostability for skin tissue engineering. *Biomaterials,*2003, 24, 4833-41.

[61]   Park CJ, Clark SG, Lichtensteiger CA, Jamison RD, Johnson AJW, Accelerated wound closure of pressure ulcers in aged mice by chitosan scaffolds with and without bFGF. *ActaBiomaterialia,*2009, 5, 1926-36.

[62]   Tsai S-, Hsieh C-, Hsieh C-, Wang D-, Huang LL-, Lai J- *et al.*, Preparation and cell compatibility evaluation of chitosan/collagen composite scaffolds using amino acids as crosslinking bridges. *J ApplPolymSci,*2007, 105, 1774-85.

[63]   Ignatova M, Starbova K, Markova N, Manolova N, Rashkov I, Electrospunnano-fibre mats with antibacterial properties from quaternised chitosan and poly(vinyl alcohol). *Carbohydr Res,*2006, 341, 2098-107.

[64]   Wang C-, Su C-, Chen C-, Water absorbing and antibacterial properties of N-isopropyl acrylamide grafted and collagen/chitosan immobilized polypropylene nonwoven fabric and its application on wound healing enhancement. *Journal of Biomedical Materials Research - Part A,*2008, 84, 1006-17.

[65]   Scherer SS, Pietramaggiori G, Matthews J, Perry S, Assmann A, Carothers A *et al.*, Poly-N-Acetyl glucosamine nanofibers: A new bioactive material to enhance diabetic wound healing by cell migration and angiogenesis. *Ann Surg,*2009, 250, 322-30.

[66]   Kubinová S, Syková E, Nanotechnologies in regenerative medicine. *Minimally Invasive Therapy and Allied Technologies,*2010, 19, 144-56.

[67]   Grant SA, Deeken CR, Hamilton SR, Grant DA, Bachman SL, Ramshaw BJ. A comparative study of the remodeling and integration of a novel AuNP-tissue scaffold and commercial tissue scaffolds in a porcine model. *Journal of Biomedical Materials Research - Part A,* 2013. 101, 2778-87.

[68]   Jin G, Prabhakaran MP, Nadappuram BP, Singh G, Kai D, Ramakrishna S, Electrospun poly(L-lactic acid)-co-poly(e-caprolactone) nanofibres containing silver nanoparticles for skin-tissue engineering. *Journal of Biomaterials Science, Polymer Edition,*2012, 23, 2337-52.

[69]   Madhumathi K, Sudheesh Kumar PT, Abhilash S, Sreeja V, Tamura H, Manzoor K *et al.*, Development of novel chitin/nanosilver composite scaffolds for wound dressing applications. *J Mater Sci Mater Med,*2010, 21, 807-13.

[70]   Zhu X, Chen J, Scheideler L, Altebaeumer T, Geis-Gerstorfer J, Kern D, Cellular reactions of osteoblasts to micron- and submicron-scale porous structures of titanium surfaces. *Cells Tissues Organs (Print),*2004, 178, 13-22.

[71]   Širc J, Hobzová R, Kostina N, Munzarová M, Juklíčková M, Lhotka M *et al.*, Morphological characterization of nanofibers: Methods and application in practice. *Journal of Nanomaterials,*2012, 2012, 121

[72]   Fu X, Li H, Mesenchymal stem cells and skin wound repair and regeneration: Possibilities and questions. *Cell Tissue Res,*2009, 335, 317-21.

[73]   Zhang S, Fabrication of novel biomaterials through molecular self-assembly. *Nat Biotechnol,*2003, 21, 1171-8.

[74]   Lo H, Ponticiello M, Leong K, Fabrication of controlled release biodegradable foams by phase separation. *Tissue Eng,*1995, 1, 15-28.

[75]   Ren L, Pandit V, Elkin J, Denman T, Cooper JA, Kotha SP, Large-scale and highly efficient synthesis of micro- and nano-fibers with controlled fiber morphology by centrifugal jet spinning for tissue regeneration. *Nanoscale,*2013, 5, 2337-45.

[76]   Edalat F, Sheu I, Manoucheri S, Khademhosseini A, Material strategies for creating artificial cell-instructive niches. *CurrOpinBiotechnol,*2012, 23, 820-5.

[77] Perán M, García MA, Lopez-Ruiz E, Jiménez G, Marchal JA, How can nanotechnology help to repair the body? Advances in cardiac, skin, bone, cartilage and nerve tissue regeneration. *Materials,*2013, 6, 1333-59.

[78] Misak H, Zacharias N, Song Z, Hwang S, Man K-, Asmatulu R *et al.*, Skin cancer treatment by albumin/5-Fu loaded magnetic nanocomposite spheres in a mouse model. *J Biotechnol,*2013, 164, 130-6.

[79] De Jong WH, Borm PJA, Drug delivery and nanoparticles: Applications and hazards. *International Journal of Nanomedicine,*2008, 3, 133-49.

[80] D'Silva J, Regulatory Aspects of Nanomedicine in Europe. *Pan Stanford Publishing, Singapore,* 2012,.

[81] Ehmann F, Sakai-Kato K, Duncan R, Pérez De La Ossa DH, Pita R, Vidal J- *et al.*, Next-generation nanomedicines and nanosimilars: EU regulators' initiatives relating to the development and evaluation of nanomedicines. *Nanomedicine,*2013, 8, 849-56.

[82] Cruz CN, Tyner KM, Velazquez L, Hyams KC, Jacobs A, Shaw AB *et al.*, CDER risk assessment exercise to evaluate potential risks from the use of nanomaterials in drug products. *AAPS Journal,*2013, 15, 623-8.

CHAPTER 9

Electrospinning: A Versatile Technique for Fabrication and Surface Modification of Nanofibers for Biomedical Applications

Hem Raj Pant[*,1,2] **and Cheol Sang Kim**[2]

[1]*Department of Engineering Science and Humanities, Pulchowk Campus, Institute of Engineering, Tribhuvan University, Kathmandu, Nepal; and* [2]*Bio-nano System Engineering Department, Chonbuk National University, Jeonju 561-756, Republic of Korea*

Abstract: Incorporation of bioactive component around the surface of synthetic polymeric fiber is essential to improve the biocompatibility of scaffold. Core-shell structured nylon-6/lactic acid (LA) nanofibers have been produced *via* single-spinneret electrospinning from the simple blending of LA and nylon-6 solution. The low evaporation rate and plasticizer property of LA was found to be responsible for the formation of point-bonded morphology whereas solvent degradation of nylon-6 with complex phase separation mechanism could give spider-web-like architecture of the mat and core-shell structure of the composite fibers. These fibers were further treated with calcium base to convert surface LA into calcium lactate (CL) which could increase the biocompatibility of composite mat. The SBF incubation test and *in vitro* cell compatibility test showed that CL/nylon-6 composite mat has far better biocompatibility compared to the pristine nylon-6 scaffold. Therefore, the novel nanofibrous composite mat may become a potential candidate for bone tissue engineering.

Keywords: Calcium lactate, calcium phosphate, core-shell fibers, electrospinning, lactic acid, mineralization, nano-nets, nylon-6, tissue scaffold.

INTRODUCTION

The fibrous component of the extracellular matrix (ECM) in the tissue is made up of protein fibers (collagens, elastin, keratin, fibronectin, *etc.*) which provide structural support to tissues and regulate many aspects of cell behavior. ECM fibers provide structural support and mechanical integrity to tissues as well as locations for cell adhesion and regulation of cell functions such as proliferation,

*Corresponding Author Hem Raj Pant: Department of Engineering Science and Humanities, Pulchowk Campus, Institute of Engineering, Tribhuvan University, Kathmandu, Nepal;
Tel: 97715543072; Fax: 97715543072; E-mail: hempant2002@yahoo.com

shape, migration, and differentiation [1]. Structural fibrous proteins can also act as storage locations for the release of small bioactive peptides and growth factors upon release by proteolytic cleavage. Remodeling of tissue involves an initial assembly of protein fibers with cells. Therefore, tissue engineering strategies utilizing fibrous components attempt to fill the role of fibrous components in natural tissue. Artificial fibrous components called scaffolds can impart mechanical strength, structure for cell attachment, and act as reservoirs for biomolecule delivery in much the same way as the natural fibrous components of the ECM. Therefore, functional nanofibers fabrication technology has great potentiality in tissue engineering.

Electrospinning, also known as electrostatic spinning, is a versatile technique which allows fabricating micro- and nanoscale fibers from polymer solutions or melts using an electrically forced fluid jet (Fig. **1a**) [2, 3]. Electrospinning is considered as a variant of the electrostatic spraying process (*i.e.* the behavior of electrically driven liquid jets) [4]. It involves the use of a high voltage to induce the formation of a liquid jet where nanofibers are formed from a liquid polymer that is feed through a capillary tube into a region of high electric field (Fig. **1a**). The electric field is commonly generated by connecting a high voltage power source in the kilovolt range to capillary tip. When electrostatic forces overcome the surface tension of the liquid, a Taylor cone is formed and a thin jet is rapidly accelerated to a grounded or oppositely charged collecting target [5]. Due to the instabilities in this jet, violent whipping motion that elongate and thin the jet allowing the evaporation of solvent to form solid nanofibers on the target site (Fig. **1b**). The size and structure of electrospun fibers can be controlled by several process/materials parameters such as solution viscosity, surface tension, applied voltage, feed rate, solution conductivity, working distance, orifice size, and physicochemical properties of used materials (type of polymer, ratio of different components in blend) [6, 7]. Different types of species (ions, molecules, particles) can be easily incorporated during the electrospinning fabrication process to produce functionalized nanofibers [8]. Electrospun fibers are collected as nonwoven membranes with randomly or aligned arranged structures.

Electrospun polymer nanofibers are excellent structures for the design of tissue engineering scaffolds because of the wide variety of biocompatible polymer

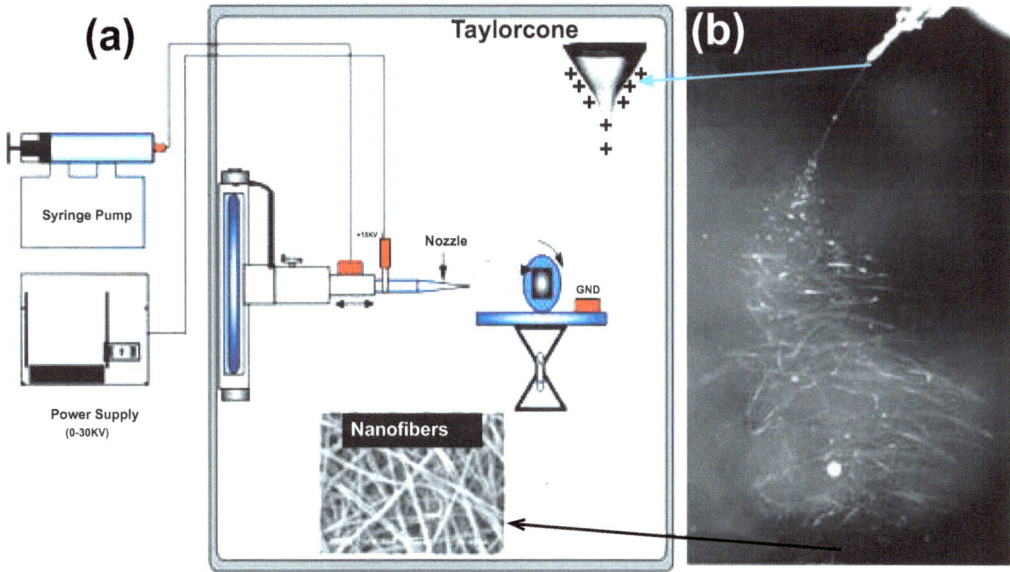

Fig. (1). Simple electrospinning system (**a**) with Taylor cone and nanofibrous mat and photograph of whipping of jet during electrospinning (**b**).

materials that can be formed into nanofibrous structures. Different types of biocompatible polymers demonstrate a variety of mechanical properties, degradation rates, and cell-material interactions, and new types of polymers are continuously being synthesized. Moreover, polymeric nanofibers of required physicochemical properties can be easily fabricated from the blend of two or more than two polymers, or polymer with other species (monomers, oligomer, ceramics, metals, drugs, genes, *etc*.). Functional polymer nanofibers can be fabricated entirely from materials found in the ECM, and a variety of biomolecules can be incorporated into polymer nanofibers during the fabrication process or by using post processing surface modification techniques.

Compared to natural polymers, synthetic polymers are cheap and can be easily fabricated into nanofibers using electrospinning. The mechanical property of electrospun synthetic polymeric fibers is also far better than that of natural polymers. However, they have low biocompatibility. Therefore, the functionalization of synthetic polymer by bioactive components is one of the suitable ways to fabricate cost effective tissue scaffold with proper mechanical strength. Generally, bone tissue scaffold needs strong mechanical properties, and nanofibrous membrane of natural polymer may not be suitable for this application. In many bone tissue engineering strategies a fibrous mesh is used as a template for subsequent mineralization in a similar way to collagen fibers in natural remodeling. The fabricated matrix forms a bonelike structure and provides an attractive microenvironment for osteogenic function in resident cells. Therefore, selection of synthetic polymer which is similar to collagen in some aspect with some incorporated functionalities required to mineralization is potential in bone tissue engineering [9, 10].

Nylon-6 shows structural and molecular similarity to the natural collagen of human bone and has good mechanical properties and nontoxicity [11, 12]. It is highly spinable in a wide range of process parameters. Moreover, two distinct types of fibers in the same mat which differs in fiber diameter by one order of magnitude (in the form of spider-web-like nano-nets) have been produced in nylon-6 electrospun mats by varying process/materials parameters [13-16]. Such spider-web-like structure could increase the effective surface area of the scaffold and promote the cell interaction. However, low hydrophilicity, brittleness, and low degradation rate of nylon-6 fibers hinder its application in bone tissue engineering. Moreover, lack of proper functionalities on nylon-6 matrix for bone regeneration hinders its application in this field. Therefore, modification of nylon-6 fibers using plasticizer bioactive component containing calcium ions, without distributing the internal structure of fiber, is essential for this application. In this chapter, we discuss our strategy of fabricating core-shell structured nylon-6 spider-web-like composite fibers using single nozzle system (core-shell structured fibers are fabricated using co-axial nozzle) in which bioactive acidic organic material such as lactic acid (LA) forms shell of the fibers which can be subsequently converted into calcium lactate (CL) by neutralization with calcium base. This simple technique not only provides a local reservoir of calcium ions on the surface of fibers for the stable nucleation sites to rapid crystal growth but also prevents from the disturbing of internal structure of polymer fibers.

FABRICATION OF LA/NYLON-6 COMPOSITE FIBERS

Nylon-6 (medium molecular weight, KN120 grade, Kolon, Korea) and lactic acid monomer (Showa, Japan) were used for this propose. Formic acid and acetic acid (analytical grade, Showa, Japan) in 4:1 ratio by weight were used as solvents. All the materials were used as obtained. A pristine nylon-6 fiber was electrospun from a 22 wt% solution. Different fibrous hybrid mats of LA/nylon-6 were prepared by mixing different amounts (1, 2, 5, and 10 gm) of LA monomer in 25 gm of 22 wt% nylon-6 solution. The electrospun mats were named M1, M2, M3, M4, and M5 to indicate the 0, 1, 2, 5, and 10 g LA containing nylon-6 mats, respectively. Electrospinning process was carried out at 18 kV electric voltage and 18 cm working distance. After vacuum dried for 24 h, the fiber mats were used for further analysis.

FE-SEM images of different electrospun mats taken by Hitachi S-7400 (Japan) field-emission scanning electron microscope (FE-SEM) are shown in Fig. (**2**). For pristine nylon-6 electrospun mat (Fig. **2a**), the fibers appear well-defined without any interconnection among the fibers. Furthermore, the presence of sub-nanofiber (spider-web- like structure) was hardly seen in the pristine nylon-6 fibers. The hybrid mats containing different amounts of LA showed some changes in fibrous morphology (Fig. **2b-d**). As the concentration of LA was increased, a slightly fused morphology (connection of fibers) was noticeable, and became even more apparent at an amount of 5 gm (M4 mat). This trend in morphology can be understood by considering that it becomes increasingly difficult for the electrospun material to completely dry before it hits the collector due to the presence of hardly volatile LA.

Attempts to electrospin nylon-6 solution at 10 gm of LA with 25 gm of 22 wt% nylon-6 resulted the film like (inset of Fig. **2d**) structure (became electrospray). The adhesive property of LA could provide the connection of two fibers at the points where they were crossing with each other (Fig. **2d**). Three different types of bonding structures named as segmented, agglomerated, and point-bonded have been identified in nonwoven fibers. Here, we found the point-bonded fiber structure caused by LA during electrospinning. Point-bonded structures represent the optimum utilization of the bonding element for reinforcement of the nonwoven fabric. The average fiber diameter of pristine nylon-6 and different hybrid mats is given in Table **1**. Our TEM observation showed that blending of LA with nylon-6 not only form point-bonded fibrous structure but also form core-shell structured fibers in which LA and nylon-6 may form shell and core of the fiber, respectively.

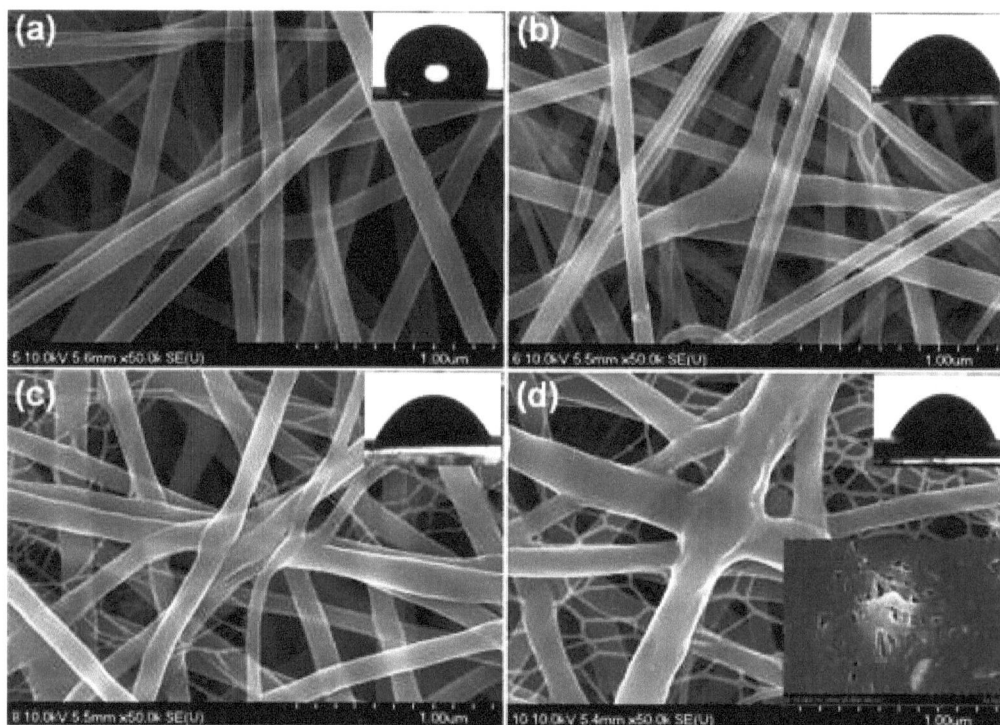

Fig. (2). FE-SEM images of M1 (**a**), M2 (**b**), M3 (**c**), and M4 (**d**) mats (upper insets are their corresponding water contact angle whereas lower inset of d is FE-SEM image of nylon-6 mat obtained from 10 g LA containing nylon-6 solution).

Table 1. Fiber diameter, tensile strength, water contact angle (at 1 s), and appearance of water droplet in different mats

Different Mats	Average Fiber Diameter (nm)		Average Tensile Strength (MPa)	Average Contact Angle (Degree)
	Thick	Thin		
M1	105	-	7.92	112.8
M2	128	-	8.46	58.8
M3	162	14	9.3	51
M4	238	16	12.34	47.6

It is well known that the nature of polymer and parameters of the polymer solution, such as molecular weight, charge density, viscosity, surface tension, conductivity, solvent evaporation rate are critical factors that affect the electrospun fiber morphology [6]. We reported that nylon-6 undergoes solvent degradation in formic acid which can produce a number of low molecular weight charged species [17, 18]. Solvent degradation might be further accelerated on the addition of LA as it decreases the viscosity of nylon-6 solution. The possible mechanism for the formation of point-bonded fibers in the form of core-shell like structure with spider-wave-like architecture can be explained with a very complex phase separation process of hybrid polymer solution during whipping of the jet (Fig. **3**). Phase inversion is based on the principle that a homogeneous multi-component system, under certain condition such as high electrical field (in this case), becomes thermodynamically unstable and tends to separate into different phases in order to lower the system free energy [19]. To understand the mechanism of formation of the core-shell fibers, it can consider that kinetic factor is more important than thermodynamic factor. Kinetically, to form phase separated core-shell structures, the molecules should have enough mobility to overcome the viscous fraction of the mixture to complete the coalescence process of phase separation prior to solidification. Solvent degraded nylon-6 molecules and LA with high mobility (low molecular weight and viscosity) will migrate to wall during the jet whipping. On the other hand, the increased charged density of solvent degraded fraction of nylon-6 not only contributes to an electric-field-induced shell-orientation [19] of LA but also forms subsidiary jets to form true (thin) nanofibers in the form of spider-web-like structure. As shown in Fig. (**3**), the partial separation of homogeneously mixed LA and nylon-6 solution should be started from Taylor cone and stable jet region, and becomes more pronounced during vibrating and whipping of the jet. During jet whipping, LA and solvent-degraded nylon-6 solution with low viscosity and high charge density forms a surface layer whereas non-degraded nylon-6 forms the core of the jet. To verify our hypothesis of increased charge density at surface compared to the core of the jet, we performed computer simulation using COMSOL® multi physics add on AD/DC module to investigate the electrical charge density of different electrospinning solution systems (pure nylon-6 and LA/nylon-6 system) during jet formation. To investigate the charge density of jet (in each system), we assumed that the jet diameter was 0.1 mm and its length was10 mm as shown in Fig. (**4**) where the jet can be considered as three layers (top, middle, and bottom) in order to know the distribution of electrical charge density during phase separation to generate core-shell nanofibers. The boundary conditions for computer simulation are given in Table **2**.

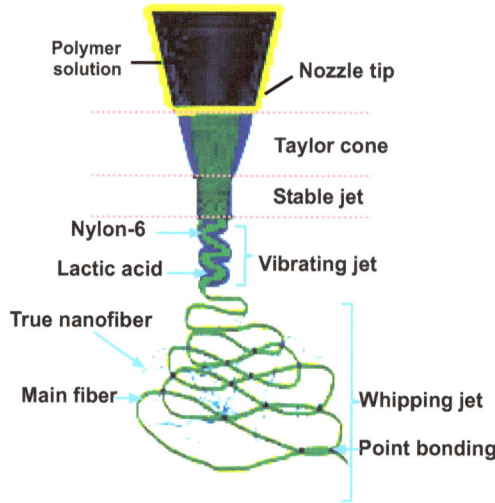

Fig. (3). Schematic representation for the formation of the core–shell structured nylon-6-lactic acid fibers with spider-wave-like architecture.

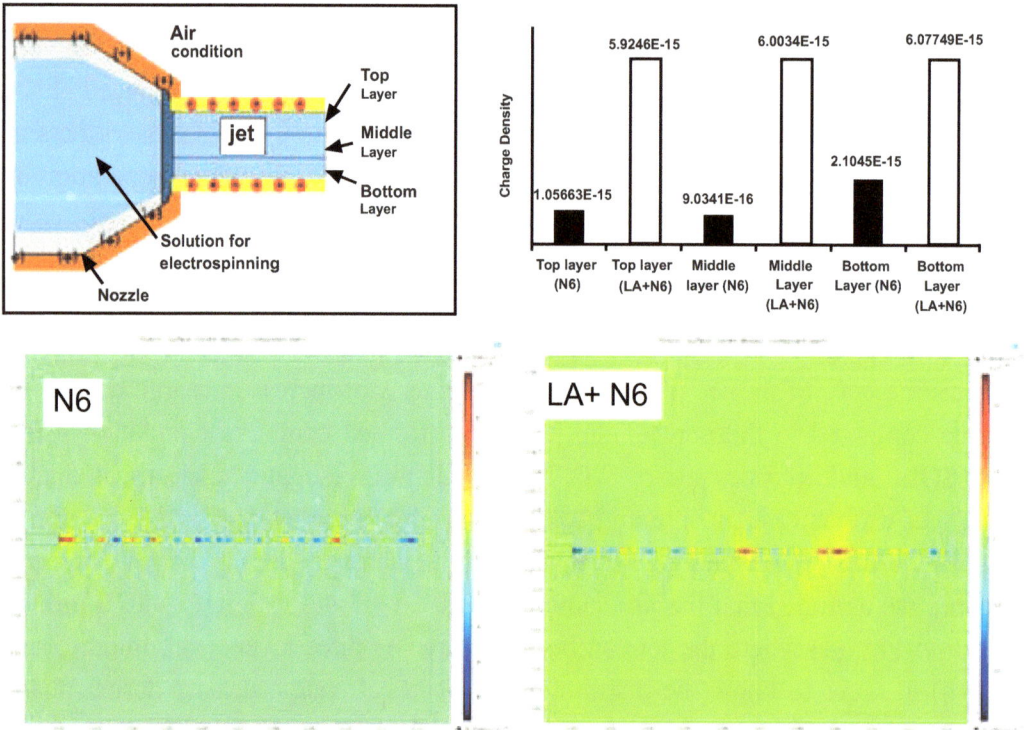

Fig. (4). Schematic diagram for phase separation and charge distribution during jet whipping for computer simulation (left upper portion), charge density graph obtained from simulation result (right upper portion), and contour graph (bottom row) for pure nylon-6 and LA/nylon-6 system.

Table 2.   Boundary Condition for Simulation

Input power magnitude	18kV
Permittivity	N6: 3.5 F/m, LA: 5.4 F/m
Needle material	Aluminum
Distance between nozzle tip and collector	20mm
Nozzle inner diameter and length	0.3mm, 10mm
Jet diameter and length	0.1mm, 10mm
Condition of electrospinning system	Air condition (permittivity: 1 F/m)

The simulation results obtained from contour graph (bottom row of Fig. **4**) are shown in Table **3** and also expressed by graph (upper right of Fig. **4**). The result indicates that the charge density of LA containing nylon-6 portion (outer layer) is higher than that of pure nylon-6 (middle layer) and support our hypothesis of core-shell and spider-wave-like structure formation mechanism.

Table 3.   The Simulation Results

Position of Materials	Magnitude of Charge Density
N6 (in the top layer)	1.0863E-15
N6 (in the middle layer)	9.0341E-16
N6 (in the bottom layer)	2.1048E-15
N6+LA (in the top layer)	5.9246E-15
N6+LA (in the middle layer)	6.0034E-15
N6+LA (in the bottom layer)	6.0779E-15

Further validation of this mechanism was carried out with the help of TEM analysis of the fibers. Fig. (**5**) shows the TEM images of electrospun fibers of nylon-6 containing different amounts of LA (0, 1, 2, and 5 g). Fig. (**5a, b**) shows that there is no phase separation on the fiber. However, Fig. (**5c, d**) clearly shows that the nanofibers consist of core-shell morphology in which LA and nylon-6 may form shell and core of the fiber, respectively. It is clearly seen from TEM images that the shell thickness is increased with the amount of LA. This result obtained from TEM images led the authors to the assumptions that the major constituent at the surface of fiber was LA and degraded portion of nylon-6, while the major constituent of the core of fiber was nylon-6. It was further supported by the TEM image of water extracted and heat treated composite (M4) fibers (Fig. **5e, f**). Fig. (**5e**) shows that most of the surface layer (made of LA) was washed away during one weak water extraction. Similarly, TEM image of heat treated (at 80 °C) fiber showed that surface LA melted during heating and agglomerated as beads on the lower surface of fiber. Existence of drop like beads on the surface of fibers without disturbing the core revealed that most of LA was present on the surface of fiber (Fig. **5f**). The formation of outer LA layer around the nylon-6 fibers and its plasticizer effect were also observed from the photograph and FE-SEM images of pristine and composite mats as given in Figs. (**6 & 7**), respectively. As shown in Fig. (**6**), composite mat (M4) collected on the surface of polyethylene sheet exhibited significant dimensional change (shrunk of its original size) while pristine nylon-6 (M1 mat) retained its original size after vacuum drying (Fig. **6b**). Furthermore, heat treatment of composite mat at 80 °C for 30 minutes showed that almost all LA was melted and point-bonding structure was destroyed without changing the other morphological features of the fibers (Fig. **7b**). This observation confirmed that almost all LA might be present on the surface of nylon-6 fiber which was melted out upon heat treatment. Therefore, surface of LA removed nylon-6 fiber became smoother compared to the unheated one. Furthermore, XPS wide energy survey scans can be performed to determine the composition of elements present on the surface of fibers. Since presence of LA on the surface of nylon-6 could decrease the concentration of nitrogen (of nylon-6) present in the outer molecular layers, the surface coverage of nylon-6 on its composite fiber can be evaluated from the [N]/[C] ratio (Fig. **8**). It was observed (from Fig. **8**) that the ratio of [N]/[C] on the surface of fibers decreased with increasing LA which also supported that most of the LA presents on the surface of fibers. Moreover, etching ion gun was carried out to clean the specimen surface for different time intervals (0, 5, and 20 min) and XPS of etched samples, water treated and heat treated samples was evaluated. Fig. (**9**) shows that the intensity of Ns1 peak of M4 mat increases with etching/heat treatment/water treatment which further supports that most of the LA presents on the surface of fibers. Therefore, all the results showed that single nozzle electrospinning not only constitutes a convenient route to polymer nanofibers, but also provides a single-step avenue by which to achieve field-driven surface enrichment of lower molecular weight species on the fiber surface for advanced textile designs.

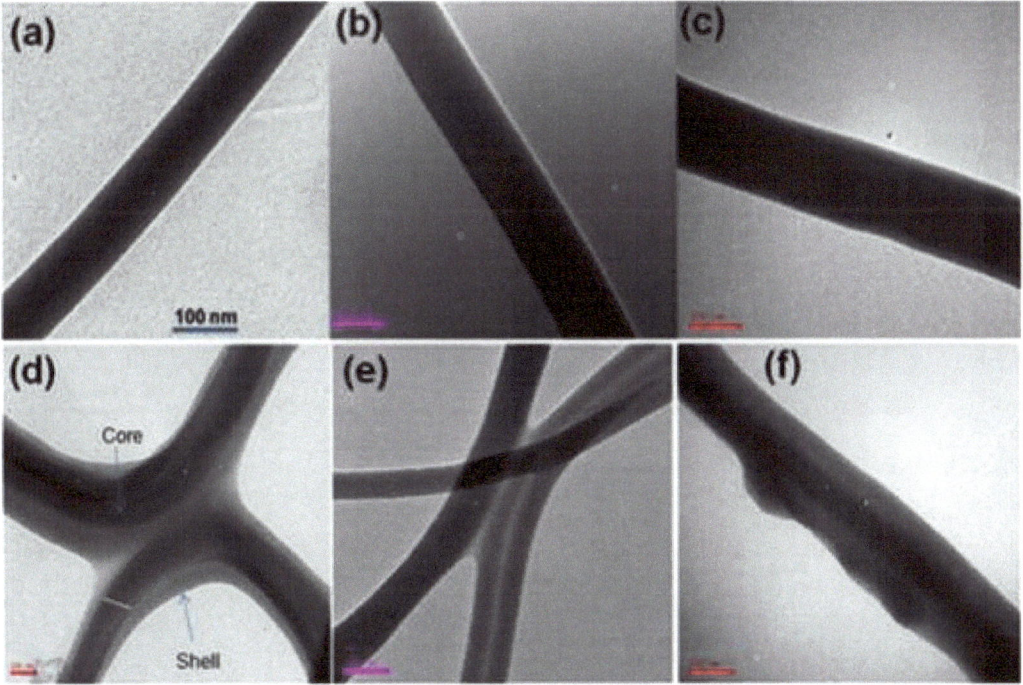

Fig. (5). TEM images of M1 (**a**), M2 (**b**), M3 (**c**), and M4 (**d**) fiber whereas (**e**) and (**f**) are the TEM images of water extracted and heat treated (at 80 °C) fibers, respectively.

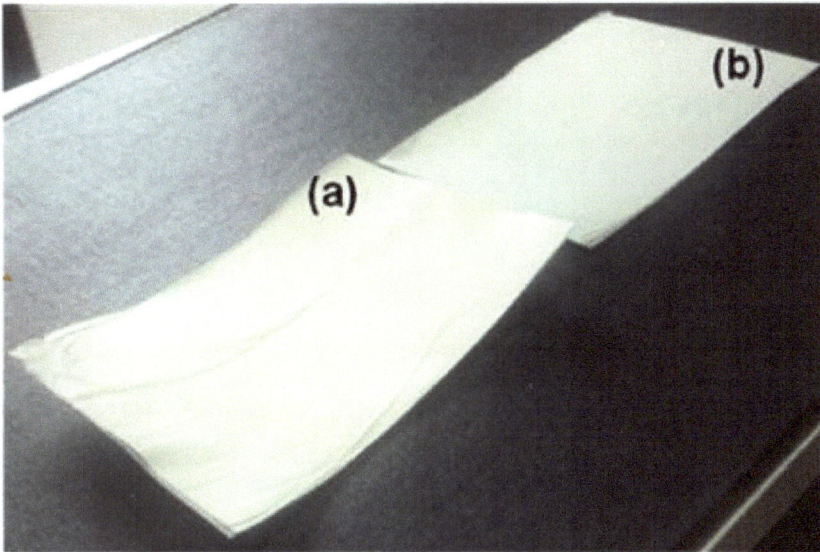

Fig. (6). Photographs of LA/nylon-6 composite (M4) mat (**a**) and pristine nylon-6 (M1) mats (**b**) after vacuum drying.

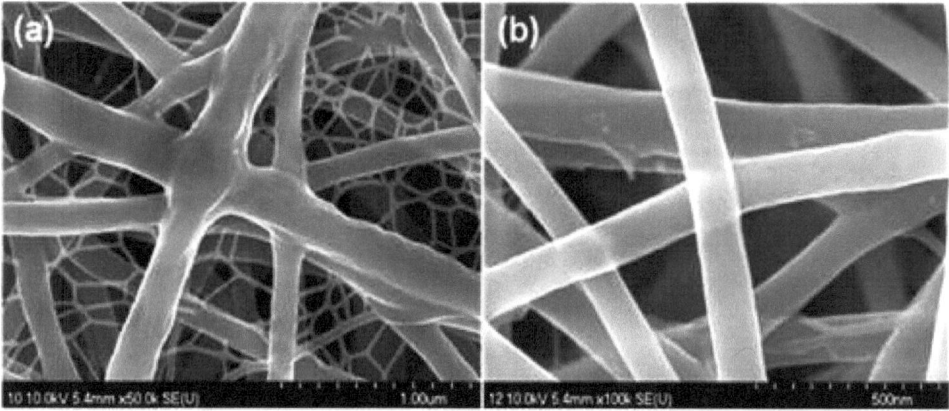

Fig. (7). FE-EM images of LA/nylon-6 composite (M4) fibers before (**a**) and after (**b**) heat treated at 80 °C for 30 minutes.

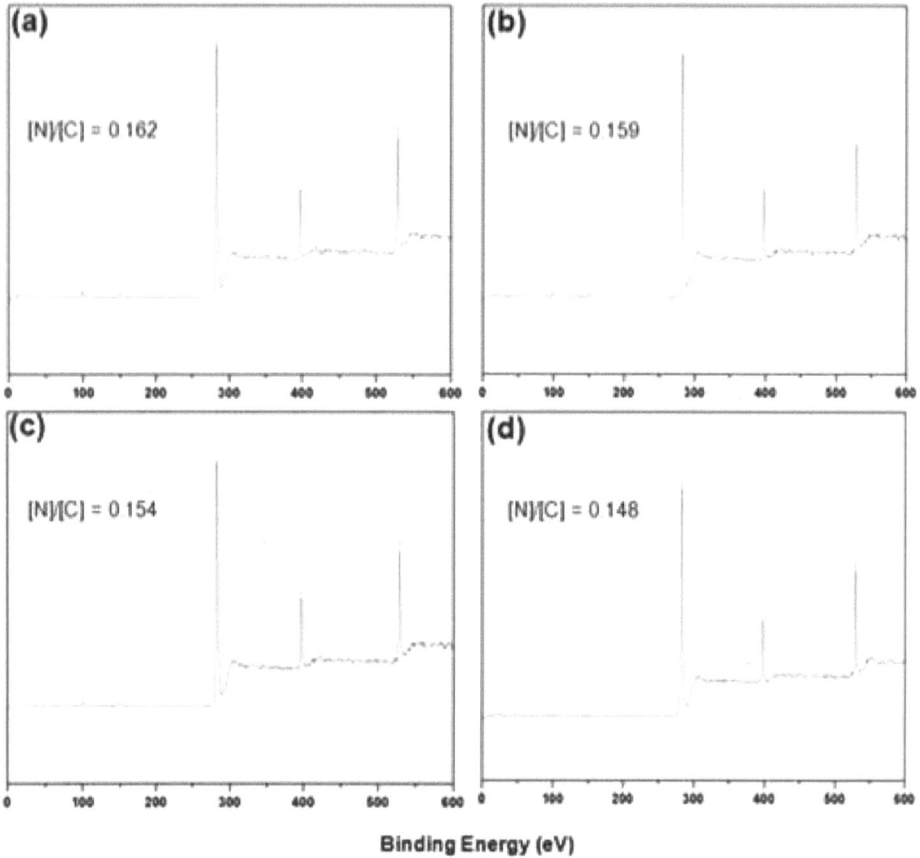

Fig. (8). XPS wide scan of nylon-6 mats containing M1 (**a**), M2 (**b**), M3 (**c**), and M4 (**d**) mats.

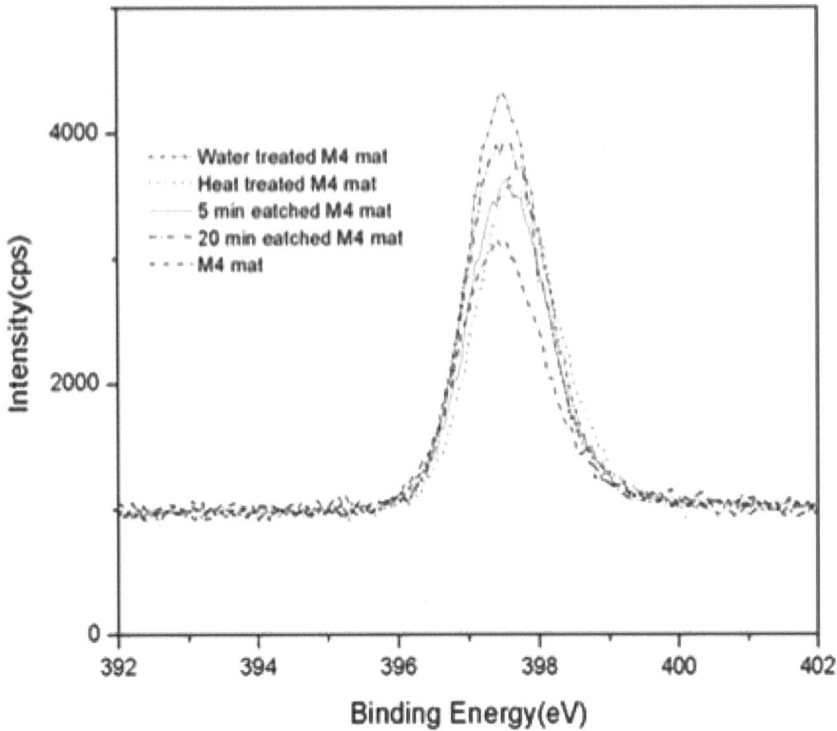

Fig. (9). XPS N1s spectra of M4 mat at different conditions.

An analysis of these hybrid mats on the molecular level showed even more dramatic changes as the amounts of LA were increased in blend solution. Information about the phase and crystallinity was obtained by using a X-ray diffractometer (XRD, Rigaku, Japan) with Cu Kα (λ = 1.54 Å) radiation over the Bragg angle ranging from 10 to 80°. Fig. (**10**) shows X-ray profiles of nylon-6 electrospun mats with different amounts of LA. It was reported that solvent cast films of nylon-6 consist primarily of the α-form, and electrospinning fibers consists mainly of the γ-form [20]. The observation of X-ray profile (Fig. **10**) clearly shows that, as the amounts of LA increase into the blending solution, the crystal structure of nylon-6 gradually transforms from γ to α-form, as seen in the clear (200) reflection at 2θ = 21.4° (γ-form) splitting into the (200) (α) and (002) (α)/(202) (α) reflections at 2θ = 20.3 and 23.5°, respectively [21]. To confirm the observed changes from X-ray profile, we performed vibrational spectroscopy, which is more sensitive to the molecular conformation of polymers [22]. It also showed similar trends to those of the X-ray profiles. The Raman spectra of different mats taken by FT- Raman spectroscopy (RFS-100S, Bruker, Germany) (Fig. **11**) showed the effect of LA on the crystalline structure of nylon-6 electrospun mats. As the amount of LA increases, the C-C stretching bands at conformation found in the α-form gradually increase in the intensity relative to the 1076 cm^{-1} band, indicative of the gauche C-C conformation typically found in the γ-form [20]. Three primary peaks at 1065, 1080, and 1130 cm^{-1} are for C-C stretching region [23]. The 1065 and 1130 cm^{-1} peaks are indicative of an all-trans C-C backbone conformation while the 1080 cm^{-1} peak is attributed to the presence of gauche bonds [23]. The linear increase in the intensity of the band at 1130 cm^{-1} (trans conformation) with the increasing amounts of LA, as compared to the band at 1080 cm^{-1} (gauche conformation) indicates to the transformation of nylon-6 from γ to α-form. It was further conformed by the significant appearance of the bands at 1280-1310 and 1440-1490 cm^{-1} attributed to the trans amide. Fourier transform infrared (FT-IR) spectra of mats were directly recorded by using an ABB Bomen MB100 Spectrometer (Bomen, Canada). Our FT-IR spectra (Fig. **12**) reveal a similar pattern to the XRD and Raman spectra. Fig. (**12**) shows the smooth increase in the CO-NH bending mode at 930 cm^{-1} (characteristic of the α-form) relative to the CO-NH bending mode at 977 cm^{-1} (characteristic of the γ-form) with the increasing amounts of LA also confirms this polymorphic behavior [24]. The bands at 930, 1040, and 1200 cm^{-1} become sharper and stronger with the increasing amounts of LA further indicated the transformation from γ to α-phase in the hybrid mat [25]. The band at 692 cm^{-1} (amide V(α)) becomes sharper and stronger, whereas the band at 712 cm^{-1} (amide V(γ)) shows no increase in the intensity further conformed the transformation from γ to α-phase [6]. Furthermore, the decrease in crystallinity with the amounts of LA in hybrid mat was also observed. The band at 1124 cm^{-1}, represents the amorphous phase which was found to be increased with LA amounts, indicated the decrease in crystallinity [25]. This result was further supported by XRD pattern in Fig. (**10**) which shows that the intensity of peak is going to be decreased with LA amounts.

Polymer crystallization chain conformation in nylon-6 *via* the addition of LA during electrospinning using above characterization technique (XRD, FT-IR and Raman) clearly showed the modification of nylon-6 in molecular level. The

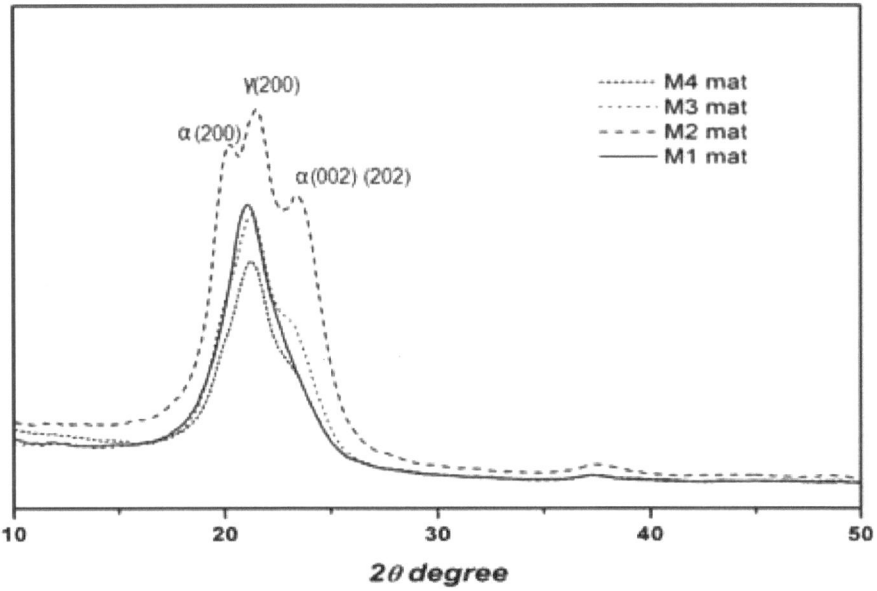

Fig. (10). X-ray profiles of nylon-6 mat containing different amounts of LA.

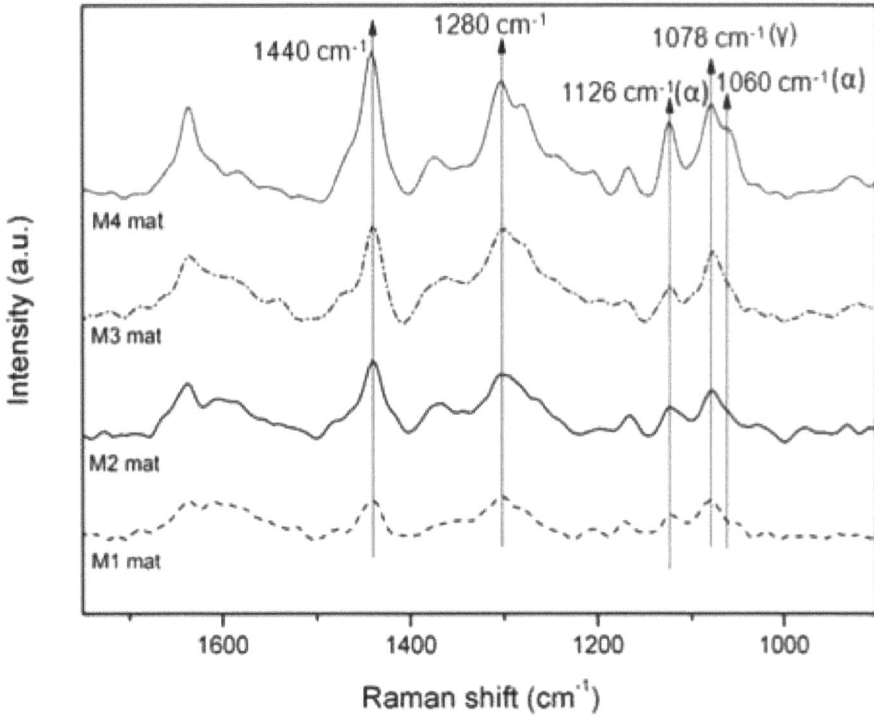

Fig. (11). Raman spectra of nylon-6 fibers containing different amounts of LA.

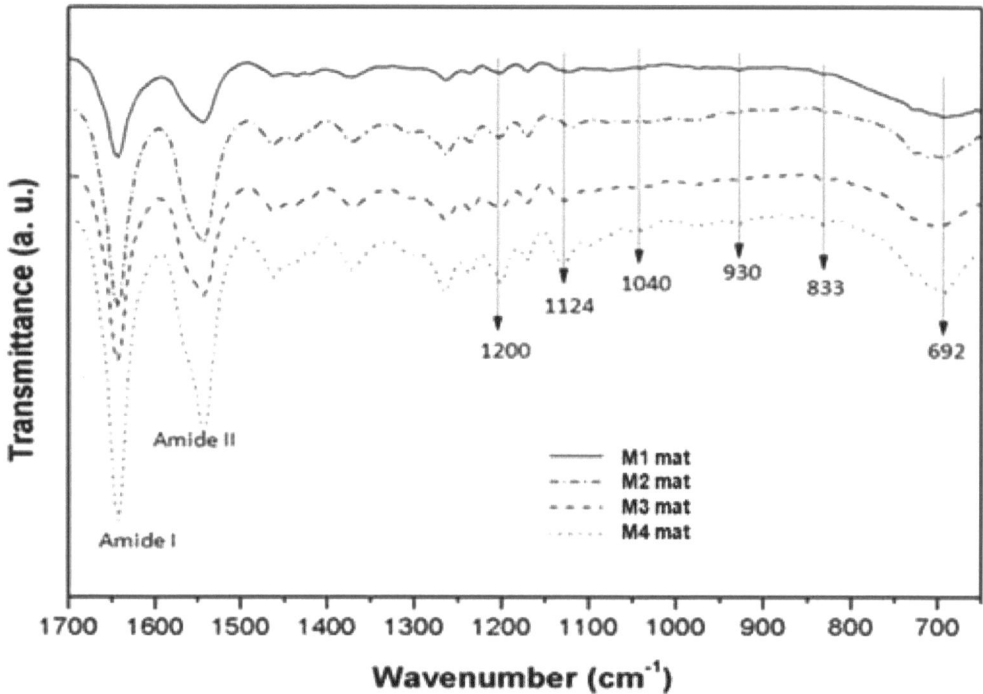

Fig. (12). FT-IR spectra of nylon-6 fibers containing different amounts of LA.

transformation of γ to α-form, with more effective hydrogen bond, makes nylon-6 fibrous mat thermodynamically more stable. The chain conformation (secondary structure) of biocompatible polymers, which are generally the materials of choice for biomedical applications, directly impacts their physiochemical as well as biological functions. Our results of an investigation of the effect of LA on the chain conformation of electrospun nylon-6 mat can offer a simple model for the protein-based polymers because their backbone structure is similar to the amino acid sequences found in polypeptides [23].

It is well known that the wettability and crystallinity of nylon-6 hinders its application for tissue scaffold. We found that the presence of LA could significantly increase the hydrophilicity of nylon-6 hybrid mat by means of simple blending. The wettability of the electrospun mats was measured with deionized water contact angle measurements using a contact angle meter (GBX, Digidrop, France). Deionized water was automatically dropped (drop diameter 6 μm) onto the mat (inset of Fig. **2**). Table **1** shows the average water contact angle (at 1 sec) of M1 mat (112.8°), M2 (58.8°), M3 (51°) and M4 (47.6°) mats. From this, it is clear that the good distribution of LA throughout the hybrid mat can sufficiently increase the hydrophilicity of nylon-6 mats. Therefore, this modified nylon-6 hybrid mat obtained by electrospinning may become a potential material for biomedical applications. Furthermore, LA, an important constituent of the living organism, is highly used in different biological systems and has no any toxicity. Therefore, the presence of LA in nylon-6 provides the positive impact in each and every aspect for making nylon-6 more biocompatible.

Along with these different proper modifications of nylon-6 mat, we further observed the effect of LA on the mechanical properties of hybrid nylon-6 mats. Using an Instron mechanical tester (LLOYD instruments, LR5K plus, UK) in tensile mode, the mechanical properties of the as-spun mats were measured. The specimen thicknesses were measured using a digital micrometer with a precision of 1 μm. The extension rate was 10 mm/min at room temperature and five specimens with dimensions of 3.5 mm and 940 mm (width and length) were tested and averaged for each fiber mat. Fig. (**13**) shows the stress strain curves of different electrospun mats and their tensile strength are given in Table **1**. We found that the mechanical strength of LA/nylon-6 hybrid mat was greater than that of pristine nylon-6 mat. Mechanical strength of hybrid mat was found to be increased with the amounts of LA into the blending mixture (Table **1**). This increased mechanical strength can be explained with the help of adhesive property of LA. At the point where polymeric nanofibers cross with each other, LA can provide the attachment of fibers by means of point bonding. Our FE-SEM images show that increasing LA amounts can provide more point-bonded sites in the mat and therefore can increase the mechanical strength of nylon-6 mats (Fig. **2**). To confirm the adhesive nature of LA for forming the point-bonded structure in electrospun nylon-6 mat, two different pieces of LA/nylon-6 (M4) mats (formed from 5 gm LA in constant wt of 22 wt% nylon-6 solution) were kept separately into the water and dichloromethane solvents (only LA (not nylon-6) miscible with water and chloromethane) for 12 hrs. After vacuum drying, the FE-SEM images of these mats were taken and it was found that the water and dichloromethane had destroyed the point bounded structure without changing the other morphology of the fibers (Fig. **14**). The destruction of point-bonded structure was found more pronounced in dichloromethane than water (caused by the miscible differences of LA in two different solvents). This transformation from point-bonded to non bonded structure of nylon-6 hybrid mat confirmed the adhesive nature of LA.

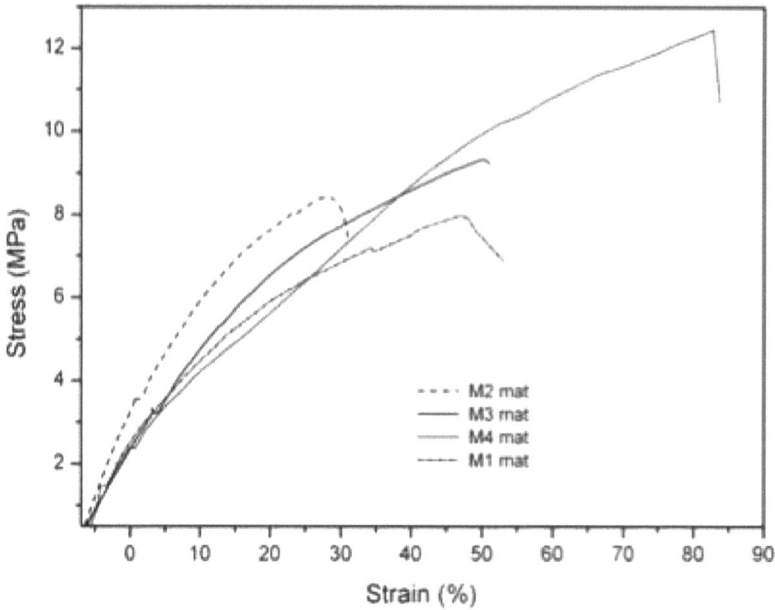

Fig. (13). Stress-strain curves of nylon-6 fibers containing different amounts of LA.

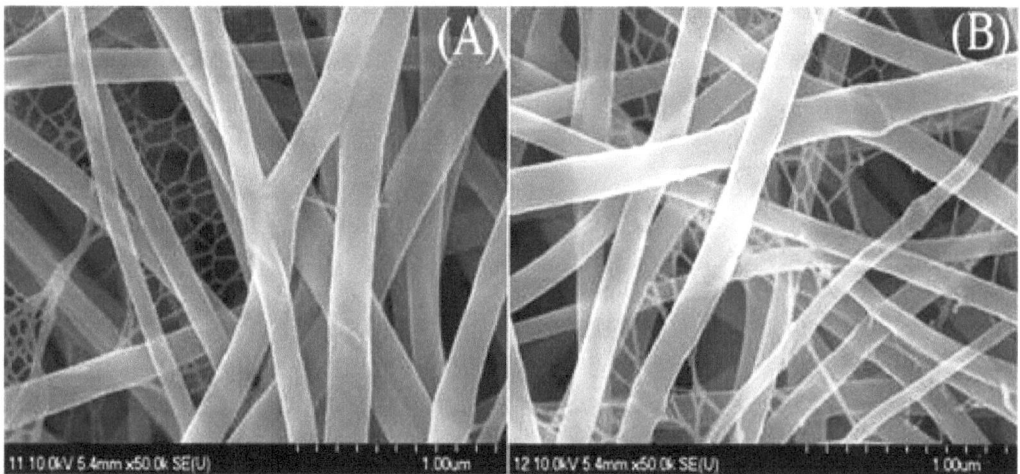

Fig. (14). FE-SEM images of LA/nylon-6 hybrid mat after washing by water (**A**) and dichloro-methane (**B**).

The increased mechanical strength was further explained with the help of polymer chains orientation and ability of maximizing hydrogen bonding interactions in α-crystalline phase. Transformation from γ- to α- crystalline phase can provide stronger hydrogen bonding between nylon-6 backbone chains in electrospun mat [21]. The shifting of different IR-bands towards lower frequency (due to the presence of LA) in FT-IR spectra was also observed, which further indicated the formation of stronger hydrogen bond in modified mat due to the presence α-crystalline form [6]. The fundamental relationship between the chemical microstructures of nylon-6 and the mechanical properties of electrospun mats can be established by means of the conversion of nylon-6 from gauche conformation to trans conformation. In crystallization (during electrospinning), the probability of polymer chain arrangement in a higher stable conformation is low enough so that they arrange in gauche conformation which ultimately give γ-form. During slow crystallization (due to LA), polymer chains get arranged themselves as far as possible, that bears a thermodynamically higher stable α-form (trans conformation) in which adjacent polymer chains oriented in opposite direction relative to each other to maximize the inter-molecular hydrogen bonding.

Lactic acid modified core-shell structured nylon-6 spider-web-like membrane showed numerous improved properties required for tissue scaffolds. However, still it has no proper nucleation sites for calcium phosphate deposition required for bone tissue engineering. Furthermore, sufficient amount of LA on fiber surface can decrease the surrounding pH and become toxic for cells when it is used for tissue scaffold. Therefore, neutralization of excess LA and deposition of Ca^{++} ions on fiber surface might be favorable for calcium phosphate nucleation and cell proliferation and differentiation.

FORMATION OF CALCIUM LACTATE/NYLON-6 NANOFIBERS AND ITS BIOMIMETIC MINERALIZATION

The increased mechanical strength and hydrophilicity, decreased crystallinity, and stable chain conformation in composite nylon-6/LA mat compared to the pristine nylon-6 mat are improved properties for biomedical application. However, cell viability result showed that composite mats were found to be fewer cells compatible than that of pristine mat (see explanation of Fig. (**18**) and Fig. (**19**)).

This result motivated us for the further modification of the composite mat. Since LA is protonic acid having pKa = 3.87 which can be sufficiently ionized in aqueous medium and can decrease the pH of the system. Therefore, neutralization of LA and subsequent deposition of calcium lactate on the surface of nylon-6 fibers (M4 mat) was carried out which was evaluated using FT-IR spectra of M4 mat before and after Ca(OH)$_2$ treatment (Fig. **15**). The comparison of FT-IR spectrum of LA/nylon-6 mat, before and after Ca(OH)$_2$ treatment (Fig. **15**), clearly shows that sufficient amount of calcium lactate was deposited on the surface of nylon-6 fibers as the intensity of different bands of LA/nylon-6 mat was sufficiently decreased. The important bands of LA/nylon-6 composite mat were explained in Fig. (**12**). The strong OH valence band of CL/nylon-6 mat appeared in the region of 3000-3700 cm^{-1} of FT-IR spectra with very low intensity as compared to the LA/nylon-6 mat clearly indicated the formation of calcium lactate [26]. In addition, a sharp new band at 3005 cm^{-1} indicated the formation of hydrate calcium lactate [26]. The presence strong C = O stretching of calcium lactate at 1745 cm^{-1}, which was also reported in previous report, further conformed the formation of calcium lactate.

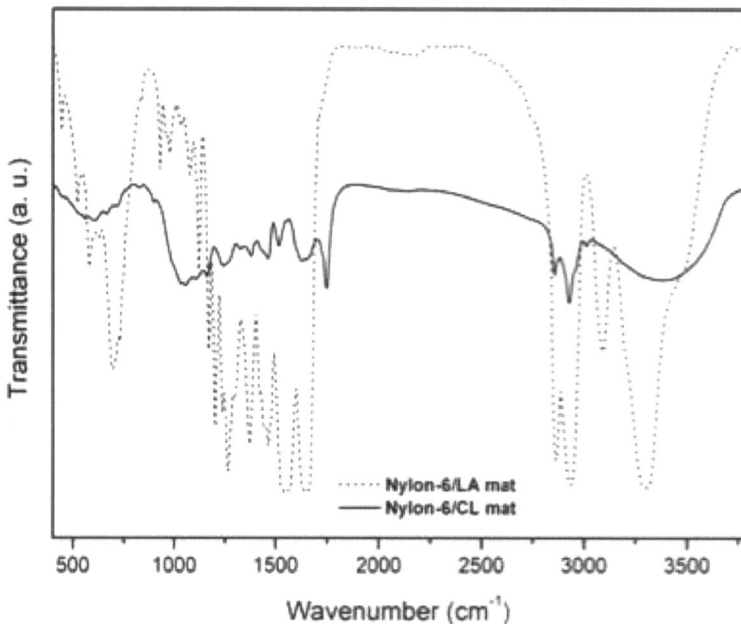

Fig. (15). FT-IR spectra of LA/nylon-6 composite mat (M4) and Ca(OH)$_2$ treated mat (CL/nylon-6 composite mat).

BIOCOMPATIBILITY OF MODIFIED NYLON-6 COMPOSITE MAT

Bone can be considered as a nanocomposite material made up of collagen protein fibers and calcium compounds, which makes up about 70 wt% of the human bone structure. Considering this biomimetic mechanism, we modified nylon-6/LA mat by calcium base to decrease the acidity of the mat caused by LA, and form surface layer of calcium compound (CL) around the nylon-6 fibers. The CL/nylon-6 composite scaffold is somewhat similar composition or molecular groups to that of natural human bone because nylon-6 resembles with collagen protein in back bone molecular structure [12] and CL is enrich in calcium ion which can act as nucleation for the deposition of bone materials (calcium phosphate). Therefore, CL containing nylon-6 matrix enable the scaffolding material to possess good biocompatibility, high bioactivity and enough mechanical strength required for bone tissue engineering.

To observe the role of CL on the surface of nylon-6 fibers for the deposition of calcium minerals after the incubation in SBF solution, FE-SEM analysis was performed. Fig. (**16**) shows the FE-SEM images of pristine nylon-6, LA/nylon-6 (M4 mat) and CL/nylon-6 composite mats after immersion in SBF solution for 7 days. As expected, the composite CL/nylon-6 mat has great potentiality to accelerate the deposition of calcium compound on the surface of fibers compared to pristine nylon-6 (Fig. **16**). The faster deposition of calcium compounds on the CL/nylon-6 fibers can be attributed to the partial dissolution of CL on the nylon-6 fibers and the subsequent release of calcium ions. The exposure of calcium ions on the nylon-6 nanofiber surfaces can provide nucleation sites for calcium compounds deposition from SBF.

The quantitative comparison of calcium deposition was carried out using Alizarin Red S (ARS) which is an anthraquinone derivative that forms a water insoluble salt with calcium [27]. Here, we stained the mineralized scaffolds with ARS, solubilized the stain in acetic acid and measured the absorbance of this solution at 550 nm (absorbance peak of ARS). Fig. (**17**) shows that composite scaffold has superior performance compared to the pristine scaffold. The intensity of staining in composite scaffold is far better than that of pristine one as observed visually

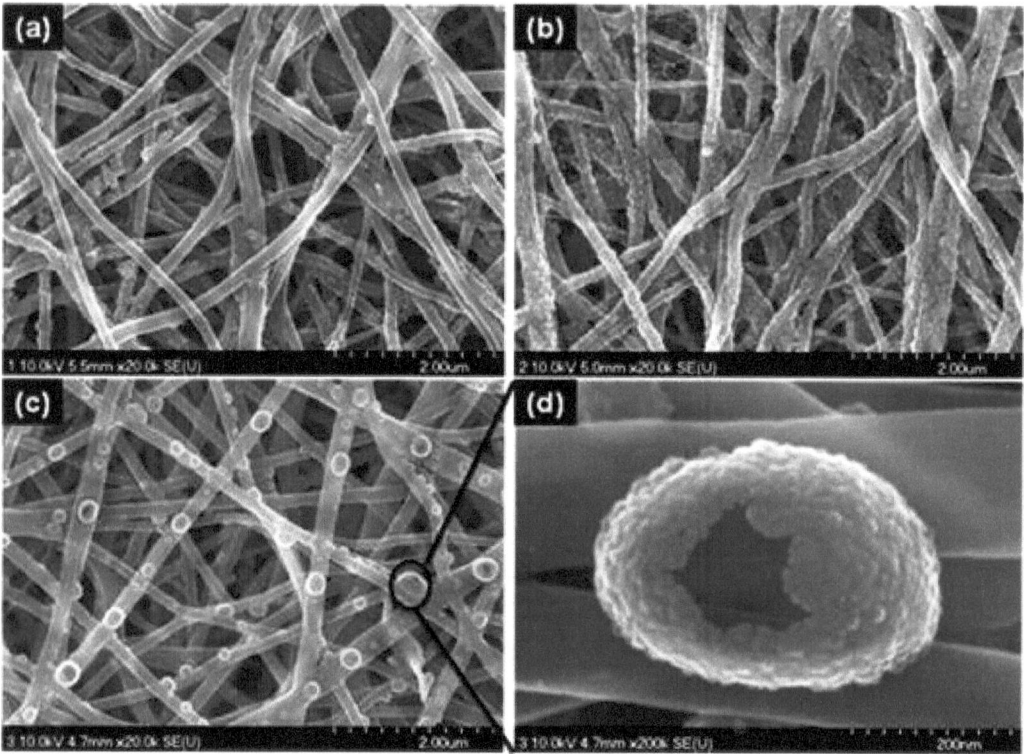

Fig. (16). FE-SEM images of pristine (**a**), LA/nylon-6 (**b**), and CL/nylon-6 (**c**) fibers after one weak SBF incubation.

from the photographs (inset of Fig. **17**). The faster deposition of calcium compounds on the composite fibers can be attributed to the partial dissolution of calcium lactate on the nylon-6 fibers and the subsequent release of calcium ions. The exposure of calcium ions on the nylon-6 nanofibers surfaces can provide nucleation sites for calcium compounds deposition from SBF. Our novel technique to incorporate calcium compound on the surface of polymer fibers is superior to the others where they blend soluble calcium compound or their nanoparticles (NPs) prior to electrospinning [28]. Homogeneous dispersion of inorganic components with polymer matrices is difficult to attain due to the particle agglomeration. Weak molecular interaction and poor dispersion consequently give rise to problems like decreased spinnability, reduced NPs loading capacity, and decreased mechanical properties of the resultant nanocomposite. Therefore, formation of surface layer of LA around the nylon-6 fibers and its subsequent conversion into calcium lactate should be the potential strategy to address the above mentioned drawback in this field. The conversion of LA into calcium lactate on the surface of core-shell structured nanofibers could form homogeneous layer of calcium compound around nylon-6 fiber which has good potentiality for the nucleation of calcium minerals. Therefore, in order to provide a local reservoir of calcium ions on the surface of fibers for the stable nucleation sites to rapid crystal growth, our technique can provide new dimension in this field. This approach may have great potential in enabling researchers to use post electrospinning surface coating strategy to engineer functional bone-like substitutes.

The most striking observation of this study was the behavior of composite scaffold compared to the pristine one with respect to mineralization potential. The superior performance of composite (nylon-6/CL) scaffold compared to the pristine one can be attributed to the fact that composite scaffold exhibited significant dimensional change (expanded almost 20% of its original size) while pristine one was unchanged (inset of Fig. **17**) up to 10 days SBF incubation. This change is accompanied by a dramatic increase in available surface area of composite scaffold for proper mineralization. Such a structural change in the nylon-6/CL composite scaffold seems to induce individual fibers mineralization and should be more suitable for bone tissue engineering. Since nylon-6 fibers take a long time for degradation in human body, the individual fibers enrich in calcium phosphate could be effectively used as artificial bone (as filler). Furthermore, the property of increase in dimension of as-synthesized bone scaffold could automatically allow it to be tightly filled on the bone defect portion after its implantation. This cumulative mineral deposition from all the individual fibers seems to account for the significantly superior performance of nylon-6/CL composite compared to pristine scaffold. The increase in dimension of this composite mat is attributed to the dissolution of calcium lactate during long time SBF incubation. Initially, the plasticizer capacity of LA can hold the fibers compatibly which is evidenced from the shrunk of composite mat on the surface of polyethylene sheet compared to the pristine one upon vacuum drying as shown in Fig. (**6**). However, fibers become free from calcium lactate or lactic acid upon its dissolution and they are expanded to increase the dimension of the mat during SBF incubation (inset of Fig. **17**).

Another possible cause of better performance of the composite scaffold may lie in the chemistry of calcium lactate present on the surface of polyamide-6 fibers. The presence of carboxyl group of calcium lactate could also initiate nucleation of calcium phosphate mineral and increase the mineralization [29].

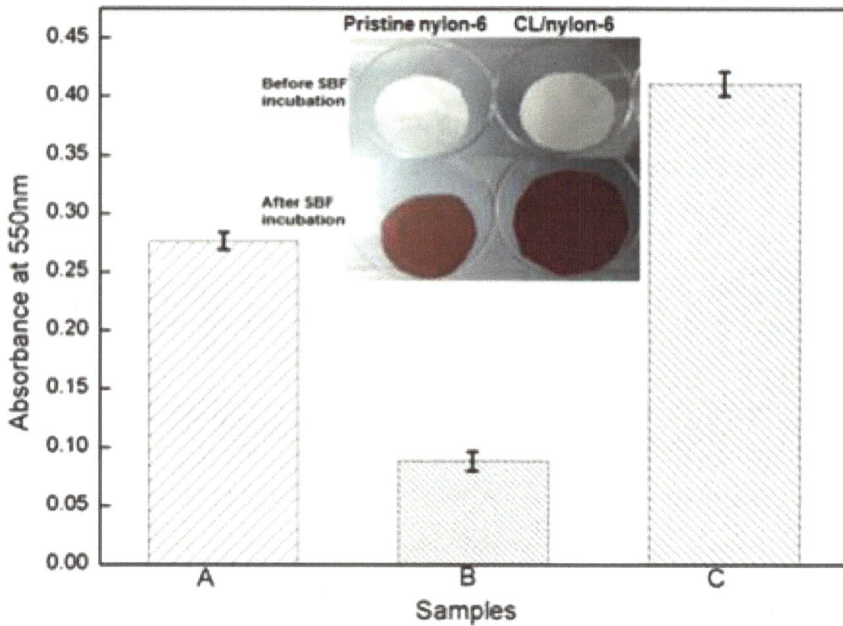

Fig. (17). Quantification of calcium compound on the surface of pristine nylon-6 after SBF incubation (a), and nylon-6/CL before (B) and after (C) SBF incubation. Inset is photograph of pristine nylon-6 and composite nylon-6/CL scaffold showing color and dimensional change before and after 10 days SBF incubation.

Another striking observation of biomimetic mineralization in this experiment was the unique morphology of deposited CaP nanoparticles on composite fibers compared to the pristine nylon-6 fibers. The superior biocompatibility of composite scaffold can be considered to the fact that the most of CaP NPs deposited on the surface of composite fibers were big hollow sphere (hole on the center) (Fig. **16d**) while they were small spherical without any hole when deposited on pristine nylon-6 or LA/nylon-6 fibers at same condition (Fig. **16**). FE-SEM EDX also revealed that the amount of CaP on composite scaffold was greater than that of pristine nylon-6 scaffold. The results showed that the amount and morphology of deposited CaP was greatly affected by the functionalities present on the surface of fibers. The binding of calcium or phosphate ions on the polar groups of electrospun fibers is one of the key factors for the first-step nucleation of CaP crystals [30]. The first-step nucleation can affect the Ca/P ratio of the deposited CaP NPs on the fiber surface. Since, pristine nylon-6 has only amide functional group with no high mineralization capacity, only few particles were deposited on the fibers (Fig. **16a**). However, LA present on the surface of nylon-6 fiber (M4 mat) can increase the density of functional groups per unit area compared to the pristine nylon-6 fibers. Moreover, its carboxylic group has higher tendency towards mineralization compared to the amide group [30]. The possible cause of interesting morphology (hollow nanosphere) of CaP on CL/nylon-6 fibers is probably due to highest mineralization affinity of Ca^{++} which can act as nucleation site for mineral deposition. The formation of hollow CaP nanosphere might be due to the high dissociation constant of CL and its solubility. Simultaneous crystallization (of CaP) and dissolution (of CL) takes place during SBF incubation and CL molecules which provide nucleation undergoes dissolution and ultimately form hole at the center of the nanosphere (Fig. **16d**). The Ca/P ratio in pristine nylon-6, LA/nylon-6, and CL/nylon-6 scaffolds was measured from FE-SEM EDX and was found 1.91, 2.16, and 1.78, respectively. This result suggested that amide group (of nylon-6) and carboxylic group (of LA) adsorbed more Ca^{++}, and the attraction of Ca^{++} was an important initial step in CaP formation on these fibers [31]. These functional groups are electron enrich and favored Ca^{++} chelating and consequently favored the higher Ca/P ratio. However, effective electrostatic attraction of Ca^{++} towards PO_4^{-3} might be initial step in CaP formation on CL/nylon-6 fibers. Therefore, amount of PO_4^{-3} becomes more as compared to the pristine and LA/nylon-6 fibers and consequently decreased the Ca/P ratio. Moreover, atomic Ca/P ratio of small particles (without hole) was observed bigger than that of hollow particles on CL/nylon-6 mat. This result revealed that bigger hollow nanosphere were nucleated by CL whereas smaller particles were nucleated by amide group of nylon-6.

Investigation of the cell viability is an important technique to evaluate the biocompatibility of biomaterials *in vitro* [32]. In this study, we cultured the osteoblast cell on the different mats for 1 and 7 days, and then the viabilities of cell were determined by MTT assay. From the MTT (Fig. **18**), we can see that the osteoblast cells proliferated on the membranes displayed a time-dependent behavior, and with comparing to the control, the nylon-6 (M1 mat) scaffolds

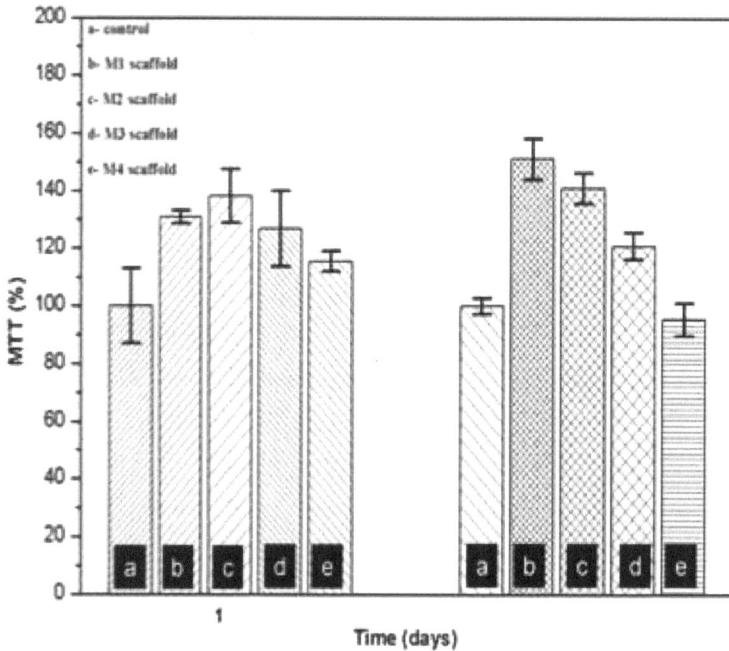

Fig. (18). MTT cytotoxicity test on different mats after 1 and 7 days culture. The viability of control cells was set at 100%, and the viability relative to the control was expressed. The data is reported as the mean ± standard deviation (n = 5 and p<0.05).

showed better cell viability. However, our hypothesis of better cell viability of nylon-6/LA (M4) composites than pristine nylon-6 was not valid from MTT experiment. For day 1, the cell viability of composite mats was more or less same to the pristine nylon-6. However, comparing the cell viability at day 7, all composite mats showed significant low cell proliferation relative to the pristine nylon-6. This is possibly related to the decreased pH of the medium due to the release of H+ ions from LA, which could cause the cell damage. The effect of Ca(OH)$_2$ treatment on the acidic property of M4 mat was also evaluated. For this equal weight of LA/nylon-6 and CL/nylon-6 mats (100 mg of each) were taken into equal volume (10 mL) of distilled water and extracted for 5 h. The pH measurement of these solution indicated that LA/nylon-6 mat sufficiently decreased the pH of distilled water (up to 3.2) while CL/nylon-6 mat maintained the pH of distilled water at 6.1. This result may also explain our observed SEM morphology of cells on different mats. Fig. (**19**) clearly shows that even though

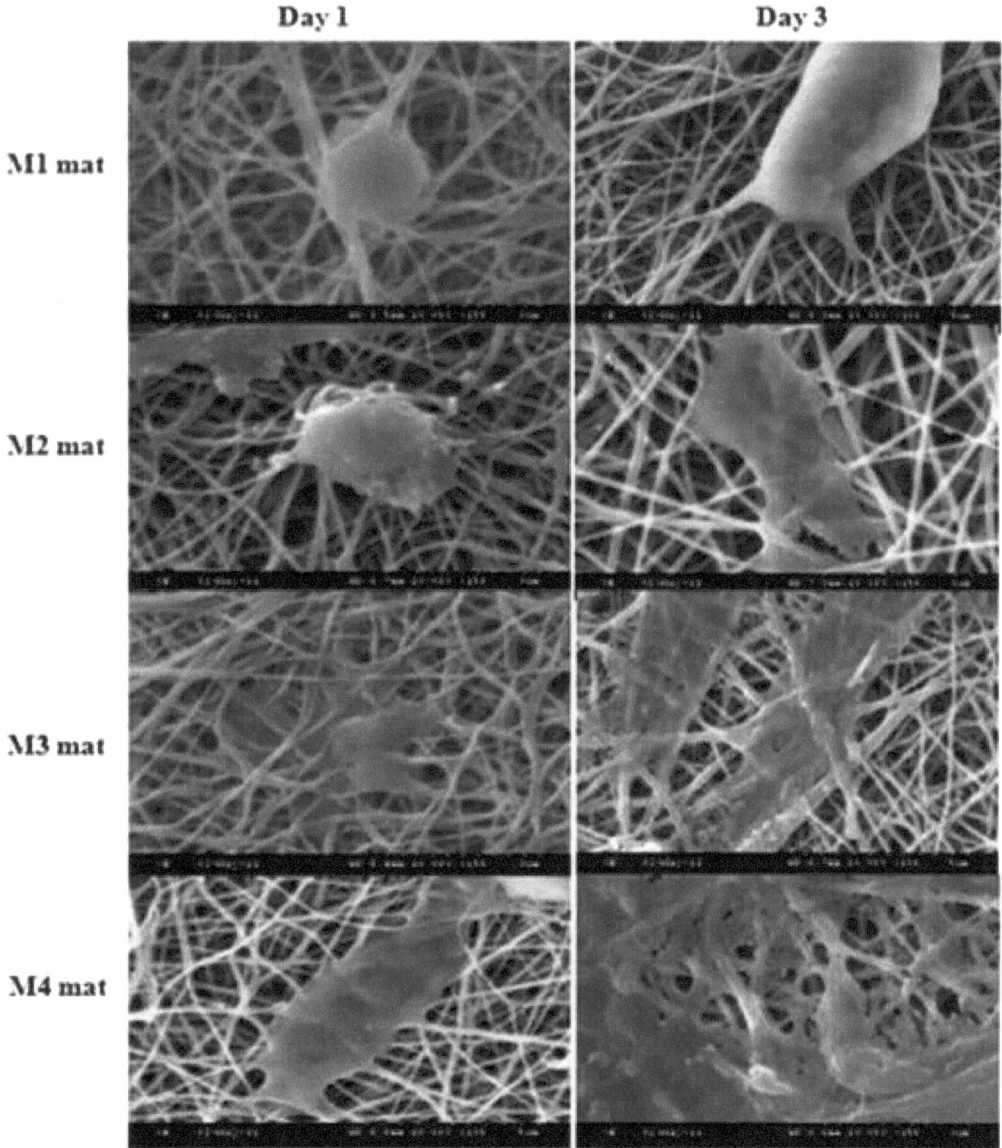

Fig. (19). SEM images of the cell growth one different electrospun mats at different time intervals.

the cell attachment is better in composite mats (M2, M3, and M4 mats) compared to pristine nylon-6 (M1) mat, the layer of cells on the composite mats looks somewhat damaged and not so healthy as compared to that of pristine nylon-6 mat. To alleviate this problem, neutralization of LA on the surface of nylon-6 is needed before cell seeding. Since composite M4 mat had not only highest mechanical strength and hydrophilicity but also sufficient spider-wave-like structure with smooth point-bonded morphology, we selected it for further modification by neutralizing with $Ca(OH)_2$ and its cell compatibility was compared with pristine nylon-6 mat.

Fig. (**20**) shows the cell viability test result of pristine and calcium hydroxide neutralized nylon-6/LA (named as CL/nylon-6) composite mat. Definitely, the viability of cells is more in CL/nylon-6 fibers than pristine one (Fig. **20**). The increased cell viability of CL/nylon-6 mat is the outcome of decreased amount of LA (less acidic) on the surface of nylon-6 fibers and subsequent deposition of CL during neutralization. Calcium lactate coated nanofibrous scaffold had remarkably favored cell growth. Fig. (**21**) shows that at 1 day the cells with a predominantly fusiform shape were smoothly distributed with their pseudopodia in CL/nylon-6

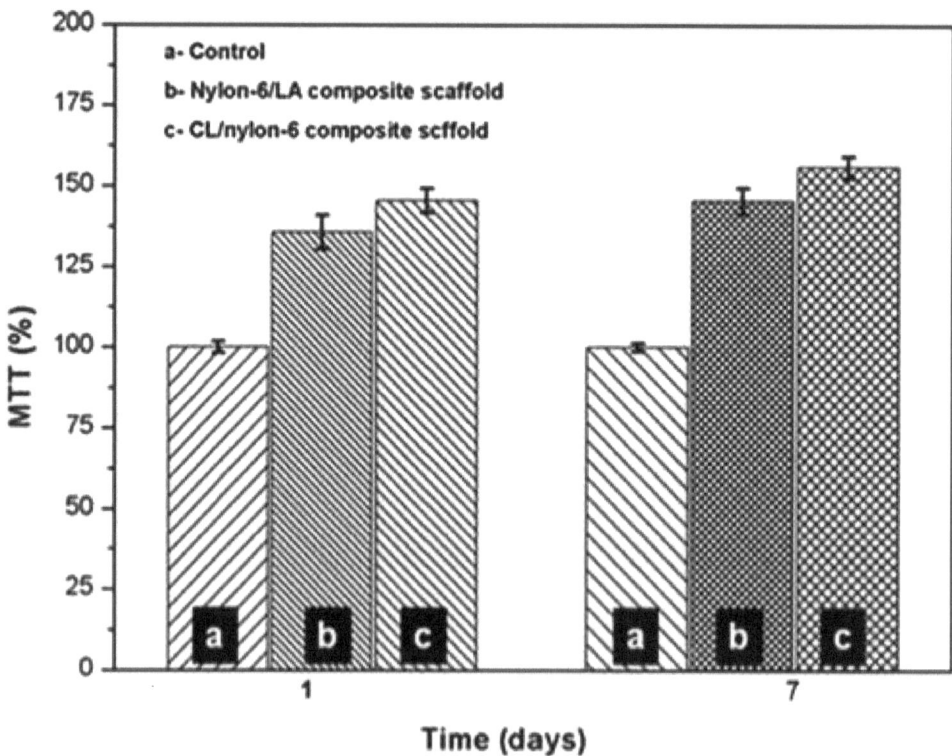

Fig. (20). MTT cytotoxicity test on pristine nylon-6 and CL/nylon-6 composite mats after 1 and 7 days culture. The viability of control cells was set at 100%, and the viability relative to the control was expressed. The data is reported as the mean ± standard deviation (n = 5 and p<0.05).

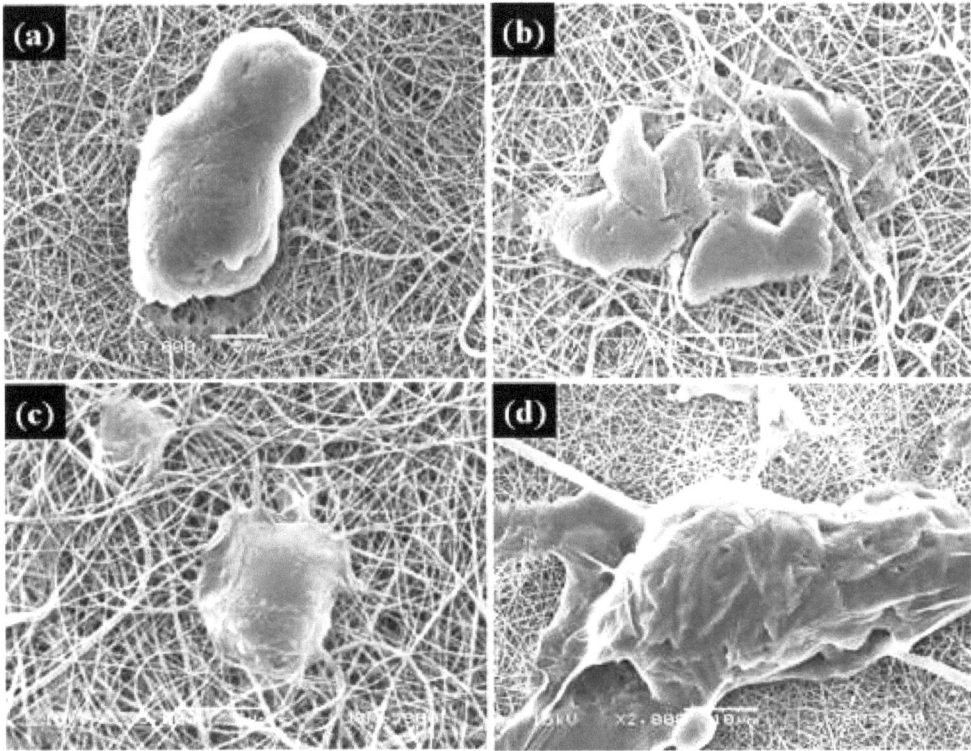

Fig. (21). SEM images of the cell growth after 1 day (**a**, **c**) and 3 days (**b**, **d**) on electrospun pristine nylon-6 and CL/nylon-6 composite mats, respectively.

mat whereas the cells were spherical shape in pristine nylon-6 mat. Similarly, in 3 days one can easily observe from Fig. (**21d**) that the cell attachment and proliferation of CL/nylon-6 composite mat are far better than that of pristine nylon-6 mat (Fig. **21b**). The CL/nylon-6 nanofibrous scaffold surface appeared to be sufficiently covered with multi-layers of cells as well as cells-secreted ECM, indicating confluence growth of osteoblast cell. Calcium lactate deposition stimulated a more significant level of bone cell formation ability because CL can absorb more proteins from the serum, which will promote better binding with integrins. Since cell adhesion, migration, proliferation, and differentiation are regulated by specific interaction of the ECM with cells, it is reasonable that the interaction of the bimodal fiber distribution in the form of spider-wave-like nano-nets and homogeneous layer of CL on their surface contributes to the good cellular responsiveness with surface modified nylon-6 fibers while used for bone tissue engineering.

CONCLUSION

In this chapter, we demonstrated a simple approach that combines an electrospinning followed by neutralization of acid on the surface of fibers to prepare a novel type calcium lactate/nylon-6 composite membrane for bone tissue engineering. Blinding of LA monomer with nylon-6 solution could produce LA coated nylon-6 fibers during electrospinning which can simply convert into calcium lactate by calcium hydroxide neutralization to get calcium lactate/nylon-6 composite fibers. As-synthesized CL/nylon-6 scaffolds appeared to have significantly stimulated the bone formation ability as shown by SBF incubation test, cell proliferation and morphology observation compared to pristine nylon-6 scaffolds. Furthermore, this work has demonstrated the mechanism of core-shell formation capacity of hybrid electrospinning solution having different molecular weight from the single-spinneret. We are able to demonstrate a simple calcium compound deposition technique around the polymer fibers without disturbing the internal structure of polymer fibers.

ACKNOWLEDGEMENTS

This work was supported by the Korean Ministry of Education, Science and Technology (MIST) through the National Research Foundation (NRF) (Project no 2012R1A1A4A01013423 and 2011-0011807).

CONFLICT OF INTEREST

The authors confirm that this chapter contents have no conflict of interest.

ABBREVIATIONS

CaP   =   Calcium phosphate

CL   =   Calcium lactate

ECM   =   Extracellular matrix

FESEM =   Field-emission scanning electron microscope

LA   =   Lactic acid

SBF   =   Simulated body fluid

TEM = Transmission electron microscope

XPS = X-ray photoelectron spectroscopy

XRD = X-ray diffractometer

REFERENCES

[1]   Beachley V, Wen X. Polymer nanofibrous structures: Fabrication, biofunctionalization, and cell interactions. *Prog Polym Sci.,* 2010; 35: 868-892.

[2]   Greiner A, Wendorff JH. Electrospinning: A fascinating method for the preparation of ultrathin fibers. *Angewandte Chemie International Edition,* 2007; 46: 5670-5703.

[3]   Huang C, Soenen SJ, Rejman J, Lucas B, Braeckmans K, Demeester J, De Smedt SC. Stimuli-responsive electrospun fibers and their applications. *Chemical Society Reviews,* 2011; 40: 2417-2434.

[4]   Li D, Xia Y. Electrospinning of nanofibers: Reinventing the wheel? *Adv Mater,* 2004; 16: 1151-1170.

[5]   Taylor G. Electrically driven jets. *Proceedings of the Royal Society of London A Mathematical and Physical Sciences* 1969; 313: 453-475.

[6]   Pant HR, Bajgai MP, Yi C, Nirmala R, Nam KT, Baek W-i, Kim HY. Effect of successive electrospinning and the strength of hydrogen bond on the morphology of electrospun nylon-6 nanofibers. *Colloids and Surfaces A: Physicochemical and Engineering Aspects,* 2010; 370: 87-94.

[7]   Fong H, Chun I, Reneker DH. Beaded nanofibers formed during electrospinning. *Polymer,* 1999; 40: 4585-4592.

[8]   Pant HR, Baek W-i, Nam K-T, Jeong I-S, Barakat NAM, Kim HY. Effect of lactic acid on polymer crystallization chain conformation and fiber morphology in an electrospun nylon-6 mat. *Polymer,* 2011; 52: 4851-4856.

[9]   Nair LS, Laurencin CT. Polymers as biomaterials for tissue engineering and controlled drug delivery. *Advances in biochemical engineering/biotechnology* 2006; 102: 47-90.

[10] Jeong SI, Lee AY, Lee YM, Shin H. Electrospun gelatin/poly(l-lactide-co-epsilon-caprolactone) nanofibers for mechanically functional tissue-engineering scaffolds. *Journal of biomaterials science Polymer edition,* 2008; 19: 339-357.

[11] Zhang X, Li Y, Lv G, Zuo Y, Mu Y. Thermal and crystallization studies of nano-hydroxyapatite reinforced polyamide 66 biocomposites. *Polym Degrad Stabil,* 2006; 91: 1202-1207.

[12] Wang H, Li Y, Zuo Y, Li J, Ma S, Cheng L. Biocompatibility and osteogenesis of biomimetic nano-hydroxyapatite/polyamide composite scaffolds for bone tissue engineering. *Biomaterials,* 2007; 28: 3338-3348.

[13] Pant HR, Bajgai MP, Nam KT, Chu KH, Park S-J, Kim HY. Formation of electrospun nylon-6/methoxy poly(ethylene glycol) oligomer spider-wave nanofibers. *Materials Letters,* 2010; 64: 2087-2090.

[14] Pant HR, Park CH, Tijing LD, Amarjargal A, Lee D-H, Kim CS. Bimodal fiber diameter distributed graphene oxide/nylon-6 composite nanofibrous mats *via* electrospinning. *Colloids and Surfaces A: Physicochemical and Engineering Aspects,* 2012; 407: 121-125.

[15]   Wang X, Ding B, Yu J, Yang J. Large-scale fabrication of two-dimensional spider-web-like gelatin nano-nets *via* electro-netting. *Colloids and Surfaces B: Biointerfaces,* 2011; 86: 345-352.

[16]   Wang X, Ding B, Sun G, Wang M, Yu J. Electro-spinning/netting: A strategy for the fabrication of three-dimensional polymer nano-fiber/nets. *Prog Mater Sci.,* 2013; 58: 1173-1243.

[17]   Pant HR, Nam K-T, Oh H-J, Panthi G, Kim H-D, Kim B-i, Kim HY. Effect of polymer molecular weight on the fiber morphology of electrospun mats. *J Colloid Interf Sci,* 2011; 364: 107-111.

[18]   Ma PX. Scaffolds for tissue fabrication. *Materials Today,* 2004; 7: 30-40.

[19]   Sun XY, Shankar R, Börner HG, Ghosh TK, Spontak RJ. Field-driven biofunctionalization of polymer fiber surfaces during electrospinning. *Adv Mater,* 2007; 19: 87-91.

[20]   Pant HR, Risal P, Park CH, Tijing LD, Jeong YJ, Kim CH. Core-shell structured electrospun biomimetic composite nanofibers of calcium lactate/nylon-6 for tissue engineering, *Chemical Engineering Journal,* 2013; 221: 90-98.

[21]   Stephens JS, Chase DB, Rabolt JF. Effect of the electrospinning process on polymer crystallization chain conformation in nylon-6 and nylon-12. *Macromolecules,* 2004; 37: 877-881.

[22]   Giller CB, Chase DB, Rabolt JF, Snively CM. Effect of solvent evaporation rate on the crystalline state of electrospun nylon 6. *Polymer,* 2010; 51: 4225-4230.

[23]   Garreau S, Leclerc M, Errien N, Louarn G. Planar-to-nonplanar conformational transition in thermochromic polythiophenes: A spectroscopic study. *Macromolecules,* 2003; 36: 692-697.

[24]   Song K, Rabolt JF. Polarized raman measurements of uniaxially oriented poly(ε-caprolactam). *Macromolecules,* 2001; 34: 1650-1654.

[25]   Vasanthan N, Salem DR. Ftir spectroscopic characterization of structural changes in polyamide-6 fibers during annealing and drawing. *Journal of Polymer Science Part B: Polymer Physics,* 2001; 39: 536-547.

[26]   Arimoto H. A–γ transition of nylon 6. *Journal of Polymer Science Part A: General Papers,* 1964; 2: 2283-2295.

[27]   Musumeci AW, Frost RL, Waclawik ER. A spectroscopic study of the mineral paceite (calcium acetate). *Spectrochimica Acta Part A: Molecular and Biomolecular Spectroscopy,* 2007; 67: 649-661.

[28]   Gregory CA, Grady Gunn W, Peister A, Prockop DJ. An alizarin red-based assay of mineralization by adherent cells in culture: Comparison with cetylpyridinium chloride extraction. *Analytical Biochemistry,* 2004; 329: 77-84.

[29]   Dinarvand P, Seyedjafari E, Shafiee A, Babaei Jandaghi A, Doostmohammadi A, Fathi MH, Farhadian S, Soleimani M. New approach to bone tissue engineering: Simultaneous application of hydroxyapatite and bioactive glass coated on a poly(l-lactic acid) scaffold. *Acs Appl Mater Inter,* 2011; 3: 4518-4524.

[30]   Kawai T, Ohtsuki C, Kamitakahara M, Hosoya K, Tanihara M, Miyazaki T, Sakaguchi Y, Konagaya S. *In vitro* apatite formation on polyamide containing carboxyl groups modified with silanol groups. *Journal of materials science Materials in medicine,* 2007; 18: 1037-1042.

[31]   Kikuchi M, Itoh S, Ichinose S, Shinomiya K, Tanaka J. Self-organization mechanism in a bone-like hydroxyapatite/collagen nanocomposite synthesized *in vitro* and its biological reaction *in vivo*. *Biomaterials,* 2001; 22: 1705-1711.

[32]   Toworfe GK, Composto RJ, Shapiro IM, Ducheyne P. Nucleation and growth of calcium phosphate on amine-, carboxyl- and hydroxyl-silane self-assembled monolayers. *Biomaterials,* 2006; 27: 631-642.

CHAPTER 10

Biocompatibility Issues of Organic and Inorganic Nanomaterials

Akhilesh Rai[1,2], Sandra Pinto[1,2], Cristiana Paulo[3], Michela Comune[1,2] and Lino Ferreira[*,1,2]

[1]*CNC-Center for Neurosciences and Cell Biology, University of Coimbra, 3004-517 Coimbra, Portugal;* [2]*Biocant, Biotechnology Innovation Center, 3060-197 Cantanhede, Portugal; and* [3]*Matera, Biocant, Biotechnology Innovation Center, 3060-197 Cantanhede, Portugal*

Abstract: Several types of nanoparticles are being evaluated for therapeutic and diagnostic applications. Although the biocompatibility of these nanoformulations has been evaluated in different models, it is of utmost importance to standardize the tests in order to advance our knowledge in this area. This book chapter summarizes experimental results related to the *in vitro* and *in vivo* toxicity of three types of nanoparticles: gold, silica and poly(lactic-*co*-glycolic acid). The chapter gives an overview about the methodologies that can be used to evaluate the toxicity of the nanoparticles. Whenever possible, a correlation between NP size, chemical composition, charge and concentration with toxicity is given. We further discuss the main mechanisms of nanomaterials toxicity including cell membrane perturbation, oxidation stress, and inflammatory response.

Keywords: Gold nanoparticles, *in vitro* cytotoxicity, *in vivo* cytotoxicity, inflammatory response, mechanism of cytotoxicity, membrane perturbation, oxidative stress, PLGA nanoparticles, silica nanoparticles, size/shape induced cytotoxicity.

INTRODUCTION

Nanoparticles (NPs) having at least one dimension in the 1 to 100 nm size range have a remarkable potential for biomedical applications. They have high surface area and physiochemical properties that cannot be observed outside of the nanometer scale. Inorganic nanomaterials such as metal, metal oxide and semiconductors, which exhibit unique optical, electronic and magnetic properties,

*Corresponding Author Lino Ferreira: CNC-Center for Neurosciences and Cell Biology, University of Coimbra, 3004-517 Coimbra, Portugal; Tel: 231249170; Fax: 231249179; E-mail: Lino@biocant.pt

Shunsheng Cao & Huijun Zhu (Eds)

offer an excellent potential for imaging and drug delivery. One type of inorganic NPs is quantum dots, which can be used for cell labeling, *in vivo* imaging and diagnostics [1]. Due to the quantum dots photophysical properties such as broad absorption spectra coupled to a narrow emission spectrum, quantum dots of different emission colors may be simultaneously excited by a single wavelength. Other examples of inorganic nanoparticles include gold (GNPs) and silica nanoparticles (SNPs). GNPs and SNPs have been used in the field of nanomedicine and therapeutics for more than 10 years [2, 3]. These NPs have been widely used to deliver various types of biomolecules for instance drugs, antigens and genetic materials. For example, GNP formulation AuroLase^{TM} is being evaluated in clinical trials to treat cancer patients [4]. In this case, the rationale is that GNPs can be activated by a near infrared laser source to thermally destroy cancer tissue without significantly damaging the surrounding healthy tissue. In addition, GNPs have been used since the 1920s to treat rheumatoid arthritis [2]. Organic NPs have also a great potential in the biomedical field as drug and gene delivery vehicles, fluorescent labels and contrast agents. These NPs can be generated from lipids, polymers and small molecules. Biodegradable polymeric NPs such as poly (D,L-glycolide) (PLG), poly(lactide-*co*-glycolide) (PLGA) [5], poly(lactic acid) (PLA) and poly(cyanoacrylate) [6] are popular choices for delivery purposes.

Despite the enormous potential of NPs in the biomedical area, they can also induce consequences and interfere with human biology. In general, the cytotoxicity of NPs depends on their size, shape, surface area, agglomeration state, chemical composition, surface chemistry and dose [7-9] (Fig. **1**). As the number of different compositions of NPs and their biological applications are rapidly expanding, cytotoxicity concerns over their usages have been raised as well, leading to an increasing number of studies on *in vitro* and *in vivo* toxicity along with bio-distribution and possible elimination in living organisms as whole or at level of cyto- and genotoxicity. Due to these challenges, "Nanotoxicology" term was coined and defined as science dealing with nature and mechanisms of toxic effects of nanomaterials/particles in living organisms and other biological organisms. The objective of this discipline is to correlate NP physiochemical properties with biological response such as kinetics of NP accumulation and elimination, and biological targeting (cells, tissues, organs). Several *in vitro* and *in vivo* tests have been proposed to evaluate the toxicology of nanomaterials. Regarding *in vitro* tests, three key factors are determinant for the toxicological evaluation of NPs: (i) physico-chemical properties of NPs, (ii) cell type and (iii) the method used to evaluate cytotoxicity. Yet, in most cases, because different cell types and assays are used to evaluate NP cytotoxicity, it is very difficult to compare the experimental data. There is a critical need to develop a "gold standard" to measure toxicity for probing *in vitro* and *in vivo* fate of various compositions of nanomaterials.

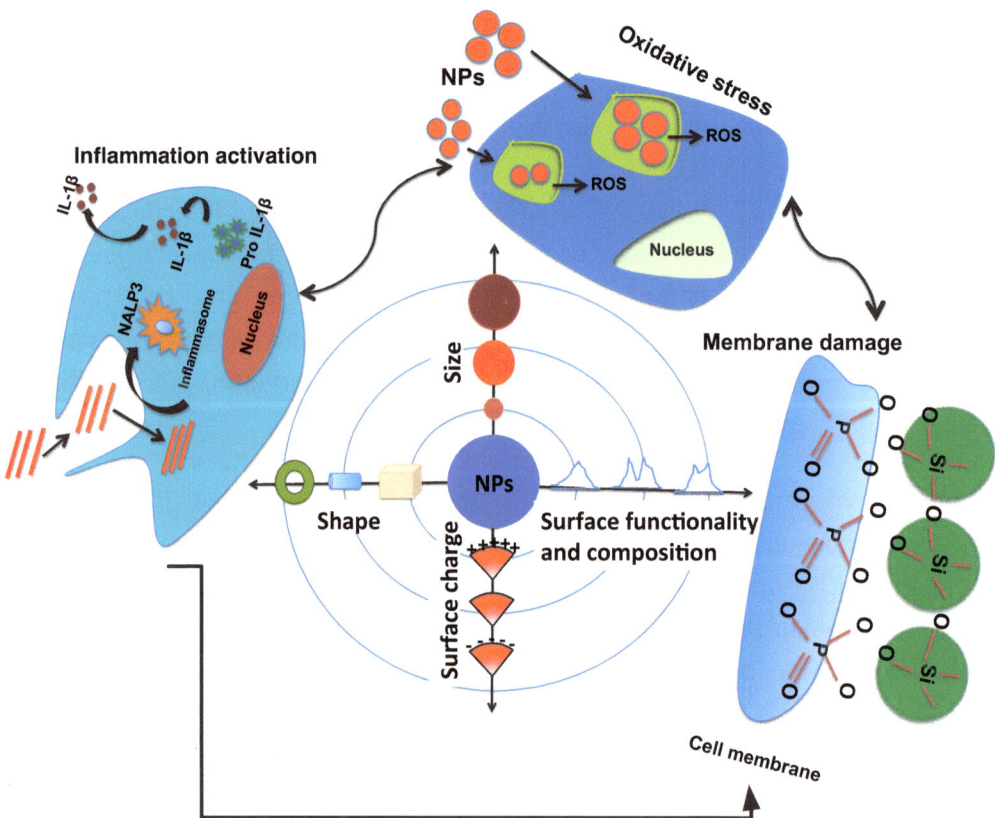

Fig. (1). Scheme illustrating the several toxicity pathways of NPs.

This chapter summarizes recent studies on *in vitro* and *in vivo* biocompatibility of inorganic (gold and silica) and organic (PLGA) NPs. These NPs were selected because they represent an important fraction of the NPs used in nanomedicine and drug delivery, and because there is a significant number of studies documenting their cytotoxic profile.

IN VITRO CYTOTOXICITY OF NANOMATERIALS

Methodologies to Assess the Cytotoxicity of Nanomaterials

The first step to evaluate the biocompatibility of nanomaterials involves cell culture studies. Compared to animal studies, cellular testing is less ethically ambiguous, is easier to control and reproduce, and is less expensive. Before the evaluation of the cytotoxic response of nanomaterials, it is important to determine the size, charge and stability of nanomaterials in the cell culture media. In a typical cytotoxicity evaluation, cells are seeded at the bottom of a culture plate and incubated with a suspension of NPs. In most cases NPs aggregate and change their physical properties when they are exposed to cell culture medium [10, 11]. Aggregation may occur when the van der Waals attractive forces between NPs are greater than electrostatic repulsive forces. Large NPs can sediment affecting the NP concentration that cells are exposed to. Because cellular uptake is directly related to the concentration of NPs, it is very important to perform stability studies of NPs in the cell culture media. In some cases, the cellular uptake of NPs depends on the ratio of sedimentation regardless of size, shape, density, surface coating and initial concentration [12].

A second important aspect to take in consideration when evaluating the cytotoxicity of nanomaterials is to determine whether the NPs interfere with the components of the assay. The NPs can react or adsorb chemicals that will have important implications for the interpretation of the assay results [13]. Therefore it is important that multiple tests should be performed to validate the conclusions. A third important aspect to consider in the cytotoxicity analysis of nanomaterials is the selection of the cell model. It is important to choose multiple cell types with differences in cell physiology, proliferation state (tumoral or resting cells), membrane characteristics, phagocyte characteristics, *etc*.

Cytotoxicity of nanomaterials is typically evaluated by calorimetric methods that can evaluate plasma membrane integrity, cell viability and cell metabolism. Cell metabolism is in most cases evaluated by a 3-(4,5-dimethylthiazol- 2-yl)-2,5-

diphenyl tetrazolium bromide (MTT) assay. Mitochondrial dehydrogenase enzymes cleave the tetrazolium ring, allowing the determination of cell metabolic activity. Only live cells have active mitochondria and thus the assessment of mitochondrial activity gives an indirect assessment of cell viability. This assay has been used for the evaluation of the cytotoxicity of SNPs [8], GNPs [9] and PLGA NPs [14] against different type of cells. The evaluation of ATP by commercial kits might be an alternative to the MTT assay. For example, the production of ATP was monitored in endothelial cells exposed to SNPs [11]. The advantage of the ATP kits is that they require a small number of cells (below 5,000 cells).

Cell viability can be assessed by several methods including annexin V/propidium iodide (PI) and a LIVE/DEAD viability test. The LIVE/DEAD viability test includes two chemicals calcein acetoxymethyl (calcein AM) and ethidiumhomodimer. Calcein AM can easily enter cells by diffusion and will be converted into calcein by live cells having intracellular esterases. In contrast, damaged or dead cells are stained by ethidiumhomodimer, a membrane-impermeable molecule. The annexin V/PI assay has the advantage of assessing early apoptotic, late apoptotic, necrotic and live cells at the same time. Annexin V is a phospholipid-binding protein with specificity for phosphatidyl serine, one of the earliest markers of cellular transition to an apoptotic state [15]. This phospholipid is translocated from the inner to outer leaflet of the plasma membrane. PI enters in necrotic cells and binds to double-stranded nucleic acids, but is excluded from cells with normal integrity [16]. The annexin V/PI assay was used to determine that SNPs were apoptotic for concentrations below 200 μg/mL [17].

Plasma cell integrity is assessed by several methods including neutral red, trypan blue and lactate dehydrogenase (LDH) release assay. Neutral red is a weak cationic dye that can cross the plasma membrane by diffusion and accumulates in lysosomes. If the cell membrane is altered, the accumulation of neutral red is affected and thus allowing for discernment between live and dead cells. Trypan blue is only permeable to cells with compromised membranes and thus dead cells stained for blue. Finally, in the LDH assay, cells damaged or lysed release LDH. LDH is an oxidoreductase enzyme that catalyses the interconversion of pyruvate and lactate. The release of LDH can be easily monitored by assessing the reduction of NAD to NADH by LDH using a colorimetric assay. The amount of LDH released is proportional to the number of cells damaged or lysed. LDH assay has been used to demonstrate a size-dependent cytotoxicity of monodisperse amorphous SNPs [8]. Concentrations leading to a 50% reduction in cell viability were 32, 89 and >1212 µg/cm^{-2} of cell culture for SNPs with 14, 19 and 104 nm in diameter.

Cellular secretion of cytokines and chemokines can be used to evaluate the pro-inflammatory activity of nanomaterials. The pro-inflammatory molecules such as IL-6, TNF-α, IL-8, IL-1β, among others can be evaluated by ELISA kits or Multiplex kits commercially available. Studies in human umbilical vein endothelial cells (HUVECs) have shown that SNPs induce the release of tissue factor, IL-6, IL-8 and MCP-1 [17]. Furthermore, we showed recently that HUVECs exposed to SNPs (50 µg/mL) for 24 hrs secrete MCP-1, IL-8, IL-6 and G-CSF, from an array of 17 cytokines/chemokines [11].

The biological impact of nanomaterials can be also evaluated at gene level. In this case, a small number of genes, typically involved in a cytotoxic response, or whole gene microarrays can be performed. Recently, we have shown the cytotoxic effect of SNPs in human umbilical vein endothelial cells (HUVECs) by microarray studies (array of 90 genes involved in cell apoptosis/necrosis) [11]. Cells incubated with SNPs (50 µg/mL) for 24 hrs showed a downregulation of genes related to cell proliferation and an upregulation of genes involved in cell arrest and senescence. In addition, our results showed that cells had impaired DNA repair mechanisms as compared to untreated cells.

Mechanisms of Nanomaterials Cytotoxicity

Cell Membrane Perturbation

Direct interaction of NPs with cells can interfere with membrane lipid bilayer and lead to the leak of cellular components (Fig. **1**). The charge of the NPs has an important effect in this process. GNPs with varying surface charges (cationic, anionic, zwitterionic and neutral) have different impact on cells [18]. Positively charged GNPs depolarize the membrane potential in a dose dependent manner on different types of cells. Furthermore, cationic GNPs increased the intracellular Ca^{2+} concentration by stimulating Ca^{2+} plasma membrane Ca^{2+} influx as well as Ca^{2+} release from the endoplasmic reticulum [19]. Cationic mixed monolayer protected gold clusters (MMNC1) have higher cytotoxicity than its anionic analogue due to strong interaction with anionic phosphatidylcholine/phosphatidyl-serine membrane and more efficiently disruption of membrane [20]. Studies on supported lipid bilayers (SLBs) have identified two general types of disruption: (1) nanoscale hole formation and (2) membrane thinning [21]. Experiments using GNPs coated with alkylamine (total diameter of 5-6 nm) showed that NPs do not directly induce defects in SLBs but instead diffuse to existing defects and expand them. In contrast, SNPs functionalized with amine groups (diameter of 50 nm) are capable of directly inducing defects in SLBs [21].

Cell membrane perturbation by SNPs depends in the number of silanol groups per NP surface area and NP porous structure. Nonporous SNPs (approximately 42 nm in diameter) cause greater membrane damage to red blood cells (RBCs) than mesoporous SNPs with the same size [22]. Higher number of silanol groups present on cell contactable nonporous SNPs than in mesoporous SNPs is likely the reason for the cell membrane perturbation [22]. Hydrogen bonding and electrostatics interaction of silanol group of SNPs aggregates with cell membrane cause membrane perturbations sensed by Nalp3 inflammation whose activation lead to secretion of cytokine IL-1β [23]. This behavior is more prominent in fumed silica having strained 3 members-ring (3MRs) as compared to colloidal silica with no 3MRs. Commercially available Ludox NPs induce severer damage to the plasma membrane of normal fibroblast cells (CCD-34 Lu) as a consequence of lipid peroxidation, resulting into translocation of phosphaditylserine to outer leaflet of plasma membrane [24].

Compared to inorganic NPs, organic NPs such as PLGA NPs do not have significant impact on structural properties of cell membrane. Smaller size PLGA NPs trigger intracellular Ca^{2+} flux in RAW 264.7 and BEAS-2B cells through ROS generation but do not cause any cell death or damage to organelles [25].

Oxidative Stress

The generation of reactive oxygen species (ROS) by cells after exposure to NPs is a common process (Fig. **1**). Either radical ROS (nitric oxide or hydroxide radicals) or non-radical ROS (hydrogen peroxide) can be generated after NP-cell interaction. ROS are released due to following factors: (1) generation of free radicals due to redox reactive property of NPs, (2) oxidative groups functionalized on surface of NPs, (3) cell-NP interaction. Typically, fluorescent probes such as dichlorodihydrofluorescein have been used to assess intracellular ROS levels. Because, ROS production is dependent on time it is important to determine the kinetics of ROS formation as well as to determine whether the effects are transient or long-lasting. Overproduction of ROS activates release of cytokines and upregulates interleukins and tumor necrosis factor-α (TNF-α) as indicators of proinflammatory signal process. In addition, overproduction of ROS leads to oxidation of proteins and lipids, leading to modulation in mitochondria function.

Cells have protective mechanisms such as the glutathione redox system, which can buffer a certain amount of ROS. It is believed that cells survive oxidative stress generated by NPs through autophagic pathways, which destroys foreign materials [26]. The link between ROS levels and the induction of toxic effects is however cell type-dependent and not very well defined [13]. For example, myeloid monocytic cell line (U937) and T cell line (Jurkat) produced low levels of ROS with SNPs while B (HMY) and prostatic cell lines (PC3) produce high levels of ROS. It is possible that the production of ROS is linked to the capacity of the cells to internalize NPs, since U937 cell line had limited capacity to internalize NPs while PC3 showed high internalization of NPs [13]. Spherical GNPs synthesized using citrate methods induce oxidative stress to lung fibroblast cells and blood serum [26, 27]. Lung is more sensitive to GNPs due to the presence of large amount of ROS producers such as inflammatory phagocytes, neutrophils and macrophages [28]. So far, it was impossible to demonstrate a direct correlation between ROS production and cell toxicity [13], ROS activity measurements should be coupled with the determination of cell viability and mitochondrial function.

ROS production depends on the size of NPs and hydrophobicity. Higher oxidation stress is induced by smaller GNPs (diameter of 1.4 nm) than larger GNPs (diameter of 15 nm) [29, 30]. GNPs with a diameter of 60 nm do not produce ROS in murine macrophage cells (RAW 264.7) at concentration of 100 µg/mL [31]. Results obtained with GNPs (diameter of 2 nm) coated with quaternary ammonium with variable (C1-C6) hydrophobic alkyl tail show that cellular production of ROS is dependent on NP hydrophobicity [29]. NPs with high hydrophobicity induce high levels of ROS.

ROS response generated by cells depends on composition of NPs. For instance, ZnO NPs induce higher oxidative stress than SNPs, carbon nanotubes and carbon black [32]. Although, ZnO and SNPs have similar crystal structures and particle size, the toxicity variation may be attributed to their different chemical composition. Similarly, amorphous TiO_2 and silver NPs induce high generation of ROS [33, 34].

SNPs induce the generation of ROS inside the cells, being this effect dependent on the concentration and chemistry of the SNPs, and type of cell. While HUVECs internalize high amounts of SNPs and suffer from generation of ROS, human dermal fibroblasts internalize low amounts of SNPs and are not affected by ROS levels [11] (Fig. **2**). The higher internalization of SNPs by HUVECs than fibroblasts was justified by the fact that HUVECs were more prone to macropinocytosis than fibroblasts. In case of HUVECs the production of ROS is time and SNP dose-dependent. The exposure of HUVECs to 100 µg/mL of SNPs (20 nm in diameter) significantly increased ROS generation at as early as 3 hrs (1.5 fold relatively to control) and continue to increase even after 24 hrs (2 fold relatively to control) [17]. This increase in ROS translated in approximately 10% of cell death after 24 hrs as assessed by a MTS test.

The generation of ROS by SNPs is affected by the corona formed around the NPs. Amorphous silica nanospheres (12 nm diameter) caused high oxidative stress and sharp decrease in metabolic activity of a human breast cancer cell line (MCF-7) at concentrations of 50 µg/mL [35]. It was observed that amorphous spherical SNPs were less cytotoxic in the presence of serum. The protein corona formed around the NPs inhibited the formation of ROS [35] and changed the strength of interaction with the cell membrane and intracellular fate of the SNPs [36].

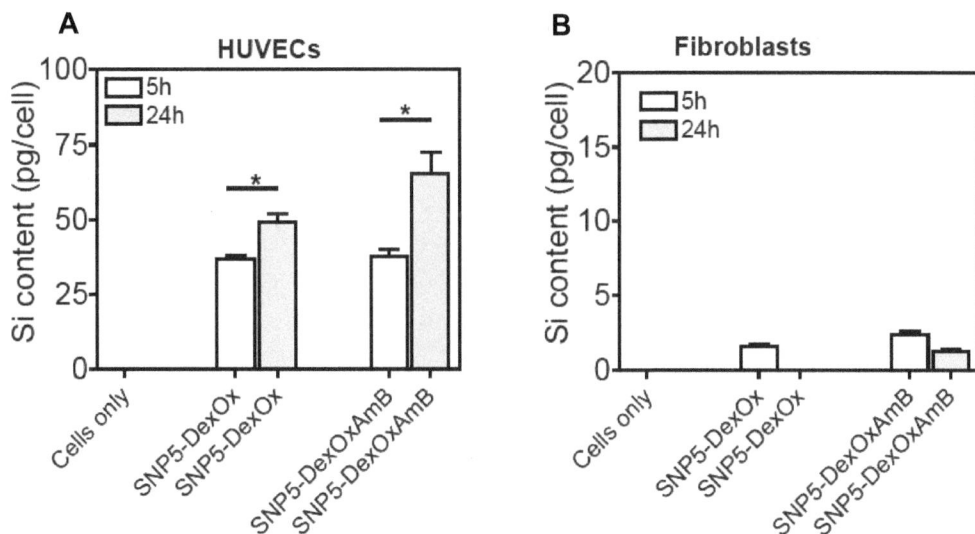

Fig. (2). Quantification of silicon in HUVECs (**A**) and human fibroblasts (**B**) as determined by ICP-MS analysis. Cells were incubated with SNP5-DexOx or SNP5-DexOxAmB (50 µg/mL) for 5 or 24 hrs. After the incubation, the cells were washed, trypsinized and finally freeze-dried. The concentration of silicon was normalized per cell. The results are expressed as Mean ± SEM (*n*=3). * Denotes statistical significance (*P*<0.05). Reprinted with permission from ref. [11].

Differences in the internalization level of the NPs might explain the lower ROS production induced by NPs with corona than without corona. NPs in serum free medium interacted more strongly with the membrane of lung epithelial A549 cells and were internalized in higher amounts than NPs with the preformed protein corona in serum supplemented medium [36].

Not only inorganic but also organic NPs such as PLGA NPs of different sizes (60, 100 and 200 nm) induce the production of ROS [25]. Mouse macrophages RAW264.7 and human bronchial epithelial BEAS-2B cells incubated for 24 hrs with bare PLGA NPs with different sizes (60, 100 and 200 nm) show a cytotoxic profile that was size dependent. The smallest NPs were the most effective in inducing cell damage, by the generation of superoxide radicals, a decrease in mitochondrial membrane potential and an increase in cytosolic Ca^{2+} [25]. Experimental results indicate that the oxidative stress induced by PLGA NPs is time and dose-dependent. The oxidative effect of PLGA and poloxamer (PLGA-PEO-NPs) NPs on rat hepatocytes was not detected at 4 hrs but detected at 24 hrs. Furthermore, ROS generation was dependent on the NP concentration [37].

Inflammatory Response

Depending on the physico-chemical properties, NPs can either activate or down-regulate inflammatory responses (Fig. **1**). Inflammatory responses are result of cascade of highly regulated events take place upon stimulation by foreign materials and are major process through which body defends itself and repair damaged tissues. The capacity of NPs to downregulate inflammatory responses has been used for biomedical applications. For example, organogold compounds have been used to treat rheumatic diseases since 1930 [2]. GNPs with a diameter of 5 nm completely down regulate the inflammatory pathways in THP-1 cells, a human myeloid leukaemia cell line [38]. This effect is dependent on the size of the NPs since GNPs with 15 or 35 nm have no effect. The anti-inflammatory activity of GNPs with a diameter of 5 nm is correlated with their capacity to interact with extracellular IL-1β and thereby neutralizing the inflammatory properties of this cytokine. Immunological responses produced after exposure to GNPs depend not only on core of the GNPs but also on surface charge, functionality and the protein corona [29, 39, 40]. For example, poly(acrylic acid) (PAA) coated GNPs bind to and induce unfolding of fibrinogen, which promotes interaction with integrin receptor (Mac-1) of monocytes, resulting in release of inflammatory cytokines [41]. GNPs with different hydrophobicities showed a direct quantitative correlation between hydrophobicity and immune activation in particular increased expression of TNF-α and IL-10 [42].

The immunomodulatory properties of NPs are, in some cases, due to their capacity to interfere with cellular toll-like receptors (TLRs). For example, GNPs cause specific inhibition of TLR9 (CpGoligodeoxynucleotides) [43]. The impaired CpG-ODN-induced TNF- α production is GNP concentration- and size-dependent in murine Raw264.7 cells. The effect is higher for GNPs of 4 nm than for diameters of 11, 19, 35 or 45 nm. Interestingly, GNPs can bind to high-mobility group box-1 inside the lysosomes, which is involved in the regulation of TLR9 signaling. Therefore, the down-regulation of inflammatory properties is due to the effect of GNPs in the translocation of TLR9 to cell membrane mediated by its binding to high-mobility group box-1 protein [43].

The exposure of SNPs of smaller (20 nm) and larger (300 nm) sizes to endothelial cells induce expression of inflammatory cytokines such as TNF-α, IL-6, MCP-1,

IL-8 and the coagulation-related protein TF [17]. The internalization of 300 nm SNPs is related to exocytosis of Weibel-Palade bodies (WPBs), which are intracellular storage sites for inflammatory cytokines and proteins and the coagulatory protein von Willebrand factor (VWF) [44]. Smaller size (60 nm) PLGA NPs of concentration up to 100 µg/ml trigger more release of TNF-α from RAW264.7 cells in comparison with 100 nm NPs of concentration 300 µg/mL [25]. However, micro size PLGA particles are potent inflammatory stimulus to cells and trigger the release of several cytokines [45, 46].

Cytotoxic Response of GNPs, SNPs and PLGA NPs

GNPs

HeLA cells incubated with GNPs with various sizes (14, 30, 50, 74 and 100 nm) and shapes (spherical and rod-shaped NPs) showed maximum uptake for NPs size of 50 nm [47]. The uptake of the NPs significantly increased for the first 2 hrs and gradually slowed and reached a plateau at 4-7 hrs [47]. Such an optimum size of NP affects the binding and activation of receptor probably due to balance between multivalent crosslinking of receptors and the process of membrane wrapping involved in receptor mediated endocytosis [48, 49]. GNPs get internalized through receptor specific or non-specific endocytosis pathways, depending on chemical composition of ligands present on NP surface, and accumulate at endocytic vesicles, cytoplasm or perinuclear regions of cells [47].

The cytotoxicity of GNPs depends on their size, geometry, charge and concentration. A summary of cytotoxicity results on both gold spherical and gold nanorods is provided in Table **1**. Cytotoxicity of GNPs is influenced by their size. Spherical GNPs of size ranging from 4 to 100 nm neither induce any cytotoxicity nor impaired the morphology of various cells such as HeLa, human leukemia, human dermal endothelial and mouse macrophage cells up to 100 µg/mL, even though they are being mostly internalized into cells based on MTT assay [30, 47, 50, 51]. In addition, large aggregates of GNPs (up to 100 nm) induce no cytotoxicity on different cells [10]. In contrast, 1.4 nm GNPs capped with triphenylphosphinemonosulfonate are more cytotoxic than 15 nm GNPs with similar surface functionality to human carcinoma cells by triggering intracellular reactive oxygen species (ROS), necrosis and mitochondrial damage [52].

Table 1.   **Summary of *In Vitro* Cytotoxicity Data of GNPs**

Cell Line	Morpho-logy of GNPs	Surface Functionali-zation	Cell Culture Conditions	GNP Concentration and Average Size		Cytotoxicity Assay	Toxicity Results	Refs.
Human liver carcinoma, HepG2 COS-1, Red blood cells	Spherical	BSA, 4 nuclear targeting peptides, NH₃ and COOH containing molecules	85% confluency 80% confluency	N/A 0.38, 0.75, 1.5 and 3 µM	20-25 nm 2 nm	LDH MTT, trypan blue, Cos-1 viability assay	95% viable LC50:anionic-1 µM and cationic> 7.5 µM	[54,60]
COS-7 cells	Spherical	PEI	3 x 10⁵ cells/well	N/A	4 nm	MTT	70-78% viability	[54]
Human breast carcinoma xenograft cells, MDA-MB 231, RAW 264.7 macrophage cells	Spherical	Coumarin-PEG thiol, m-PEG-thiol Lysine, PLL	10⁵ cells/well 10⁵ cells/well	50-200 µg/mL 10, 25, 50 and 100 µM	10 nm 4 nm	Cell titer MTT	Non-toxic up to 200 µg/mL Toxic 85 % viable, 100 µM after 72 hrs	[80]
Human dermal fibroblast	Spherical	Citrate	N/A	0-0.8 mg/mL	13 nm	Microscopy	Viability decreases with dose	[81]
Human dermal microvascular endothelial cells	Spherical	Glucosamine, ethanediamine, hydroxylpropy leamine,	N/A	10-250 µg/mL	20-63 nm	MTS	99 % cell viable after 24 hrs	[50]
Human embryonic kidney	Rod	AEDP, plasmid, rhodamine	3x10⁵ cells/well	44 µg/mL	200 nm	WST	LD50= 750 µg/mL	[82]
HeLa cells	Rod	CTAB, PEG	5x10³ cells/well	0.01-0.5 mM,	65±5 nm	WST	CTAB-Rod: 80% cell died at 0.05 mM, PEG-Rod: 10/ died at 0.05 mM	[83, 84]
HeLa cells	Rod	Phosphatidylc holine	5x10³ cells/well	0.09-1.45 mM	65±5 nm	MTT	20% cell died at 1.45 mM	[84]

Surface chemistry/charge also plays a key role in internalization and cytotoxicity of GNPs. Positively charged GNPs functionalized with long carbon chains are generally more toxic to cells at a lower concentration due to combined effect of strong electrostatic interaction with negatively charged cell membrane and hydrophobicity induced toxicity [42]. In addition, a high degree of hydrophobicity of GNP surface elicits increased immune response with up-expression of various cytokines in comparison with the GNPs without any surface coatings [42, 51]. On the other hand, negatively charged, and short carbon chain functionalized GNPs have low internalization and exert no toxicity effect on cells [42]. Importantly, the ligand present at the surface of the NP has an important role in their cytotoxicity. It was found that cetyltrimethylammonium bromide (CTAB) capped gold nanorods are cytotoxic to HeLa cells [53]; however, the level of cytotoxicity was reduced after being modified with poly(ethylene glycol) (PEG), phosphatidylcholine, poly(acrylic acid) or poly(allylamine hydrochloride), indicating that the chemicals involved in the synthesis of gold nanorods play a role in their cytotoxicity [53].

The shape of gold nanomaterials seems also very important for their internalization and likely cytotoxicity response. The uptake of rod-shaped GNPs is lower than their spherical counterpart [47]. For example, HeLa cells took up 500 and 375% more 74 and 14 nm spherical GNPs than 74 × 14 nm rod-shaped GNPs, respectively. The reason for the differences might be due to differences in the curvature of the nanomaterials. The rod-shaped NPs have larger contact area with the cell receptors than the spherical NPs. Another reason might be due to differences in the surface chemistry either from the synthesis process of both nanomaterials or the adsorption of proteins from cell culture media. Unfortunately, the authors are not aware of a direct cytotoxicity comparison between rod-shaped and spherical-shaped GNPs using the same *in vitro* conditions. It is likely that for the same original concentration of GNPs (concentration added to the cell culture medium), the spherical-shaped GNPs will have higher cytotoxicity than the rod-shaped GNPs because the first ones are higher internalized than the second ones. However, the density of ligands at the surface of GNPs (which might be different for rod-shaped and spherical-shaped GNPs) might have an important effect in the cytotoxicity profile, and not only shape aspects. Recent results indicate that poly(acrylic acid) or poly(allylamine hydrochloride) gold nanorods at 1.0 nM resulted in significant toxicity to endothelial cells, while poly(ethylene glycol) gold nanorods had no significant toxicity against the same cells, indicating that the ligand might have a significant role in the overall cytotoxicity profile [54].

SNPs

The cytotoxicity of SNPs depends on their physiochemical properties. The IC_{50} of smaller SNPs (14 nm) is lower than larger SNPs (335 nm) for endothelial cells [8]. HUVECs exposed to 20 nm SNPs with concentration of 200 µg/mL suffer the increased cell membrane damage, necrosis and apoptosis, although the latter could be reversed by addition of antioxidant [17]. On contrary to this study, a low amount of larger size SNP (304 nm) in serum free media is toxic to HUVECs than smaller size SNPs [44]. Similarly, the death of HepG2 cells after exposure to amorphous SNPs (127 nm) is due to apoptosis induced by mitochondrial damage and ROS generation [55].

Subcellular localization of the SNPs influences their cytotoxicity. Perinuclear localization affects endothelial cell migration and proliferation, leading to cell necrosis [44]. SNPs with sizes around or below 70 nm can penetrate the nucleus, which promotes protein aggregates [56]. Additionally, positively charged spherical SNPs and silica nanotubes of small size are toxic to Caco-2 cells and HUVECs respectively due to easier internalization of large amount of nanoparticles [57, 58]. A summary of results on toxicity of SNPs is provided in Table **2**.

PLGA NPs

PLGA is a biodegradable polymer approved as drug delivery system in humans by the FDA and the EMA (European Medicine Agency). The rate and extent of PLGA NPs (average diameter of 100 nm) uptake differs among epithelial cell lines [59, 60]. The uptake reaches a plateau after 2-6 hrs. Confocal microscopy studies as well as internalization inhibition studies indicate that endocytosis is the main internalization mechanism of PLGA NPs. These NPs are then trafficked to subcellular compartments such as early endosomes, Golgi apparatus and endoplasmic reticulum [59]. NPs first encounter endosomes followed by retrieval or escape from the compartment and subsequent interaction with the exocytic organelles of the cell such as endoplasmic reticulum, the Golgi apparatus and secretory vesicles.

Table 2.   Summary of *In Vitro* Cytotoxicity Data of SNPs

Cell Line	Morphology of SNPs	Surface Functional -ization	Cell Culture Conditions	SNP Concentration and Average Size		Cytotoxicity Assay	Toxicity Results	Refs.
endothelial EAHY926	Spherical, amorphous	Bare	66,000 cells/well	33 to 47 μg/mL	14, 15, and 16 nm	MTT and LDH	50% reduction in cell viability	[8]
endothelial EAHY926	Spherical, amorphous	Bare	66,000 cells/well	89 and 254 μg/mL	19 and 60 nm,	MTT and LDH	50% reduction in cell viability	[8]
endothelial EAHY926	Spherical, amorphous	Bare	66,000 cells/well	1095 and 1087 μg/mL	104 and 335nm	MTT and LDH	50% reduction in cell viability	[8]
HUVEC	Spherical, amorphous	Bare	15000 cells/well	1000, 15000, 30000 NP/cell	16, 41, 80, 212, 304 nm	MTT and LDH Caspase 3/7 assay PI staining	At the highest concentration 304 nm NPs cause > 50% decrease in reduction of MTT, along with LDH leakage Cell death by necrosis	[44]
HUVEC	Spherical, amorphous	Bare	15000 cells/well	30000 NP/cell	304 nm	Scratch test. Confocal microscopy.	Slower migration and proliferation. Exocytosis of vasoactive VWF and inflammatory cytokines.	[44]
HUVEC	Hollow, mesoporous	Bare	10^5 cells per well	1.25 ng/cell	300-430 nm	Confocal microscopy. Quantification of Si content in medium by ICP-OES.	After 48 and 96h mostly lysosomal localization. Rapid uptake of NPs: 30 min. Si accumulation in medium fastest in the first two days, but continues increasing for at least 7 days.	[73]
A549 human lung epitlelial cell line	Spherical, amorphous	Bare	2.5×10^5 cells	250 μg/mL	50 nm	Flourescence measurement. ATP quantification.	Medium without serum: stronger interaction with cells and higher internalization rate. Cellular ATP content lower in cells incubated with NP in serum-free medium.	[36]
Caco-2, human epithelial colon carcinoma	Spherical, amorphous	Bare SiNP: -45,7 mV; PAA-SiNP: -53.6 mV; PDHA-SINP: -9,08 mV; PAEA-SiNP: 22.4 mV; PNIPAM-SiNP: -2.58 mV; PEG-SiNP: -3.66 mV	2.5×10^4 cells/well	200 to 1000 μg/mL	50 nm	MTT	Neutral polymers with high grafting density on SiNPs effectively protect cells from toxicity of silica core. Cationic polymer-SiNPs: high cytotoxicity. Neutral and anionic polymer-SiNPs: limited cytoxicity.	[58]

(Table 2) contd.....

Cell Line	Morphology of SNPs	Surface Functional-ization	Cell Culture Conditions	SNP Concentration and Average Size		Cytotoxicity Assay	Toxicity Results	Refs.
MDA-MB-231 and HUVEC	Nanotubes	Bare or amine-functionalized (APTMS) surface	1000 cells/well	0.005 to 5 μg/mL	50 nm diameter. 200 or 500 nm length	MTT	500 nm are more toxic than 200 nm nanotubes. Amine Funtionalized are more toxic than bare nanotubes.	[57]
HEp-2, RPMI 2650, A549, RLE-6TN, N2a	Spherical, amorphous	Bare	Sub confluence	25 μg/mL	50, 70, 200 and 500 nm	Fluorescence microscopy. Trypan blue exclusion. BrdU and Fl-U incorporation.	NPS with 50 and 70 nm: Formation of intranuclear protein aggregates. Inhibition of cell proliferation. No significant redution of cell viability.	[46]

PLGA NPs (with an average diameters around 100 nm) are substantially non-cytotoxic against several types of cells for concentrations up to 100 μg/mL. PLGA NPs with surface area between 3 and 10 m^2/g and concentration ranging from 1 to 100 μg/mL are non-toxic to Caco-2 and HeLa cells [61]. PLGA NPs coated with chitosan, poloxamer, poly(vinyl alcohol), and cetyltrimethyl-ammonium bromide having positive, neutral and negative charges do not induce cytotoxicity to cells [62, 63]. However, it have been shown that PLGA NPs coated with Tween-20 and poly (beta-amino esters) (PBAE) exhibit toxicity to brain endothelial and COS-7 cells respectively with the increasing concentration of functionalized ligands and NP doses [64, 65].

In vivo Biocompatibility of Nanomaterials

The *in vivo* evaluation of NP biodistribution, circulation, toxicity and elimination is of utmost importance to determine their biological impact. Typically, these studies are performed in mice or rats [4]. In some cases, it is difficult to predict the *in vivo* toxicity of NPs based on the *in vitro* toxicity results of NPs. To evaluate *in vivo* toxicity of NPs, the administration routes, dose of NPs and biodistribution of NPs in various tissues and organs need to be considered. Generally, systemically administrated NPs are taken up by liver and spleen in a large amount and small amounts distributed in kidney, lung, heart and brain after single administration [66, 67]. Different routes of administration can result in various effects on biodistribution of NPs in body. For instance, oral and intraperitonial administration of GNPs showed the highest toxicity while tail vein injection showed the lowest toxicity [68]. Similarly, the repeated dose of NPs can trigger immune response and toxicity to animals [69].

In vivo toxicity is generally evaluated by changes in blood serum chemistry and histological analysis. Serum protein from blood can be separated using electrophoresis and quantified using protein specific labeling methods. Some of typical biochemical indicators examined are amino transferase, albumin, glucose, creatinine, hemoglobin, urea and total protein. Toxicity assessment can be performed using probing inflammation and tissue/organ histology. Histological analysis is performed on tissues that have been fixed after exposure to animal and changes in cells or tissues morphology are observed using light or transmission electron microscope (TEM). Weight loss and animal behavior are other indicators for NP intolerance and toxicity. Moreover, the analysis of biomarkers for inflammation, oxidative stress and cell viability would provide mechanistic study into NP toxicity. Biodistribution studies usually perform in tandem to examine localization of NPs in tissues or organs and follow the transport of NPs through animal over time. Overall biodistribution of NPs in blood and various organs can be analyzed by inductively coupled plasma-mass spectrometry (ICP-MS) and conjugating NPs with dye or radiolabel materials [4]. As with *in vitro* studies, it is also be important to consider many aspects prior to *in vivo* studies such as choice of suitable NPs and characterizations prior to exposure and relevant model systems.

In vivo studies are complicated in terms of what is happening inside animal after short/long exposure and the facile assessment of localized concentration and trafficking of NPs. *In vivo* nanotoxicology studies could get benefit from dynamic *in vivo* tests such as microfluidics and microeletrochemistry where samples are taken from live animals through implanted probe. This section summarizes the effect of GNPs, SNPs and PLGA NPs on various animal models.

GNPs

The size dictates the biodistribution of GNPs. The various sizes of GNPs (15, 50, 100 and 200 nm) administered intravenously in mice were mainly accumulated in liver, lung and spleen [4]. A large amount of small GNPs (15 nm) was also accumulated in blood, liver, lung, spleen, kidney, and stomach and was able to pass blood-brain barrier, however, a tiny amount of 200 nm GNPs was found in brain, stomach and kidney. In another study, 1.4 nm GNP can be translocated through air-blood barrier of respiratory tract while 18 nm GNPs are completely trapped in lung [4, 70]. Citrate stabilized GNPs help to downregulate interleukin induced inflammatory response in C57BL/6 mice and do not promote platelet aggregation and coagulation [42, 70].

The biodistribution of GNPs is influenced by surface charge. Neutral and zwitterionic GNPs (2 nm in diameter core; overall hydrodynamic diameter of 9-10 nm) have longer circulation time *via* both intraperitoneal and intravenous injections, whereas negatively and positively charged NPs have relatively short half-lives [67] (Fig. **3**). The surface functionalization of GNPs is also a key player in governing the fate of GNPs and in inducting immune response in animal. Large size of GNPs (80 nm) functionalized with PEG is cleared from blood within a minute is relocated to liver and spleen after administration, which could cause acute inflammation and apoptosis [4]. On the other hand, smaller GNPs (20 nm) take approximately 40 min to clear from blood. PEG coated GNPs (13 nm) induced acute inflammation and apoptosis in liver and accumulated in liver and spleen up to 7 days after injection (Fig. **4**) [71]. Interestingly, no apparent histopathological abnormalities or lesions are found in near-infrared (NIR) exposed PEG-GNPs coated silicon nanowires (PEG-GNPs@SiNWs) exposed organs (Fig. **4**) [72]. In addition, hydrophobic moieties functionalized GNPs induces immune response in mouse with an increasing hydrophobicity [42]. GNPs functionalized with glutathione are voided through the renal system within 1 hr and 60% of the NPs are excreted within 8 hrs [73]. Mice injected with glutathione-coated GNPs did not experience any clinical signs of illness, stress, or discomfort, nor did any expire over the course of the entire 6-week study [73].

According to FDA guidelines, pharmaceutical drugs and nanomaterials should be eliminated *via* metabolism or excretion process once they have been administered in the body. No long-term studies of GNPs on *in vivo* system have been reported yet. GNPs are generally larger than renal filtration cutoff (5 nm), it was found that GNPs were eliminated from the blood by reticuloendotelial system (RES) and thus to accumulate in spleen and liver [74]. While the most of studies are based on animal models (such as mice, rats and pigs), Zebrafish and Daniorerio have also been used as *in vivo* model to assess toxicity of NPs. Zebrafish is an excellent *in vivo* model due to its high degree of homology with human genome. GNPs of different size ranging from 3 to 100 nm are not cytotoxic to both Zebrafish and Daniorerio embryos in dose and time dependent manner [4].

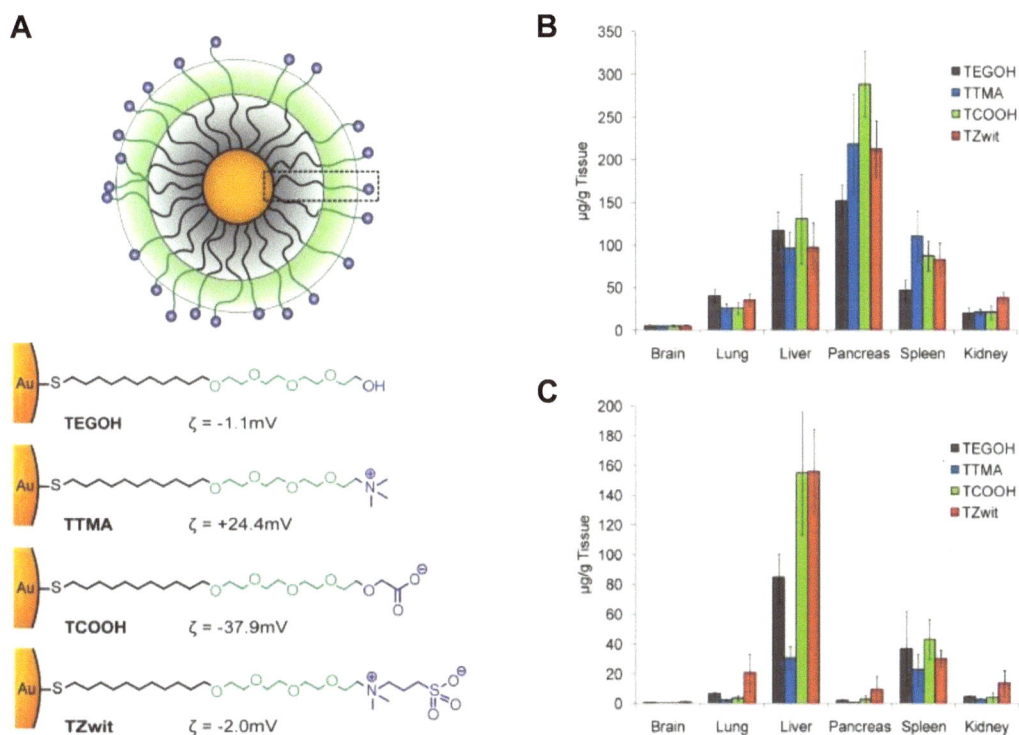

Fig. (3). (A) GNPs of different surface charges were generated by chemical modification of the terminal portion of the ligand bonded to the NP core. Four types of GNPs were used: neutral (TEGOH), positive (TTMA), negative (TCOOH) and zwitterionic (TZwit). The surface charge was measured by zeta potential. (B-C) *In vivo* mean gold concentration (µg) per gram of organ 24 hrs post **(B)** IP injection and **(C)** IV injection. The mode of administration and the ligand end group of GNPs affects the level of gold uptake in different tissues with the RES being the dominant mode of clearance. Data points are the mean +/- SEM from n=5 animals. Results are reported as gold concentration (µg) per gram of organ. Reprinted with permission from ref. [44].

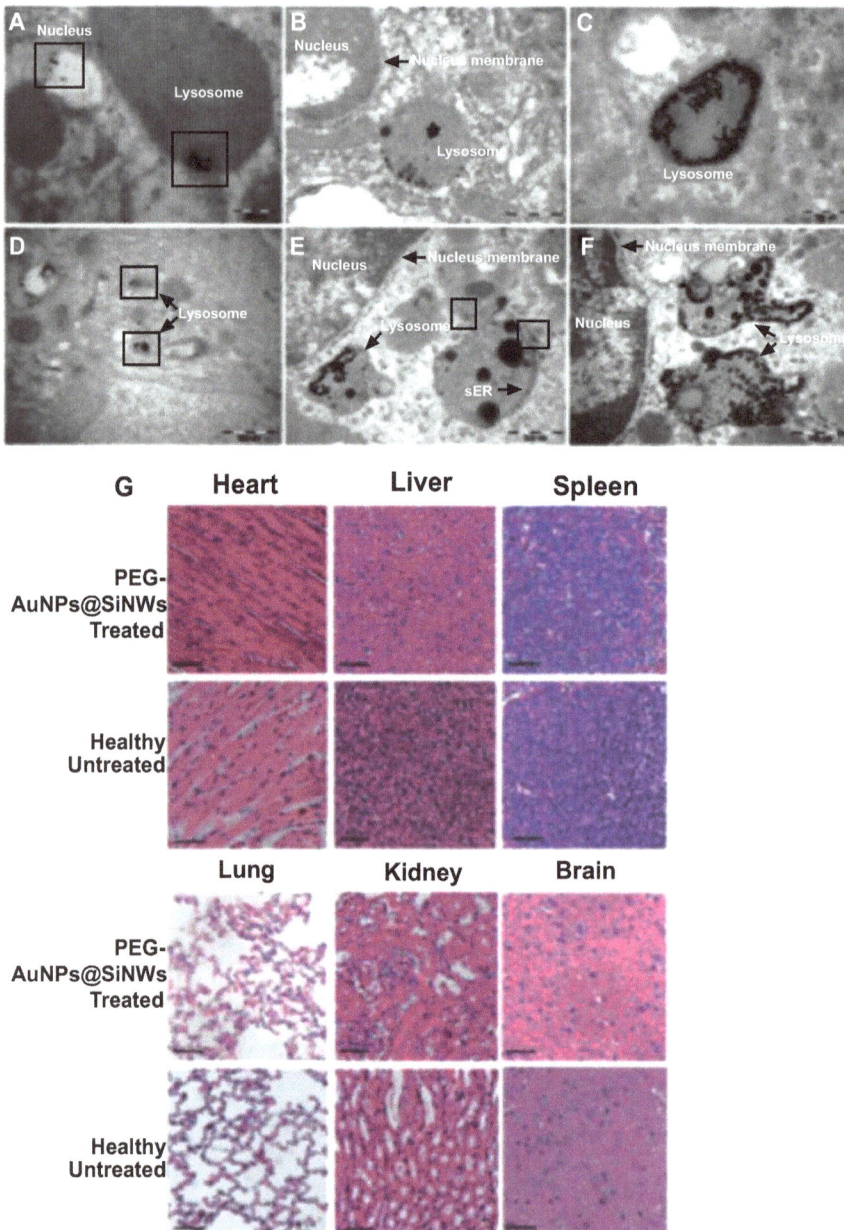

Fig. (4). Thin section TEM images of mouse liver and spleen tissues at 24 hrs or 7 days after intravenous injection of PEG-coated Au NPs. Kupffer cells at (**A**) 24 hrs and (**B, C**) 7 days post injection at scope magnifications of (**A**) 100,000x (**B**) 50,000x and (**C**) 100,000x. Spleen macrophages at (**D**) 24 hrs or (**E, F**) 7 days after injection at scope magnifications of (**D**) 50,000x, (**E**) 50,000x and (**F**) 50,000x. (**G**) H&E stain photos of major organs harvested from the mice treated with the SiNW based nanoagents. Reprinted with permission from refs. [71, 72].

SNPs

The ease to synthesize various sizes and shape SNPs and their surface functionalization provides plethora of opportunities for applications in nanomedicine. However, concerns remain about potential toxic effect of these NPs after exposure to animals. Porous SNPs of size 126 nm functionalized with doxorubicin (ζ = -39 mV) injected at dose of 20 mg/kg into tail vain of BALB/c mice were degraded into non-toxic orthosilicic acid and small particles and were rapidly excreted by kidney. Porous SNPs were accumulated in liver and spleen during initial period of administration however, the level of silicon in these organs returned to normal after 4 weeks. No significant change in body mass of mice was detected over 4-week period using inductively coupled plasma-optical emission spectrometry ICP-OES) [75]. On the other hand, hexagonal mesoporous NPs (50 to 100 nm) injected at a dose of 16 mg/Kg into the tail vein of Sprague-Dawley rats were accumulated in liver, stomach and intestines after 3 hrs of administration. Moreover, highly charged (34.4 mV) NPs were excreted faster in the bile, and the peak levels of excretion in feces were reached 2 days after injection. Particles with a low charge density (-17.6 mV) were retained in the liver [76]. *In vivo* cytotoxicity of SNPs is also greatly influenced by NP porosity and aspect ratio. The maximum tolerated dose (MTD) of mesoporous SNPs (aspect ratio 1, 2, 8) is lower in comparison with either amine modified or nonporous SNPs of same aspect ratio when exposed intravenously to animal. Mesoporous SNPs exerted considerable systemic toxicity irrespective of the geometrical features [77]. It is found that bare SNPs of size 70 nm can cross placenta barrier of pregnant mice after intravenous administration while such observation is not found with the amine and carboxyl groups modified SNPs (70 nm) and larger size (300 nm) bare SNPs [78].

PLGA NPs

PLGA NPs with surface area ranging from 3 to 10 m^2/g and size from 200 to 350 nm show no specific pathological effects in mice, however the NPs were detected in brain, liver, long, kidney, heart and spleen after 7 days [61]. After intravenous injection, NPs should be present in blood circulation for longer time in order to reach the target. NPs must be able to escape from the clearance function of macrophages of the reticuloendothelial system (RES) located in the liver (Kupffer cells) and in the spleen (mononuclear phagocyte system, MPS). The increasing dose of 0.1 to 20 mg PLGA-PEG NPs does not alter the rate of blood clearance of NPs, although the level of IgM increases proportionally, meaning that threshold of IgM level is required for enhanced clearance of NPs [79]. PLGA NPs conjugated with anticancer drugs such as cisplatin, doxorubicin, paclitaxel, 5-fluorouracil, 9-nitrocamptothecin, triptorelin, dexamethasone, xanthone, and PE38KDL have been successfully used for treatment of cancer in *in vivo* model [80]. Furthermore, numerous antigens for instances proteins, peptides, lipopeptides, cell lysates, viruses or plasmid DNA have been formulated in PLGA NPs for the treatment of inflammation, infections, cerebral and cardiovascular diseases, osteoporosis and diabetes [5]. Recently, miRNA delivery using PLGA NPs is tested for proangiogenic effect in both *in vitro* and *in vivo* models [14].

FUTRURE PERSPECTIVES

A considerable number of studies have analyzed the toxic profile of a single type of NP with a limited range of properties. Large-scale comparative studies need to be performed for further understanding the toxicity of NPs under the same conditions. It is important to perform these studies using different cell lines and exposure conditions (cell confluency, exposure duration, NP concentration, *etc.*). In addition, it is important to define very well the end-points of cytotoxicity. In many studies, the toxicity of the nanomaterials is evaluated by cell death; however, nanomaterials might affect cell activity/function without inducing cell death. For example nanomaterials might induce cell senescence. Therefore, it will be important to evaluate cellular signaling alterations for sub-lethal concentrations of NPs. In addition, it will be important to evaluate the toxicity of NPs against an universal NP standard. GNPs have been suggested as a reference NP for low toxicity [7], because only 15% reduction in cell viability has been observed for concentrations up to 200 μg/mL.

Few studies have quantified the real concentration of NPs internalized by the cells. Typically, the initial dose of NPs added to cells is used to evaluate the cytotoxicity of NPs. Future studies should monitor cellular NP internalization by recording the intracellular levels of NPs. In addition, it will be important to study in more detail the intracellular trafficking of the NPs since the cytotoxicity profile may be related to their accumulation in specific cellular organelles.

Further studies are needed to establish a direct correlation between *in vitro* and *in vivo* results. In order to set the standard rules for safe delivery of NPs, it is required the accurate physiochemical characterization of NPs in biological environments and the study of their toxicity mechanism either *in vitro* or *in vivo*. Additionally the development of *in situ* techniques for real time dynamic characterization of toxicity of NPs in living animals and computer simulation to interpolate *in vitro* data to *in vivo* metabolism will boost our understanding on toxicity, which would help in designing clinically relevant and safer NPs.

A thorough understanding of biological behavior and safety aspect of NPs requires how different compositions of NPs interact with biological membrane, organelles, and biomolecules, these generally lack systematic investigation so far. *In vivo*, NP's surface is in direct contact with the biological milieu and therefore in dynamic exchange with biomolecules capable of changing NP properties. A major challenge is to identify crucial relationship between physiochemical properties of NPs and their *in vivo* toxicities. The appropriate modulation of surface functionality of NPs is crucial in determining their cellular transport, overall biodistribution and pharmacokinetics.

ACKNOWLEDGEMENTS

This work was funded by FEDER through the "ProgramaOperacionalFactores de Competitividade- COMPETE" and by Portuguese funds through FCT in the context of the project PTDC/ Qui-Qui / 105000 / 2008, and COMPETE funding (Project "Stem cell based platforms for Regenerative and Therapeutic Medicine", Centro-07-ST24-FEDER-002008). The authors would like to thank the financial support of Marie Curie Initial Training Network (project 289454).

CONFLICT OF INTEREST

The authors confirm that this chapter contents have no conflict of interest.

ABBREVIATIONS

3MRs   =   3 members-ring

CTAB   =   Cetyltrimethylammonium bromide

EMA   =   European Medicine Agency

GNPs   =   Gold nanoparticles

HUVECs   =   Human umbilical vein endothelial cells

ICP-MS   =   Inductively coupled plasma-mass spectrometry

LDH   =   Lactate dehydrogenase

MTD   =   Maximum tolerated dose

MTT   =   3-(4,5-dimethylthiazol- 2-yl)-2,5-diphenyl tetrazolium bromide

NPs   =   Nanoparticles

PC3   =   Prostatic cell lines

PEG   =   Poly(ethylene glycol)

PLA   =   Poly(lactic acid)

PLG   =   Poly(D,L-glycolide)

PLGA   =   Poly(lactide-co-glycolide)

RBCs   =   Red blood cells

ROS   =   Reactive oxygen species

SNPs   =   Silica nanoparticles

TEM   =   Transmission electron microscope

TNF-α   =   Tumor necrosis factor-α

VWF   =   Willebrand factor

REFERENCES

[1]   Michalet, X.; Pinaud, F. F.; Bentolila, L. A.; Tsay, J. M.; Doose, S.; Li, J. J.; Sundaresan, G.; Wu, A. M.; Gambhir, S. S.; Weiss, S., Quantum dots for live cells, *in vivo* imaging, and diagnostics. *Science* 2005, *307* (5709), 538-44.

[2]   Thakor, A.; Jokerst, J.; Zavaleta, C.; Massoud, T.; Gambhir, S., Gold nanoparticles: a revival in precious metal administration to patients. *Nano Lett* 2011, *11* (10), 4029-4036.

[3]   Bitar, A.; Ahmad, N. M.; Fessi, H.; Elaissari, A., Silica-based nanoparticles for biomedical applications. *Drug Discov Today* 2012, *17* (19-20), 1147-54.

[4]   Khlebtsov, N.; Dykman, L., Biodistribution and toxicity of engineered gold nanoparticles: a review of *in vitro* and *in vivo* studies. *ChemSoc Rev* 2011, *40* (3), 1647-1671.

[5]   Danhier, F.; Ansorena, E.; Silva, J. M.; Coco, R.; Le Breton, A.; Preat, V., PLGA-based nanoparticles: an overview of biomedical applications. *J Control Release* 2012, *161* (2), 505-22.

[6]   Vauthier, C.; Dubernet, C.; Chauvierre, C.; Brigger, I.; Couvreur, P., Drug delivery to resistant tumors: the potential of poly(alkyl cyanoacrylate) nanoparticles. *J Control Release* 2003, *93* (2), 151-60.

[7]   Lewinski, N.; Colvin, V.; Drezek, R., Cytotoxicity of nanoparticles. *Small* 2008, *4* (1), 26-49.

[8]   Napierska, D.; Thomassen, L. C.; Rabolli, V.; Lison, D.; Gonzalez, L.; Kirsch-Volders, M.; Martens, J. A.; Hoet, P. H., Size-dependent cytotoxicity of monodisperse silica nanoparticles in human endothelial cells. *Small* 2009, *5* (7), 846-53.

[9]   Pan, Y.; Neuss, S.; Leifert, A.; Fischler, M.; Wen, F.; Simon, U.; Schmid, G.; Brandau, W.; Jahnen-Dechent, W., Size-dependent cytotoxicity of gold nanoparticles. *Small* 2007, *3* (11), 1941-9.

[10]   Albanese, A.; Chan, W. C., Effect of gold nanoparticle aggregation on cell uptake and toxicity. *ACS Nano* 2011, *5* (7), 5478-89.

[11]   Paulo, C. S.; Lino, M. M.; Matos, A. A.; Ferreira, L. S., Differential internalization of amphotericin B--conjugated nanoparticles in human cells and the expression of heat shock protein 70. *Biomaterials* 2013, *34* (21), 5281-93.

[12]   Cho, E. C.; Zhang, Q.; Xia, Y., The effect of sedimentation and diffusion on cellular uptake of gold nanoparticles. *Nat Nanotechnol* 2011, *6* (6), 385-91.

[13]   Diaz, B.; Sanchez-Espinel, C.; Arruebo, M.; Faro, J.; de Miguel, E.; Magadan, S.; Yague, C.; Fernandez-Pacheco, R.; Ibarra, M. R.; Santamaria, J.; Gonzalez-Fernandez, A., Assessing methods for blood cell cytotoxic responses to inorganic nanoparticles and nanoparticle aggregates. *Small* 2008, *4* (11), 2025-34.

[14]   Gomes, R. S.; das Neves, R. P.; Cochlin, L.; Lima, A.; Carvalho, R.; Korpisalo, P.; Dragneva, G.; Turunen, M.; Liimatainen, T.; Clarke, K.; Yla-Herttuala, S.; Carr, C.; Ferreira, L., Efficient pro-survival/angiogenicmiRNA delivery by an MRI-detectable nanomaterial. *ACS Nano* 2013, *7* (4), 3362-72.

[15]   Koopman, G.; Reutelingsperger, C. P.; Kuijten, G. A.; Keehnen, R. M.; Pals, S. T.; van Oers, M. H., Annexin V for flow cytometric detection of phosphatidylserine expression on B cells undergoing apoptosis. *Blood* 1994, *84* (5), 1415-20.

[16]   Waring, M. J., Complex formation between ethidium bromide and nucleic acids. *J MolBiol* 1965, *13* (1), 269-82.

[17]   Liu, X.; Sun, J., Endothelial cells dysfunction induced by silica nanoparticles through oxidative stress *via* JNK/P53 and NF-kappa B pathways. *Biomaterials* 2010, *31* (32), 8198-8209.

[18]   Arvizo, R. R.; Miranda, O. R.; Thompson, M. A.; Pabelick, C. M.; Bhattacharya, R.; Robertson, J. D.; Rotello, V. M.; Prakash, Y. S.; Mukherjee, P., Effect of nanoparticle surface charge at the plasma membrane and beyond. *Nano Lett* 2010, *10* (7), 2543-8.

[19]   Monteith, G. R.; McAndrew, D.; Faddy, H. M.; Roberts-Thomson, S. J., Calcium and cancer: targeting Ca2+ transport. *Nat Rev Cancer* 2007, *7* (7), 519-530.

[20]   Goodman, C. M.; McCusker, C. D.; Yilmaz, T.; Rotello, V. M., Toxicity of gold nanoparticles functionalized with cationic and anionic side chains. *Bioconjugate Chem* 2004, *15* (4), 897-900.

[21]   Leroueil, P. R.; Berry, S. A.; Duthie, K.; Han, G.; Rotello, V. M.; McNerny, D. Q.; Baker, J. R.; Orr, B. G.; Holl, M. M. B., Wide varieties of cationic nanoparticles induce defects in supported lipid bilayers. *Nano Lett* 2008, *8* (2), 420-424.

[22]   Lin, Y. S.; Haynes, C. L., Impacts of Mesoporous Silica Nanoparticle Size, Pore Ordering, and Pore Integrity on Hemolytic Activity. *J Am Chem Soc* 2010, *132* (13), 4834-4842.

[23]   Zhang, H. Y.; Dunphy, D. R.; Jiang, X. M.; Meng, H.; Sun, B. B.; Tarn, D.; Xue, M.; Wang, X.; Lin, S. J.; Ji, Z. X.; Li, R. B.; Garcia, F. L.; Yang, J.; Kirk, M. L.; Xia, T.; Zink, J. I.; Nel, A.; Brinker, C. J., Processing Pathway Dependence of Amorphous Silica Nanoparticle Toxicity: Colloidal *vs* Pyrolytic. *J Am ChemSoc* 2012, *134* (38), 15790-15804.

[24]   Fede, C.; Selvestrel, F.; Compagnin, C.; Mognato, M.; Mancin, F.; Reddi, E.; Celotti, L., The toxicity outcome of silica nanoparticles (Ludox (R)) is influenced by testing techniques and treatment modalities. *Anal BioanalChem* 2012, *404* (6-7), 1789-1802.

[25]   Xiong, S. J.; George, S.; Yu, H. Y.; Damoiseaux, R.; France, B.; Ng, K. W.; Loo, J. S. C., Size influences the cytotoxicity of poly (lactic-co-glycolic acid) (PLGA) and titanium dioxide (TiO2) nanoparticles. *ArchToxicol* 2013, *87* (6), 1075-1086.

[26]   Li, J.; Hartono, D.; Ong, C.-N.; Bay, B.-H.; Yung, L.-Y. L., Autophagy and oxidative stress associated with gold nanoparticles. *Biomaterials* 2010, *31* (23), 5996-6003.

[27]   Jia, H.; Liu, Y.; Zhang, X.; Han, L.; Du, L.; Tian, Q.; Xu, Y., Potential oxidative stress of gold nanoparticles by induced-NO releasing in serum. *J Am ChemSoc* 2009, *131* (1), 40-41.

[28]   Li, J.; Muralikrishnan, S.; Ng, C.-T.; Yung, L.-Y. L.; Bay, B.-H., Nanoparticle-induced pulmonary toxicity. *ExpBiolMed* 2010, *235* (9), 1025-1033.

[29]   Chompoosor, A.; Saha, K.; Ghosh, P.; Macarthy, D.; Miranda, O.; Zhu, Z.-J.; Arcaro, K.; Rotello, V., The role of surface functionality on acute cytotoxicity, ROS generation and DNA damage by cationic gold nanoparticles. *Small* 2010, *6* (20), 2246-2249.

[30]   Connor, E.; Mwamuka, J.; Gole, A.; Murphy, C.; Wyatt, M., Gold nanoparticles are taken up by human cells but do not cause acute cytotoxicity. *Small* 2005, *1* (3), 325-327.

[31]   Zhang, Q.; Hitchins, V. M.; Schrand, A. M.; Hussain, S. M.; Goering, P. L., Uptake of gold nanoparticles in murine macrophage cells without cytotoxicity or production of pro-inflammatory mediators. *Nanotoxicology* 2011, *5* (3), 284-95.

[32]   Yang, H.; Liu, C.; Yang, D. F.; Zhang, H. S.; Xi, Z. G., Comparative study of cytotoxicity, oxidative stress and genotoxicity induced by four typical nanomaterials: the role of particle size, shape and composition. *J ApplToxicol* 2009, *29* (1), 69-78.

[33]   Carlson, C.; Hussain, S. M.; Schrand, A. M.; Braydich-Stolle, L. K.; Hess, K. L.; Jones, R. L.; Schlager, J. J., Unique Cellular Interaction of Silver Nanoparticles: Size-Dependent Generation of Reactive Oxygen Species. *J PhysChem B* 2008, *112* (43), 13608-13619.

[34]   Jiang, J.; Oberdorster, G.; Elder, A.; Gelein, R.; Mercer, P.; Biswas, P., Does nanoparticle activity depend upon size and crystal phase? *Nanotoxicology* 2008, *2* (1), 33-42.

[35]   Shi, J.; Karlsson, H. L.; Johansson, K.; Gogvadze, V.; Xiao, L.; Li, J.; Burks, T.; Garcia-Bennett, A.; Uheida, A.; Muhammed, M.; Mathur, S.; Morgenstern, R.; Kagan, V. E.; Fadeel, B., Microsomal Glutathione Transferase 1 Protects Against Toxicity Induced by Silica Nanoparticles but Not by Zinc Oxide Nanoparticles. *ACS Nano* 2012, *6* (3), 1925-1938.

[36]   Lesniak, A.; Fenaroli, F.; Monopoli, M. R.; Aberg, C.; Dawson, K. A.; Salvati, A., Effects of the Presence or Absence of a Protein Corona on Silica Nanoparticle Uptake and Impact on Cells. *ACS Nano* 2012, *6* (7), 5845-5857.

[37]   Aranda, A.; Sequedo, L.; Tolosa, L.; Quintas, G.; Burello, E.; Castell, J. V.; Gombau, L., Dichloro-dihydro-fluorescein diacetate (DCFH-DA) assay: a quantitative method for oxidative stress assessment of nanoparticle-treated cells. *Toxicol In Vitro* 2013, *27* (2), 954-63.

[38]   Sumbayev, V.; Yasinska, I.; Garcia, C.; Gilliland, D.; Lall, G.; Gibbs, B.; Bonsall, D.; Varani, L.; Rossi, F. o.; Calzolai, L., Gold nanoparticles downregulate interleukin-1ΠΞ-induced pro-inflammatory responses. *Small* 2013, *9* (3), 472-477.

[39]   Albanese, A.; Tang, P. S.; Chan, W. C. W., The Effect of Nanoparticle Size, Shape, and Surface Chemistry on Biological Systems. *Annu Rev Biomed Eng* 2012, *14*, 1-16.

[40]   Kim, S. T.; Saha, K.; Kim, C.; Rotello, V. M., The Role of Surface Functionality in Determining Nanoparticle Cytotoxicity. *AccChem Res* 2013*46*(3), 681-691.

[41]   Deng, Z.; Liang, M.; Monteiro, M.; Toth, I.; Minchin, R., Nanoparticle-induced unfolding of fibrinogen promotes Mac-1 receptor activation and inflammation. *Nat Nanotechnol* 2011, *6* (1), 39-44.

[42]   Moyano, D.; Goldsmith, M.; Solfiell, D.; Landesman-Milo, D.; Miranda, O.; Peer, D.; Rotello, V., Nanoparticle hydrophobicity dictates immune response. *J Am ChemSoc* 2012, *134* (9), 3965-3967.

[43]   Tsai, C.-Y.; Lu, S.-L.; Hu, C.-W.; Yeh, C.-S.; Lee, G.-B.; Lei, H.-Y., Size-depnedent attenuation of TLR9 signaling by gold nanoparticles in macrophages. *J Immunol* 2012, *188*.

[44]   Bauer, A. T.; Strozyk, E. A.; Gorzelanny, C.; Westerhausen, C.; Desch, A.; Schneider, M. F.; Schneider, S. W., Cytotoxicity of silica nanoparticles through exocytosis of von Willebrand factor and necrotic cell death in primary human endothelial cells. *Biomaterials* 2011, *32* (33), 8385-8393.

[45]   Sy, J. C.; Seshadri, G.; Yang, S. C.; Brown, M.; Oh, T.; Dikalov, S.; Murthy, N.; Davis, M. E., Sustained release of a p38 inhibitor from non-inflammatory microspheres inhibits cardiac dysfunction. *Nat Mater* 2008, *7* (11), 863-868.

[46]   Nicolete, R.; dos Santos, D.; Faccioli, L., The uptake of PLGA micro or nanoparticles by macrophages provokes distinct *in vitro* inflammatory response. *Int Immunopharmacol* 2011, *11* (10), 1557.

[47]   Chithrani, B.; Ghazani, A.; Chan, W., Determining the size and shape dependence of gold nanoparticle uptake into mammalian cells. *Nano Lett* 2006, *6* (4), 662-668.

[48]   Jiang, W.; Kim, B.; Rutka, J.; Chan, W., Nanoparticle-mediated cellular response is size-dependent. *Nat Nanotechnol* 2008, *3* (3), 145-150.

[49]   Nel, A.; M√§dler, L.; Velegol, D.; Xia, T.; Hoek, E.; Somasundaran, P.; Klaessig, F.; Castranova, V.; Thompson, M., Understanding biophysicochemical interactions at the nano-bio interface. *Nat Mater* 2009, *8* (7), 543-557.

[50]   Freese, C.; Gibson, M.; Klok, H.-A.; Unger, R.; Kirkpatrick, C., Size- and coating-dependent uptake of polymer-coated gold nanoparticles in primary human dermal microvascular endothelial cells. *Biomacromolecules* 2012, *13* (5), 1533-1543.

[51]   Shukla, R.; Bansal, V.; Chaudhary, M.; Basu, A.; Bhonde, R.; Sastry, M., Biocompatibility of gold nanoparticles and their endocytotic fate inside the cellular compartment: a microscopic overview. *Langmuir* 2005, *21* (23), 10644-10654.

[52]   Pan, Y.; Leifert, A.; Ruau, D.; Neuss, S.; Bornemann, J. r.; Schmid, G. n.; Brandau, W.; Simon, U.; Jahnen-Dechent, W., Gold nanoparticles of diameter 1.4 nm trigger necrosis by oxidative stress and mitochondrial damage. *Small* 2009, *5* (18), 2067-2076.

[53]   Murphy, C.; Gole, A.; Stone, J.; Sisco, P.; Alkilany, A.; Goldsmith, E.; Baxter, S., Gold nanoparticles in biology: beyond toxicity to cellular imaging. *AccChem Res* 2008, *41* (12), 1721-1730.

[54]   Alkilany, A. M.; Shatanawi, A.; Kurtz, T.; Caldwell, R. B.; Caldwell, R. W., Toxicity and cellular uptake of gold nanorods in vascular endothelium and smooth muscles of isolated rat blood vessel: importance of surface modification. *Small* 2012, *8* (8), 1270-8.

[55]   Sun, L.; Li, Y.; Liu, X.; Jin, M.; Zhang, L.; Du, Z.; Guo, C.; Huang, P.; Sun, Z., Cytotoxicity and mitochondrial damage caused by silica nanoparticles. *Toxicology in Vitro* 2011, *25* (8), 1619-1629.

[56]   Chen, M.; von Mikecz, A., Formation of nucleoplasmic protein aggregates impairs nuclear function in response to SiO2 nanoparticles. *Exp Cell Res* 2005, *305* (1), 51-62.

[57]   Nan, A.; Bai, X.; Son, S. J.; Lee, S. B.; Ghandehari, H., Cellular uptake and cytotoxicity of silica nanotubes. *Nano Lett* 2008, *8* (8), 2150-2154.

[58]   Lin, I. C.; Liang, M.; Liu, T.-Y.; Jia, Z.; Monteiro, M. J.; Toth, I., Effect of polymer grafting density on silica nanoparticle toxicity. *Bioorg MedChem* 2012, *20* (23), 6862-6869.

[59]   Cartiera, M. S.; Johnson, K. M.; Rajendran, V.; Caplan, M. J.; Saltzman, W. M., The uptake and intracellular fate of PLGA nanoparticles in epithelial cells. *Biomaterials* 2009, *30* (14), 2790-8.

[60]   Qaddoumi, M. G.; Ueda, H.; Yang, J.; Davda, J.; Labhasetwar, V.; Lee, V. H., The characteristics and mechanisms of uptake of PLGA nanoparticles in rabbit conjunctival epithelial cell layers. *Pharm Res* 2004, *21* (4), 641-8.

[61]   Semete, B.; Booysen, L.; Lemmer, Y.; Kalombo, L.; Katata, L.; Verschoor, J.; Swai, H. S., *In vivo* evaluation of the biodistribution and safety of PLGA nanoparticles as drug delivery systems. *Nanomedicine: Nanotechnology, Biology and Medicine* 2010, *6* (5), 662-671.

[62]   Mura, S.; Hillaireau, H.; Nicolas, J.; Le Droumaguet, B.; Gueutin, C.; Zanna, S.; Tsapis, N.; Fattal, E., Influence of surface charge on the potential toxicity of PLGA nanoparticles towards Calu-3 cells. *IntJ Nanomedicine* 2011, *6*, 2591.

[63]   Basarkar, A.; Devineni, D.; Palaniappan, R.; Singh, J., Preparation, characterization, cytotoxicity and transfection efficiency of poly (DL-lactide-co-glycolide) and poly (DL-

lactic acid) cationic nanoparticles for controlled delivery of plasmid DNA. *Int J Pharm* 2007, *343* (1), 247-254.

[64]   Chang, J.; Jallouli, Y.; Kroubi, M.; Yuan, X.-b.; Feng, W.; Kang, C.-s.; Pu, P.-y.; Betbeder, D., Characterization of endocytosis of transferrin-coated PLGA nanoparticles by the blood-brain barrier. *Int J Pharm* 2009, *379* (2), 285-292.

[65]   Fields, R. J.; Cheng, C. J.; Quijano, E.; Weller, C.; Kristofik, N.; Duong, N.; Hoimes, C.; Egan, M. E.; Saltzman, W. M., Surface modified poly (beta amino ester)-containing nanoparticles for plasmid DNA delivery. *J Control Release* 2012.

[66]   Yildirimer, L.; Thanh, N. T. K.; Loizidou, M.; Seifalian, A. M., Toxicological considerations of clinically applicable nanoparticles. *Nano Today* 2011, *6* (6), 585-607.

[67]   Arvizo, R. R.; Miranda, O. R.; Moyano, D. F.; Walden, C. A.; Giri, K.; Bhattacharya, R.; Robertson, J. D.; Rotello, V. M.; Reid, J. M.; Mukherjee, P., Modulating Pharmacokinetics, Tumor Uptake and Biodistribution by Engineered Nanoparticles. *Plos One* 2011, *6* (9).

[68]   Zhang, X. D.; Wu, H. Y.; Wu, D.; Wang, Y. Y.; Chang, J. H.; Zhai, Z. B.; Meng, A. M.; Liu, P. X.; Zhang, L. A.; Fan, F. Y., Toxicologic effects of gold nanoparticles *in vivo* by different administration routes. *Int J Nanomedicine* 2010, *5*, 771-81.

[69]   Park, E. J.; Bae, E.; Yi, J.; Kim, Y.; Choi, K.; Lee, S. H.; Yoon, J.; Lee, B. C.; Park, K., Repeated-dose toxicity and inflammatory responses in mice by oral administration of silver nanoparticles. *Environ Toxicol Phar* 2010, *30* (2), 162-168.

[70]   Semmler-Behnke, M.; Kreyling, W.; Lipka, J.; Fertsch, S.; Wenk, A.; Takenaka, S.; Schmid, G. n.; Brandau, W., Biodistribution of 1.4- and 18-nm gold particles in rats. *Small* 2008, *4* (12), 2108-2111.

[71]   Cho WS, Cho M, Jeong J, *et al.* Acute toxicity and pharmacokinetics of 13 nm-sized PEG-coated gold nanoparticles. *ToxicolApplPharmacol* 2009; 236(1): 16-24.

[72]   Su Y, Peng F, Ji X, *et al.* Silicon nanowire-based therapeutic agents for *in vivo* tumor near-infrared photothermal ablation. *J MaterChemB* 2014; 2(19): 2892.

[73]   Simpson, C. A.; Salleng, K. J.; Cliffel, D. E.; Feldheim, D. L., *In vivo* toxicity, biodistribution, and clearance of glutathione-coated gold nanoparticles. *Nanomedicine* 2013, *9* (2), 257-63.

[74]   De Jong, W.; Hagens, W.; Krystek, P.; Burger, M.; Sips, A. n.; Geertsma, R., Particle size-dependent organ distribution of gold nanoparticles after intravenous administration. *Biomaterials* 2008, *29* (12), 1912-1919.

[75]   Zhai, W.; He, C.; Wu, L.; Zhou, Y.; Chen, H.; Chang, J.; Zhang, H., Degradation of hollow mesoporous silica nanoparticles in human umbilical vein endothelial cells. *Journal of Biomedical Materials Research Part B-Applied Biomaterials* 2012, *100B* (5), 1397-1403.

[76]   Souris, J. S.; Lee, C.-H.; Cheng, S.-H.; Chen, C.-T.; Yang, C.-S.; Ho, J.-a. A.; Mou, C.-Y.; Lo, L.-W., Surface charge-mediated rapid hepatobiliary excretion of mesoporous silica nanoparticles. *Biomaterials* 2010, *31* (21), 5564-5574.

[77]   Yu, T.; Greish, K.; McGill, L. D.; Ray, A.; Ghandehari, H., Influence of Geometry, Porosity, and Surface Characteristics of Silica Nanoparticles on Acute Toxicity: Their Vasculature Effect and Tolerance Threshold. *ACS Nano* 2012, *6* (3), 2289-2301.

[78]   Yamashita, K.; Yoshioka, Y.; Higashisaka, K.; Mimura, K.; Morishita, Y.; Nozaki, M.; Yoshida, T.; Ogura, T.; Nabeshi, H.; Nagano, K.; Abe, Y.; Kamada, H.; Monobe, Y.; Imazawa, T.; Aoshima, H.; Shishido, K.; Kawai, Y.; Mayumi, T.; Tsunoda, S.-i.; Itoh, N.; Yoshikawa, T.; Yanagihara, I.; Saito, S.; Tsutsumi, Y., Silica and titanium dioxide

nanoparticles cause pregnancy complications in mice. *Nat Nanotechnol* 2011, *6* (5), 321-328.

[79]   Saadati, R.; Dadashzadeh, S.; Abbasian, Z.; Soleimanjahi, H., Accelerated Blood Clearance of PEGylated PLGA Nanoparticles Following Repeated Injections: Effects of Polymer Dose, PEG Coating, and Encapsulated Anticancer Drug. *Pharma Res* 2013, 1-11.

[80]   Kumari, A.; Yadav, S. K.; Yadav, S. C., Biodegradable polymeric nanoparticles based drug delivery systems. *Colloids and Surfaces B: Biointerfaces* 2009, *75* (1), 1-18.

[81]   Pernodet, N.; Fang, X.; Sun, Y.; Bakhtina, A.; Ramakrishnan, A.; Sokolov, J.; Ulman, A.; Rafailovich, M., Adverse effects of citrate/gold nanoparticles on human dermal fibroblasts. *Small* 2006, *2* (6), 766-73.

[82]   Salem, A. K.; Searson, P. C.; Leong, K. W., Multifunctional nanorods for gene delivery. *Nat Mater* 2003, *2* (10), 668-71.

[83]   Niidome, T.; Yamagata, M.; Okamoto, Y.; Akiyama, Y.; Takahashi, H.; Kawano, T.; Katayama, Y.; Niidome, Y., PEG-modified gold nanorods with a stealth character for *in vivo* applications. *J ControlRelease* 2006, *114* (3), 343-7.

[84]   Takahashi, H.; Niidome, Y.; Niidome, T.; Kaneko, K.; Kawasaki, H.; Yamada, S., Modification of gold nanorods using phosphatidylcholine to reduce cytotoxicity. *Langmuir* 2006, *22* (1), 2-5.

CHAPTER 11

Silica-Based Scaffolds: Fabrication, Synthesis and Properties

Juanrong Chen[1,3], Long Fang[2], Ying Zhang[2], Huijun Zhu[3] and Shunsheng Cao[*,2,3]

[1]*School of Environment and Safety Engineering, Jiangsu University, Xuefu Road 301, Zhenjiang, 212013, P.R. China;* [2]*School of Materials Science and Engineering, Jiangsu University, Xuefu Road 301, Zhenjiang, 212013, P.R. China; and* [3]*Cranfield Health, Vincent Building, Cranfield University, Cranfield, Bedfordshire, MK43 0AL, UK*

Abstract: Considerable endeavors have been devoted to the synthesis of biocompatible scaffolds with tunable new structures and improved bioactivities. Within the field of bioceramics, silica-based ordered porous materials are receiving increasing attention by the biomaterials scientific community because silica is the main constituent of many biocompatible porous scaffold materials. In addition, dietary silicon plays an important role in bone formation and is markedly present in active calcification sites, stimulating the expression of genes involved in bone and cartilage formation and concurrently, inducing osteogenic differentiation and cell mineralization. More importantly, silica-based scaffolds hold their capability to host different guest molecules, representing a new generation of structurally unique materials. This chapter collects and discusses the current advances in silica-based scaffolds. The synthetic methods of tailoring scaffolding chemical composition and architecture are highlighted.

Keywords: Biomaterials, scaffold, silica materials, tissue engineering.

INTRODUCTION

Tissue engineering is an interdisciplinary field describing a set of tools at the interface of the biomedical and engineering sciences that apply the principles of engineering and life sciences to aid tissue formation or regeneration and thereby produce therapeutic or diagnostic benefits [1-3]. Among the different methods integrated in the tissue engineering, one of the most employed techniques aimed at the construction of new tissue involves the initiation of the regeneration process *in vitro* by soaking the scaffold in a suitable cell culture and in the presence of tissue-inducting substances such as certain peptides, hormones or growth factors,

*Corresponding Author Shunsheng Cao: School of Materials Science and Engineering, Jiangsu University, Xuefu Road 301, Zhenjiang, 212013, P.R. China; Tel: +86(0)-511-88790181; Fax: +86(0)-511-88790181; E-mail: sscaochem@hotmail.com

(*e.g.*, bone morphogenetic protein), and then, the scaffold is implanted in the patient [4]. Another method could be used to chemically graft the tissue-inducting substances, *i.e.* peptides, hormones and growth factors, alone or in combination into the three-dimensional (3D) scaffold to be directly implanted in the patient [4, 5]. Generally, for any type of tissue, a scaffold should have the following characteristics [1, 6-11].

- A three-dimensional interconnected porous hierarchical architecture that should be open and interconnected to allow cell growth, migration, and nutrient flow.

- A bio-acceptable surface chemistry and topography that facilitates the ingrowth of cells and vascular tissue.

- Designed substances whose tunable release may aid the integration of the scaffolds without any adverse reactions.

- Good biocompatibility and biorestorability.

- Sufficient and appropriate mechanical properties that maintain the three-dimensional architecture in order to facilitate, replace or match those of the tissue during the reconstruction process. These scaffolds should be consistent enough to allow their manipulation during the cell seeding or surgical implantation procedures and even to be adapted *in situ* to fit odd shaped defects.

- Full reproducibility under large-scale manufacturing conditions.

Besides, developing highly reactive materials is very important in tissue engineering because the faster the osteointegration process, the quicker the patient will recover and the smaller is the risk of fibrous capsule formation with the subsequent implant failure [12]. Especially, each type of tissue demands unique features depending on its functions, components, cell populations, *etc.* [13]. For example, bone and dental substitution materials should encompass many different characteristics for consideration in clinical use. Not only should the material be porous hierarchical architecture to serve as a scaffold for capillary growth, the material should have good biocompatibility, osteoconductivity, and a complete lack of antigenicity [14, 15]. Therefore, the selection of the biomaterial component and surface properties is a critical step that defines the functionality and, ultimately, the success of all tissue engineering ventures. Clearly, biomaterials which most closely mimic natural bone structure or offer specific and suitable surface chemistry functions and topography are most promising for bone replacement/repair applications [13]. In the last decade, tissue engineering has developed as a discipline of increasing importance in the world as a result of an aging population and a related increase in diseases. In that context, a wide range of substitute materials including organic polymers [16], hydroxyapatite-based ceramics [17] and bioactive glasses [18], have been developed for repair and preservation of tissue function a recent review of inorganic materials used in this way see the article by Bruce *et al.* [19] Silicon has been proven to be a very important trace element in bone and connective tissue formation and can effectively stimulate biological activity by improving the solubility of the material, offering a more electronegative surface and creating a finer microstructure resulting in transformation of the material surface to a biologically equivalent apatite [14, 20]. Since the development of silica-based mesoporous material [21], its study has been one of the most energetic research areas in tissue engineering. This chapter collects and discusses the main advances occurred during the last decade, regarding silica-based scaffolds intended for tissue engineering. Furthermore, the synthetic strategies to prepare biofunctionalized scaffolds, for bone grafting and tissue engineering, are also described with many details.

SILICA-BASED MATERIALS

Polymeric Hydrogels

Hydrogels are highly biocompatible three-dimensional (3D) networks of cross-linked polymers [22]. They have received growing interest as ideal vehicles for cell encapsulation and biomolecular delivery [23]. Moreover, hydrogels have proven to be very effective for tissue regeneration because of their high water content, physical properties that mimic native extracellular matrices (ECMs), and their ability to facilitate mass transfer [23-25]. Although these polymeric hydrogels offer some chemical and biological features that mimic biological tissue, gel are facing challenges in providing synthetic connective tissues that serve a predominantly biomechanical role in the body, such as articular cartilage, semilunar cartilage, tendons, and ligaments [26-30]. However, in order to substitute the natural tissues with hydrogels, a lot of significant engineering questions should be addressed, such as the provision of low surface friction and wear, a suitable elastic modulus, and high mechanical strength, both *in vivo* and *in vitro*, limiting their further application as ideal scaffolds [30]. During past decade, considerable efforts have been made to enhance the mechanical strength of hydrogels [24, 30, 31]. Gong *et al.* [30] introduced a general method of preparing very strong hydrogels by inducing a double-network structure consisting of a tightly-crosslinked first network and asparsely-crosslinked second network for various combinations of hydrophilic polymers. Kaneko *et al.* [32] reported on a novel method to obtain hydrogels with extremely high mechanical toughness. Besides, using nanoparticles is an effective method to improve the properties of hydrogels [23]. The nanoparticles can either be used as a cross-linker or as filler entrapped within the hydrogel network [33]. For instance, silica nanoparticles have been used as nanoscale cross-linkers to prepare gels, which not only provide the final hydrogel products with high mechanical performance, but also promote cell adhesion [23, 34-36]. Besides, nanocomposite approaches have shown potential in overcoming the limitations of hydrogel networks because polymer nanocomposites offer several novel property combinations such as high toughness, elastomeric properties, gas barrier, and control release due to the molecular interaction of fillers with polymers at the nano scale beyond macro- and micro-composites [37-40] silicate nanoplatelets can be used as physical cross-linkers to form hydrogel networks [34, 35, 41].

Mesoporous Materials

The fabrication of three-dimensional (3-D) macroporous scaffolds for bone tissue engineering is receiving great attention by the biomedical scientific community [2, 3]. Synthetic scaffolds to regenerate functional tissues must satisfy requirements similar to those that nature has fabricated to build and regenerate natural hard tissues, providing specific environments and interconnected porous architectures to facilitate cellular attachment, growth and differentiation [42].

Therefore, considerable endeavor has being devoted to the development of such functional scaffolds with pores similar in size and number to those in natural bone [43]. The necessary range of porosity is from 1 μm to several hundreds of microns.

Mesoporous silica (MPS) is one of the important members of nanomaterials in biomedical fields, also is a special class of synthetically modified colloidal silica, in which highly ordered pores in the meso-scale (2-50 nm) are introduced [44]. Since Beck *et al.* [21, 45] first developed the silica-based MCM-41 molecular sieve in 1991, highly ordered mesoporous silica materials are receiving increasing interest by the biomaterials scientific community due to their capability to host different guest molecules. Flexible shell, high mechanical stability, high surface area, pore volume, and pore size, with narrow pore diameter distribution as well as low cost production of silica microspheres are important in a variety of applications [46, 47]. Due to their unique textural features of surface and porosity, ordered mesoporous silica materials have proved to be excellent candidates for tissue regeneration [48, 49]. When silica-based ordered mesoporous materials are used as drug delivery systems, a host-guest interaction occurs between the silanol groups covering the surface of the mesoporous channels and the functional groups of the drug [4]. The parameters that conducted drug adsorption and release processes mainly depend on the textural and structural features of the host-matrix, enabling adaptation of their properties to specific clinical needs [4]. For example, these materials can bond to living bone when implanted through the formation of a nonstoichiometric carbonated hydroxyapatite of nanometrical size (CHA) [50]. This bioactiVe bond makes sure the implant osteo-integration, and its degradation products increase the bone tissue regeneration. Moreover, these materials can be loaded with osteogenic agents acting as signals to attract bone-forming cells to the site of injury and can also be used as scaffolds for bone tissue engineering [2, 51, 52]. However, pure porous silica (PS) scaffolds generally have too slow *in vitro* mineralization to be considered as bioactive bone graft materials and their cytocompatibility is far from optimal [51, 53]. Although PS scaffolds have been widely used as a drug delivery support, it remains unclear whether the delivery of drug from PS scaffolds will have a positive effect on the proliferation and differentiation of bone forming cells. Consequently, it is of interest to modify and functionalize porous scaffolds materials not only at the outer surface but also inside the porous structure [54, 55]. For example, Durrieu *et al.* [56] modified hydroxyapatite with oligopeptides to improve the interactions with several plasma and extracellular matrix proteins. Wang *et al.* [57] investigated the biomineralization properties and drug release properties of a mesoporous silica-hydroxyapatite composite material which was used as drug vehicle and filler for polymer matrices. However, development of MPS nanoparticles for biomedical applications requires close attention to safety issues, because extremely high surface area of MPS could exert different effects on human health and environment [44]. Previous reports concerning biocompatibility of MPS investigated the general conditions of nanomaterials, such as size, surface charge, and morphology and have shown that the surface area of nanomaterials may also greatly affect on biocompatibility due to high reactivity [58-61]. Recently, Kim and Yun [44] investigated in more detail the effect of MPS nanoparticles on the cytotoxicity and the relationship between pore structural properties (surface area) and the biological response, as compared with colloidal silica nanoparticles in macrophages. They found that the characteristics of pore structure of silica nanoparticles were close related with their biocompatibility and thus should be carefully designed and controlled for use in biomedical applications.

Smart Materials

Modern nanomedicine is devoted to present new strategies by combining robust materials with functional properties (*e.g.* thermal, electric, magnetic, superconducting, optical and biological properties), driving a striking development of a wide range of multi-functional materials. These materials could further have one or more properties that can be significantly changed in a tunable way by external stimuli, such as stress, temperature, pH, electric or magnetic fields, offering improved performance for *in vivo* applications [12, 62]. Spadaro JA [63] explored the electrical-sensitive materials due to the presence of electrical potentials in mechanically loaded bones. Nakamura *et al.* [64] introduced two new and important items of information on polarized HA surface characteristics and cell behavior on polarized HA and found that a residual permanent charge on the material surface, positive or negative, as well as a direct electrical stimulation can promote the attraction of charged ions from the environment to the cells, although the electrical polarization had no effect on the surface roughness, crystallinity, and constituent elements according to contact-angle measurements. Obviously, this would modify their protein adsorption with the subsequent influence on the cells metabolic activity. Therefore, the use of electrical stimulation after biomaterial implantation to favor cell adhesion and differentiation and thus induce bone healing seems a smart approach to speed up the osteointegration process [12].

As one of the natural organic-inorganic composite materials, silica finds its way to develop smart structures and materials because it exhibits an excellent combination of elastic modulus, strength, and toughness, offering a prime microstructural design model for the construction of new materials [65, 66]. In addition, silica has a high surface area and smooth nonporous surface, which could promote strong physical contacts between the filler and the polymer matrix [67-69]. More importantly, the presence of silanol and siloxane groups on the silica surface results in the hydrophilic nature of the particles, increasing strong physical contacts and a stress transfer interface between the filler and hydrophilic polymer matrix without aggregation or sedimentation [67, 70].

SCAFFOLD FABRICATION TECHNIQUES

An intensive research endeavor is aimed at increasing the behavior of implantable materials through better understanding and application of surface modifications (*e.g.*, chemistry, hydrophobicity, roughness, eluting coatings) to enhance integration as well as resistance to infections [71]. Most established strategies of surface coating implant materials include surface roughening techniques, plasma spraying, sputter deposition, electrophoretic deposition, biomimetic precipitation, and sol-gel coating [72-74].

Sol-Gel Processing Method

It has been proved that the sol-gel processing method is becoming an increasingly popular approach for various surface modifications because it offers a simple method to control composition and structure. This technique has exhibited many advantages by increasing the compatibility of inorganic-organic materials without affecting the organic polymer features [75]. The most investigated nanosol systems are silica sols by hydrolyzing metal alkoxides following condensation, a dispersion of nanosized alkoxide particles is formed [6, 76]. During the sol-gel process, sol-gel materials are formed when the solvent is removed from a colloidal suspension of precursors (sol) and the material is allowed to solidify (gel). In the presence of water, the alkoxide groups are hydrolyzed, creating silanol groups and releasing ethanol. Condensation-polymerization between silanol groups then occurs, producing Si-O-Si bonds. Extension of this reaction results in a silica network with pores resulting from the removal of water and ethanol molecules [71]. The potential processing methods are illustrated in Fig. (**1**).

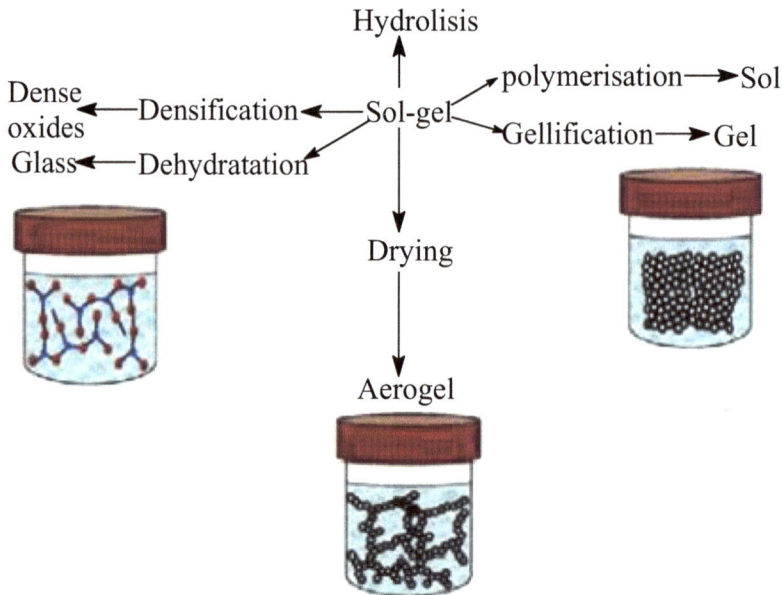

Fig. (1). Sol-gel processing and potential processing methods (Reproduced with permission from Ref [48]).

Silica-based composites represent one such class of hybrid organic/inorganic material with many applications including catalysis, sensors, biomaterials, biotechnology and medicine [77-80]. Conventionally, most such hybrid materials are prepared by a sol-gel process based on template substrate [81]. Ihara *et al.* [82] fabricated novel hybrid polymer hydrogels in a facile manner by simply mixing of a water-soluble copolymer having trimethoxysilyl side chains with silica nanoparticles used as multiple crosslinkers. Up to date, a number of biocompatible components including polyethylene glycol, gelatin, alginate, cellulose, chitosan, and collagen have been reported in combination with silica [6, 37, 83-85]. Snyder *et al.* [71] introduced a novel nebulizer deposition system to generate vaporized sol-gel nanoparticles for the controlled surface modification of biomaterial substrates at ambient temperatures and pressures. Recently, Cai J [83] and co-workers prepared cellulose-silica nanocomposite aerogels with high mechanical strength and flexibility, large surface area, and low thermal conductivity by *in situ* formation of silica in cellulose gel. Yang *et al.* [84] reported a facile technique to develop physically cross-linked hydrogels from silica nanoparticles and poly(acrylic acid), and demonstrated that physical cross-linking between silica nanospheres and polymer resulted in the formation of highly stable networks. Gaharwar *et al.* [37] developed photocrosslinkable PEG (Polyethylene glycol) -silica nanocomposites and evaluated the effect of silica on some physical, chemical, and biological properties of PEG hydrogels, making it more potential to be used in drug delivery and biomaterials engineering applications.

Template-Directed Method

Templating has been explored as a powerful pathway to produce hollow materials, and it has led to great progress in developing hollow spherical and polycrystalline shells, such as inorganic ceramics, organic polymer, inorganic-organic hybrids, as well as hollow non-spherical and single crystalline shells, such as alloy and metal oxide [86-89]. Mesoporous materials represent a new class of structurally unique materials. The synthesis of mesoporous materials, which was introduced for the first time at the beginning of the 1990s [4, 21], is based in the use of surfactants as templates of the mesostructure for the assembly and subsequent condensation of inorganic precursors. After that, template removal leaves a network of cavities within the silica framework that will determine the physico-chemical properties of the resulting materials [4, 86]. This is more clearly illustrated in Fig. (**2**).

Besides the synthesis of mesoporous materials, the design and development of macroporous bioceramics or hierarchically meso-macroporous scaffolds with

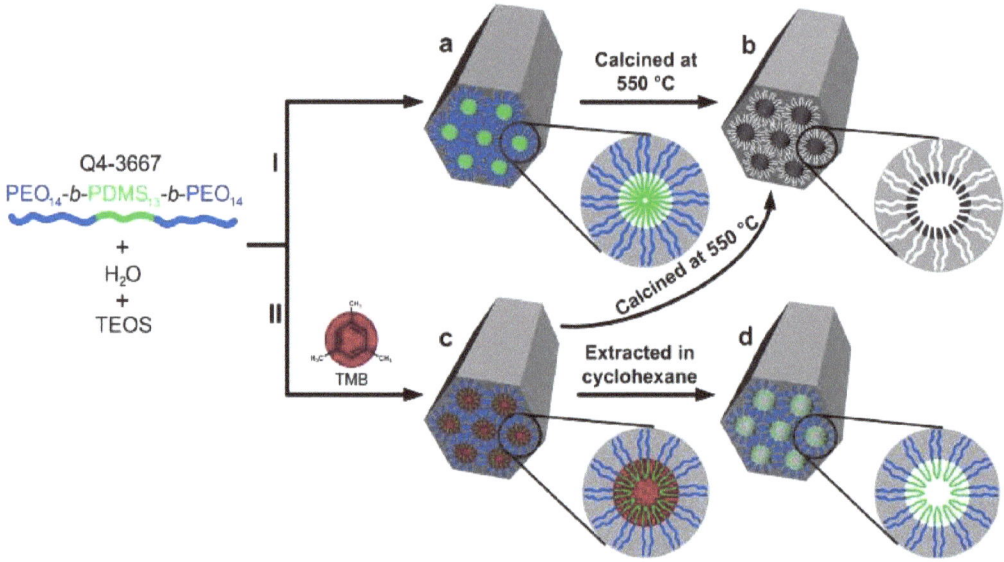

Fig. (2). Schematic illustration of the synthetic routes to the formation of Q4-3667 directed mesostructure (**a**), mesoporous silica with thick wall (**b**), organo-functionalized mesoporous silica with addition of TMB (**c**) and subsequent extraction (**d**). The black part of the cross section view in (**b**) denoted the deoxidized product of the PDMS chains ((Reproduced with permission from Ref. [90]).

additional ordered mesoporosity would represent an improved value in bone tissue engineering applications due to the possibility of incorporating different therapeutic agents into the mesoporous cavities to be subsequently locally released [42, 91-93]. Generally, macroporous bioceramics can be fabricated by techniques such as porogen leaching, hard template conversion, and foaming, and the synthesized macroporous bioactive glasses (BGs) with disordered macropore structures and internal architecture [94, 95]. Yu *et al.* [94] prepared mesoporous bioactive glass materials with tunable macropores in a wide range (0.6-200 µm) by using a nonionic block copolymer surfactant as the mesostructure directing agent, polystyrene colloidal particles or polyester (Terylene) fibers as the macropore templates, and investigated in more detail their bioactivities *in vitro*. Shi *et al.* [96] synthesized hierarchically porous BG (CaO-SiO2-P2O5) scaffolds by using nonionic block copolymer EO20PO70EO20 (P123) and polyurethane (PUF) as cotemplates. It offered a hierarchical structure with interconnected macropores (about 200-400 or 500-700 µm), giving the potential for tissue ingrowth and the neovascularization, and uniform mesopores (3.68 nm), resulting in an increased specific surface area and enhanced bioactivity and release of ionic products. Zhu *et al.* [53] developed hierarchically 3D porous mesoporous bioactive glasses scaffolds with four different chemical compositions by a combination of polyurethane sponge and non-ionic block copolymer EO20PO70EO20 (P123) surfactant as co-templates and evaporation-induced self-assembly process. Garca *et al.* [97] reported a SiO_2-P_2O_5 binary system as good bioceramics that have also shown an ability to load and release antiosteoporotic drugs, exhibiting accelerated bioactive behavior compared to pure silica matrices due to their improved biocompatible response by inducing less cellular damage than pure silica materials. Recently, they further prepared three-dimensional scaffolds in the binary system SiO2-P2O5 with different scales of porosity, making them more suitable for bone tissue engineering applications [42]. The preparation method is shown in Fig. (**3**).

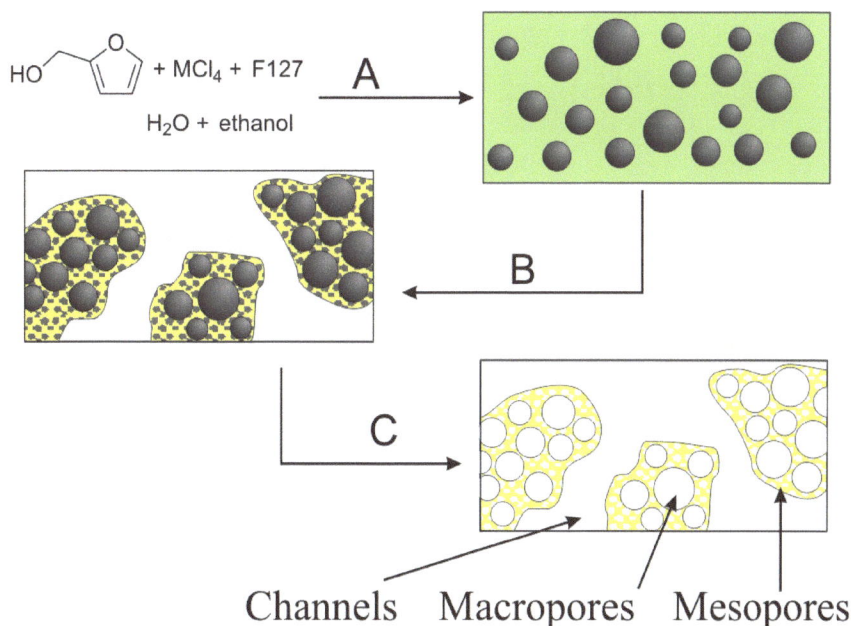

Fig. (3). Synthesis Mechanism of Hierarchically Porous Metal Oxide Monoliths: (**A**) polymerization of FA leads to the formation of PFA nanoparticles (depicted by black spheres) dispersed in an aqueous suspension of metal oxide/Pluronic F127/ethanol (green); (**B**) evaporation of ethanol and water causes the metal oxide sol to condense into a mesostructured network around the PFA particles; solvent channels (white) exist between the mesostructured metal oxide (dotted yellow); (**C**) calcination removes the Pluronic F127 and the PFA to leave a mesoporous and bimodal macroporous framework (Reproduced with permission from [91]).

Electro-Spinning Technique

The template-directed method utilizes specific interactions such as hydrogen bonding and/or electrostatic interactions between the hydrolyzing sol-gel precursor and the substrate to generate the organic and inorganic components [98]. Besides such template transcription, electro-processing (or electrospinning) offers the potential to prepare ceramic and hybrid nanocomposites [98]. A number of electrospun ceramic nano-fibers, including silica (SiO_2) and titanium (TiO_2) nanofibers, have been developed [76, 99]. Silica (SiO_2) is the most convenient and widely used due to its mild reactivity and good chemical properties. Sol-gel-derived bioactive silica glass nanofibers have been recently reported as scaffolding materials for bone-tissue regeneration [77, 100]. Two techniques of developing silica electrospun nanofibers *via* solutions (spin dopes) are frequently used: the first method is the direct spinning of aged (partially reacted) sol-gel precursor solutions or their blends with polymers to generate ceramic or composite nanofibers [101]. In this method, pH and concentrations of the sol-gel constituents are the main factors influencing the gelation and the solution viscosity, the direct method is difficulty controlled. By contrast, the second is more suitable method by using the solutions containing organic polymers, producing nanofibers of controllable size and uniformity [76].

Biomimetic Precipitation

In comparison to electrospinning technique, biomimetic synthesis is usually executed under mild conditions of near-neutral or slightly acidic pH and is rapid, thus giving many advantages to the fabrication and development of silica-based scaffolds [98, 102]. Numerous studies have already provided insight to simpler alternative biomimetic strategies for silica formation, creating the potential for construction of nano-structured composite materials at biocompatible conditions and higher rates [98, 103-106]. The organic matrix silicatein (proteins), silaffin (peptides) and long-chain polyamines in marine organisms play a decisive role in the synthesis and morphology of inorganic materials [107, 108]. In a proposed mechanism, the polyamines catalyze the silica formation because of the alternating presence of protonated and nonprotonated amine groups in the polyamine chains, which allows hydrogen bond formation with the oxygen adjacent to silicon in the precursor and thus facilitate -Si-O-Si- bond formation [109]. The importance of polyamines in silica precipitation has led to the development of various bio-inspired molecules, synthetic proteins, polypeptides, block copolypeptides, and small functional molecules containing polyamines that catalyzes silica [110]. The majority of biomimetic silica formation has been investigated in the presence of a pre-hydrolyzed precursor, usually by acid/base catalysis rather than directly from pure alkoxysilanes [98].

FINAL REMARKS

Although the conventional fabrication methods are widely used to develop silica-based scaffolds such as sol-gel foaming, gel casting, plasma spraying, sputter deposition, electrophoretic deposition, and biomimetic precipitation due to their potential application in tissue engineering, such these technologies will be inevitable suffer some challenges derived from the difficulty in precisely controlling pore size, geometry and spatial distribution, creating internal channels within the scaffold for vascularisation, as well as generating scaffolds within arbitrary and complex 3-D anatomical shapes. This chapter has summarized and discussed the current progress in silica-based scaffolds and highlighted the synthetic methods of tailoring scaffolding chemical composition, and architecture. As evidenced by the described and discussed literature, a better understanding of the construction procedures for silica-based materials has enabled the design and creation of various scaffolds with good biocompatibility and biorestorability. However, the nature of the support synthetic steps should be understood and considered, to make full use of these strategies for the fabrication and application of such silica-based materials. This understanding will drive the processes to continue to evolve and provide more facile preparation approaches.

ACKNOWLEDGEMENTS

The authors would like to thank Jiangsu Natural Science Fund of China (No. BK20141299) and the Research Directorate-General of European Commission for financial support to carry out this work under the framework of Marie Curie Action FP7-People-IIF-2010 (No. 275336).

CONFLICT OF INTEREST

The authors confirm that this chapter contents have no conflict of interest.

ABBREVIATIONS

3-D   =   Three-dimensional

BGs   =   Bioactive glasses

CHA   =   Carbonated hydroxyapatite

ECMs   =   Extracellular matrices

MPS   =   Mesoporous silica

P123   =   EO20PO70EO20

PEG   =   Polyethylene glycol

PS   =   Porous silica

PUF   =   Polyurethane

REFERENCES

[1]   Pena J. Román J. Cabanas, M. V. Vallet-Regí M. An alternative technique to shape scaffolds with hierarchical porosity at physiological temperature. Acta Biomaterialia 2010, 6: 1288-1296.
[2]   Langer R. J. P. Vacanti, Tissue engineering, *Science*, 1993, 260: 920-926.
[3]   Griffith, L. G. Naughton, G. Tissue engineering--current challenges and expanding opportunities. *Science*, 2002, 295: 1009-1014.
[4]   Vallet-Regi, M. Colilla, M. Gonzalez. B. Medical applications of organic-inorganic hybrid materials within the field of silica-based bioceramics. *Chem. Soc. Rev.*, 2011, 40: 596-607.
[5]   Xia, L. Zeng, D. Sun, X. Xu, Y. Xu, L. Ye, D. Zhang, X. Jiang, X. Zhang. Z. Engineering of bone using rhBMP-2-loaded mesoporous silica bioglass and bone marrow stromal cells for oromaxillofacial bone regeneration. *Micropor. Mesopor. Mater.* 2013, 173:155-165.
[6]   Heinemann, S. Heinemann, Jager, C. M. Neunzehn, J. Wiesmann, H. P. Hanke. T. Effect of Silica and Hydroxyapatite Mineralization on the Mechanical Properties and the Biocompatibility of Nanocomposite Collagen Scaffolds. *ACS Appl. Mater. Interfaces* 2011, 3:4323-4331.
[7]   Chung HJ, Park TG. Surface engineered and drug releasing pre-fabricated scaffolds for tissue engineering. *Adv Drug Deliv Rev* 2007, 59: 249-262.

[8]   Liu C, Xia Z, Czernuszka JT. Design and development of three-dimensional scaffolds for tissue engineering. *Chem Eng Res Des* 2007, 85:1051-1064.

[9]   Vallet-Regi M. Current trends on porous inorganic materials for biomedical applications. *Chem Eng J* 2008, 137:1-3.

[10]   Stevens M, George JH. Exploring and engineering the cell surface interface. *Science* 2005, 310:1135-1138.

[11]   Harley, B. A.; Leung, J. H.; Silva, E. C.; Gibson, L. J. echanical characterization of collagen-glycosaminoglycan scaffolds. *Acta Biomater*. 2007, 3 : 463-474.

[12]   Vila, M. Cicuendez, M. Sanchez-Marcos, Fal-Miyar, J. V. Manzano, M. Prieto, C. Vallet-Regi. M. Electrical stimuli to increase cell proliferation on carbon nanotubes/mesoporous silica composites for drug delivery. *J Biomed Mater Res Part A*: 2013, 101A: 213-221.

[13]   Hertz, A. FitzGerald, V. Pignotti, E. Knowles, J. C. Sen, T. Bruce. I. J. Preparation and characterisation of porous silica and silica/titania monoliths for potential use in bone replacement. *Micropor. Mesopor. Mater,* 2012, 156: 51-61.

[14]   Fielding, G. A. Bandyopadhyay, A. Bose. S. Effects of silica and zinc oxide doping on mechanical and biological properties of 3D printed tricalcium phosphate tissue engineering scaffolds. *Dent. Mater,* 2012, 28:113-122.

[15]   Neamat A, Gawish A, Gamal-Eldeen AM. B-Tricalcium phosphate promotes cell proliferation, osteogenesis and bone regeneration in intrabony defects in dogs. *Arch. Oral Biology* 2009; 54: 1083-1090.

[16]   Cheung, H.Y. Lau, K.T. Lu, T.P. Hui, D. A critical review on polymer-based bio-engineered materials for scaffold development. *Compos. Part B* 2007, 38: 291-300.

[17]   Vallet-Regi, M. JM, G.C. Calcium phosphates as substitution of bone tissues. *Prog. Solid State Chem.* 2004, 32:1-31.

[18]   Jones, J.R. Sehrenfried, L.M. Hench, L.L. Optimising bioactive glass scaffolds for bone tissue engineering. *Biomaterials* 2006, 27: 964-973.

[19]   Hertz, A. Bruce, I.J. Inorganic materials for bone repair or replacement applications. *Nanomedicine* 2007, 2: 899-918.

[20]   Pietak A, Reid J, Stott M, Sayer M. Silicon substitution in the calcium phosphate bioceramics. *Biomaterials* 2007; 28: 4023-4032.

[21]   Kresge, C. T.; Leonowicz, M. E.; Roth, W. J.; Vartuli, J. C.; Beck, J. S. Ordered Mesoporous Molecular Sieves Synthesized by a Liquid-Crystal Template Mechanism. *Nature* 1992, 359: 710–712.

[22]   Van der Manakker, F. Braeckmans, K. Morabit, N. El. De Smedt, S. C. Van Nostrum C. F. Hennink, W. E. Protein-Release Behavior of Self-Assembled PEG-β-Cyclodextrin/PEG-Cholesterol Hydrogels. *Adv. Funct. Mater.*, 2009, 19:2992-3001.

[23]   Yang, S. Wang, J. Tan, H. Zeng, F. Liu. C. Mechanically robust PEGDA-MSNs-OH nanocomposite hydrogel with hierarchical meso-macroporous structure for tissue engineering. *Soft Matter*, 2012, 8: 8981-8989.

[24]   Hoffman, A. S. Hydrogels for biomedical applications. *Adv. Drug Delivery Rev.*, 2002, 54: 3-12.

[25]   Peppas, N. A. Hilt, J. Z. Khademhosseini A. Langer, R. Hydrogels in Biology and Medicine: From Molecular Principles to Bionanotechnology. *Adv. Mater.*, 2006, 18: 1345-1360.

[26]   Lin C. C. Metters, A. T. Hydrogels in controlled release formulations: network design and mathematical modeling. *Adv. Drug Delivery Rev.*, 2006, 58: 1379-1408.

[27] Ong, S. M. Zhang, C. Toh, Y. C. Kim S. H. Foo, H. L. A gel-free 3D microfluidic cell culture system. *Biomaterials*, 2008, 29: 3237-3244.

[28] Williams, C. G. Malik, A. N. Kim, T. K. Manson P. N. Elisseeff, J. H. Variable cytocompatibility of six cell lines with photoinitiators used for polymerizing hydrogels and cell encapsulation. *Biomaterials*, 2005, 26: 1211-1218.

[29] Ding, Y. Hu, Y. Zhang, L. Chen Y. Jiang, X. Synthesis and magnetic properties of biocompatible hybrid hollow spheres. *Biomacromolecules*, 2006, 7: 1766-1772.

[30] Gong, J. P. Katsuyama, Y. Kurokawa T. Osada, Y. Double-Network Hydrogels with Extremely High Mechanical Strength. *Adv. Mater.,* 2003, 15: 1155-1158.

[31] Haraguchi K. Takeshita, T. Nanocomposite Hydrogels: A Unique Organic-Inorganic Network Structure with Extraordinary Mechanical, Optical, and Swelling/De-swelling Properties. *Adv. Mater.,* 2002, 14: 1120-1124.

[32] Daisaku K, Tada T, Gong JP, Osada Y. Mechanically strong hydrogels with an ultra low frication coefficient. *Adv Mater,* 2005, 17: 535-538.

[33] Schexnailder, P. Schmidt, G. Nanocomposite polymer hydrogels. *Colloid Polym. Sci.* 2009, 287 :1-11.

[34] Gaharwar, A. K. Schexnailder, P. Kaul, V. Akkus, O. Zakharov, D. Seifert S. Schmidt, G. Highly Extensible Bio-Nanocomposite Films with Direction-Dependent Properties. *Adv. Funct. Mater.*, 2010, 20: 429-436.

[35] Gaharwar, A. K. Schexnailder, P. Jin, Q. Wu C. J. Schmidt, G. Addition of chitosan to silicate cross-linked PEO for tuning osteoblast cell adhesion and mineralization. *ACS Appl. Mater. Interfaces,* 2010, 2: 3119-3127.

[36] Gaharwar, A. K. Dammu, S. A. Canter, J. M. Wu C. J. Schmidt, G. Highly extensible, tough, and elastomeric nanocomposite hydrogels from poly(ethylene glycol) and hydroxyapatite nanoparticles. *Biomacromolecules*, 2011, 12: 1641-1650.

[37] Gaharwar, A. K. Rivera, C. Wu, C. Chan, B. K. Schmidt. G. Photocrosslinked nanocomposite hydrogels from PEG and silica nanospheres: Structural, mechanical and cell adhesion characteristics. *Mater. Sci. Eng. C* 2013, 33: 1800-1807.

[38] Das, D. Kar, T. Das, P.K. Gel-nanocomposites: materials with promising applications. *Soft Matter* 2012, 8: 2348-2365.

[39] Karen I. Winey, Richard A. Vaia, Polymer Nanocomposites. *MRS Bull.* 2007, 32: 314-322.

[40] Hule, R.A. Pochan, D.J. Polymer Nanocomposites for Biomedical Applications. *MRS Bull.* 2007,32: 354-359.

[41] Gaharwar, A.K. Schexnailder, P.J. Dundigalla, A. White, J.D. Matos-Pérez, C.R. Cloud, Seifert. J.L. Wilker J J. Schmidt G. Highly extensible bio-nanocomposite fibers. *Macromol. Rapid Commun.* 2011, 32: 50-57.

[42] García, A. Izquierdo-Barba, I. Colilla, M. López de Laorden, C. Vallet-Regí. M. Preparation of 3-D scaffolds in the SiO2-P2O5 system with tailored hierarchical meso-macroporosity. *Acta Biomaterialia* 2011,7: 1265-1273

[43] Hollister SJ. Porous scaffold design for tissue engineering. *Nat Mater* 2005; 4: 518-24.

[44] Lee, S. Yun, H. Kim. S. The comparative effects of mesoporous silica nanoparticles and colloidal silica on inflammation and apoptosis. *Biomaterials* 2011, 32: 9434-9443.

[45] Beck, J. S.; Vartulli, J. C.; Roth, W. J.; Leonowicz, M. E.; Kresge, C. T.; Schmitt, K. D.; Chu, C. T. W.; Olson, D. H.; Sheppard, E. W.; McCullen, S. B.; Higgings, J. B.; Schlenker, J. L. A new family of mesoporous molecular sieves prepared with liquid crystal templates. *J. Am. Chem. Soc.*1992, 114: 10834-10843.

[46]   Cao, S. Fang, L. Zhao, Z. Ge, Y. Piletsky, S. Turner. A. P. F. Hierachically Structured Hollow Silica Spheres for High Efficiency Immobilization of Enzymes. *Adv. Funct. Mater*, 2013, 23:2162-2167.

[47]   Cao, S. Zhao, Z. Jin, X. Sheng, W. Li, S. Ge, Y. Dong, M. Fang. L. Unique double-shelled hollow silica microspheres: template-guided self-assembly, tunable pore size, high thermal stability, and their application in removal of neutral red. *J. Mater. Chem.* 2011, 21: 19124-19131.

[48]   Arcos, D. Vallet-Regí. M. Sol-gel silica-based biomaterials and bone tissue regeneration. *Acta Biomate*rialia 2010, 6: 2874-2888.

[49]   Sowjanya, J.A. Singh, J. Mohita, T. Sarvanan, S. Moorthi, A. Srinivasan, N. Selvamurugan.N. Biocomposite scaffolds containing chitosan/alginate/nano-silica for bone tissue engineering. Colloid. Surfaces B: 2013, 109: 294- 300.

[50]   Vallet-Regı', M. Ceramics for medical applications. *J. Chem. Soc., Dalton Trans.* 2001, 2: 97-108.

[51]   Wu, C. Fan, W. Chang, J. Xiao. Y. Mussel-inspired porous SiO2 scaffolds with improved mineralization and cytocompatibility for drug delivery and bone tissue engineering. *J. Mater. Chem.,* 2011, 21: 18300-18307.

[52]   Hench, L. L.; Polack, J. M. Third-generation biomedical materials. *Science* 2002, 295: 1014-1017.

[53]   Zhu, Y. Wu, C. Ramaswamy, Y. Kockrick, E. Simon, P. Kaskel S. Zreiqat, H. Preparation, characterization and *in vitro* bioactivity of mesoporous bioactive glasses (MBGs) scaffolds for bone tissue engineering. *Micropor. Mesopor. Mater.*, 2008, 112: 494-503.

[54]   Peter A.L. Jacobsen, Jens Rafaelsen, Jeppe L. Nielsen, Maria V. Juhl, Naseem Theilgaard, Kim L. Larsen. Distribution of grafted b-cyclodextrin in porous particles for bone tissue engineering. *Micropor. Mesopor. Mater.* 2013, 168: 132-141.

[55]   Lan, P.X. Lee, J.W. Seol, Y.J. Cho, D.W. Development of 3D PPF/DEF scaffolds using micro-stereolithography and surface modification. *J. Mater. Sci.: Mater. Med.* 2009,20: 271-279.

[56]   Durrieu, M.C. Pallu, S. Guillemot, F. Bareille, R. Amedee, J. Baquey, C. Labrugere, C. Dard, M. Grafting RGD containing peptides onto hydroxyapatite to promote osteoblastic cells adhesion. *J. Mater. Sci.: Mater. Med.* 2004, 15: 779-786.

[57]   Shi, X. Wang, Y. Ren, L. Zhao, N. Gong, Y. Wang. D. Novel mesoporous silica-based antibiotic releasing scaffold for bone repair. *Acta Biomaterialia* 2009, 5 :1697-1707.

[58]   Chung TH, Wu SH, Yao M, Lu CW, Lin YS, Hung Y, *et al*. The effect of surface charge on the uptake and biological function of mesoporous silica nanoparticles in 3T3-L1 cells and human mesenchymal stem cells. *Biomaterials* 2007; 28:2959-2966.

[59]   Fadeel B, Garcia-Bennett AE. Better safe than sorry: understanding the toxicological properties of inorganic nanoparticles manufactured for biomedical applications. *Adv Drug Deliv Rev* 2010;62: 362-374.

[60]   Lu F, Wu SH, Hung Y, Mou CY. Size effect on cell uptake in well-suspended, uniform mesoporous silica nanoparticles. *Small* 2009; 5:1408-1413.

[61]   Witasp E, Kupferschmidt N, Bengtsson L, Hultenby K, Smedman C, Paulie S, *et al*. Efficient internalization of mesoporous silica particles of different sizes by primary human macrophages without impairment of macrophage clearance of apoptotic or antibody-opsonized target cells. *Toxicol Appl Pharmacol* 2009; 239:306-319.

[62] Mieszawska, A. J. Nadkarni, L. D. Perry, C. C. Kaplan. D. L. Nanoscale Control of Silica Particle Formation *via* Silk-Silica Fusion Proteins for Bone Regeneration. *Chem. Mater.* 2010, 22: 5780-5785.

[63] Spadaro JA. Mechanical and electrical interactions in bone remodeling. *Bioelectromagnetics* 1977; 18:193-899.

[64] Nakamura M, Nagai A, Hentunen T, Salonen J, Sekijima Y, Okura T, Hashimoto K, Toda Y, Monma H, Yamashita K. Surface electric fields increase osteoblast adhesion through improved wettability on hydroxyapatite electret. *Appl Mater Interfac* 2009; 1:2181-2189.

[65] Wang, Q. Hou, R. X. Cheng Y. J. Fu, J. Super tough double network hydrogels reinforced by covalently compositing with silica-nanoparticles, *Soft Matter*, 2012, 8: 6048-6056.

[66] Zou, H. Wu S. S. Shen, J. Polymer/silica nanocomposites: preparation, characterization, properties, and applications. *Chem. Rev.*, 2008:108, 3893-3957.

[67] Yang, J.. Deng, L Han, C. Duan, J. Ma, M. Zhang, X. Xu, F. Sun. R. Synthetic and viscoelastic behaviors of silica nanoparticle reinforced poly(acrylamide) core-shell nanocomposite hydrogels. *Soft Matter*, 2013, 9: 1220-1230.

[68] Norton, J. C. S. Han, M. G. Jiang, P. Shim, G. H. Ying, Y. R. Creager S. Foulger, S. H. Poly(3,4-ethylenedioxythiophene) (PEDOT)-Coated Silica Spheres: Electrochemical Modulation of the Optical Properties of a Hydrogel-Stabilized Core−Shell Particle Suspension. *Chem. Mater.*, 2006, 18:4570-4575.

[69] Yoon, J. Lee K. J. Lahann, J. Multifunctional Polymer Particles with Distinct Compartments. *J. Mater. Chem.*, 2011, 21:8502-8510.

[70] Taylor-Pashow, K. M. L. Rocca, J. D. Huxford R. C. Lin, W. B. Hybrid nanomaterials for biomedical applications. *Chem. Commun.,* 2010, 46: 5832-5849.

[71] Katherine L. Snyder, Hallie R. Holmes, Michael J. VanWagner, Natalie J. Hartman, Rupak M. Rajachar. Development of vapor deposited silica sol-gel particles for use as a bioactive materials system. *J Biomed Mater Res Part A* 2013:101A:1682-1693.

[72] Elias C, Oshida Y, Lima J, Muller C. Relationship between surface properties (roughness, wettability and morphology) of titanium and dental implant removal torque. *J Mech Behav Biomed Mater* 2008;1: 234-242.

[73] Schuler M, Owen G, Hamilton D, de Wild M, Textor M, Brunette D, Tosatti S. Biomimetic modification of titanium dental implant model surfaces using the RGDSP-peptide sequence: A cell morphology study. *Biomaterials* 2006; 27: 4003-4015.

[74] Vasudev D, Ricci J, Sabatino C, Li P, Parsons J. *In vivo* evaluation of a biomimetic apatitie coating grown on titanium surfaces. *J Biomed Mater Res A* 2004; 69: 629-636.

[75] Cho, J. W.; Sul, K. I. Characterization and properties of hybrid composites prepared from poly(vinylidene fluoride-tetrafluoroethylene) and SiO2. *Polymer* 2001, 42: 727-736.

[76] Toskas, G. Cherif, C. Hund, R. Laourine, E. Fahmi, A. Mahltig B.. Inorganic/Organic (SiO2)/PEO Hybrid Electrospun Nanofibers Produced from a Modified Sol and Their Surface Modification Possibilities. *ACS Appl. Mater. Interfaces* 2011, 3: 3673-3681.

[77] Kim, H. W.; Kim, H.-E.; Knowles, J.C. Production and Potential of Bioactive Glass Nanofibers as a Next-Generation Biomaterial. *Adv. Funct. Mater.* 2006, 16: 1529-1535.

[78] Patel AC, Li S, Wang C, Zhang W, Wei Y. Electrospinning of Porous Silica Nanofibers Containing Silver Nanoparticles for Catalytic Applications. *Chem. Mater.*2007;19:1231-1238.

[79]   Patel AC, Li S, Yuan J-M, Wei Y. *In Situ* Encapsulation of Horseradish Peroxidase in Electrospun Porous Silica Fibers for Potential Biosensor Applications. *Nano Lett.* 2006; 6:1042-6.

[80]   Zhang Y, Lim CT, Ramakrishna S, Huang Z-M. *J. Mater. Sci: Mater. Medi.*2005; 16:933-46.

[81]   Douglas AL. Sol-gel processing of hybrid organic-inorganic materials based on polysilsesquioxanes. In: Prof. Dr. Guido K, editor. *Hybrid materials*; 2007. p. 225-254.

[82]   Takafuji, M. Yamada, S.-Y. Ihara, H. Strategy for preparation of hybrid polymer hydrogels using silica nanoparticles as multifunctional crosslinking points. *Chem. Commun.* 2011,47: 1024-1026.

[83]   Cai, J. Liu, S. Feng, J. Kimura, S. Wada, M. Kuga, S. Zhang. L. Cellulose-silica nanocomposite aerogels by *in situ* formation of silica in cellulose gel. *Angew. Chem. Int. Ed.* 2012, 51: 2076-2079.

[84]   Yang, J. Wang, X.-P. Xie, X.-M. *In situ* synthesis of poly(acrylic acid) physical hydrogels from silicananoparticles. *Soft Matter* 2012,8: 1058-1063.

[85]   Desimone, M. F.; Helary, C.; Rietveld, I. B.; Bataille, I.; Mosser, G.; Giraud-Guille, M. M.; Livage, J.; Coradin, T. Silica-collagen bionanocomposites as three-dimensional scaffolds for fibroblast immobilization. *Acta Biomater.* 2010, 6: 3998-4004.

[86]   Cao, S. Chen, J. Hu. J. Yuan. X. The Fabrication and Progress of Hollow Materials. *Polym. Polym. Compos.* 2010,18 : 227-235.

[87]   Kamata K., Lu, Y. Xia Y., Synthesis and Characterization of Monodispersed Core–Shell Spherical Colloids with Movable Cores. *J. Am. Chem. Soc.* 2003, 125: 2384-2385.

[88]   Yang J.H., Qi L.M., Lu C.H., Ma J.M. and Cheng H.M., Morphosynthesis of rhombododecahedral silver cages by self-assembly coupled with precursor crystal templating. *Angew.Chem. Int. Ed.* 2005,44: 598-603.

[89]   Wang W.Z., Poudel B., Wang D.Z, and Ren Z.F., Synthesis of PbTe Nanoboxes Using a Solvothermal Technique. *Adv. Mater.* 2005,17: 2110-2114.

[90]   Ji Feng, Bo Sun, Yuan Yao, Shunai Che. Silicone surfactant templated mesoporous silica. *Micropor. Mesopor. Mater.* 2013,172: 30-35.

[91]   Drisko GL, Zelcer A, Luca V, Caruso RA, Soler-Illia GJAA. One-pot synthesis of hierarchically structured ceramic monoliths with adjustable porosity. *Chem Mater* 2010; 22:4379.

[92]   Mortera R, Onida B, Fiorilli S, Cauda V, Vitale Brovarone C, Baino F, *et al*. Synthesis and characterization of MCM-41 spheres inside bioactive glass- ceramic scaffold. *Chem Eur J* 2008; 137:54-61.

[93]   Cauda V, Fiorilli S, Onida B, Verne E, Vitale Brovarone C, Viterbo D, *et al*. SBA-15 ordered mesoporous silica inside a bioactive glass-ceramic scaffold for local drug delivery. *J Mater Sci: Mater Med* 2008; 19:3303-10.

[94]   Wei, G. Yan, X. Yi, J. Zhao, L. Zhou, L. Wang, Y. Yu. C. Synthesis and in-vitro bioactivity of mesoporous bioactive glasses with tunable macropores. *Micropor. Mesopor. Mater.* 2011, 143: 157-165.

[95]   Jones, J.R. Tsigkou, O. Coates, E.E. Stevens, M.M. Polak, J.M. Hench, L.L. Extracellular matrix formation and mineralization on a phosphate-free porous bioactive glass scaffold using primary human osteoblast (HOB) cells. *Biomaterials* 2007, 28: 1653-1663.

[96] Li, X. Wang, X.P. Chen, H.R. Jiang, P. Dong, X.P. Shi, J.L. Hierarchically Porous Bioactive Glass Scaffolds Synthesized with a PUF and P123 Cotemplated Approach. *Chem. Mater.* 2007 19: 4322-4326.

[97] García A, Colilla M, Izquierdo-Barba I, Vallet-Regí M. Incorporation of phosphorus into mesostructured silicas: a novel approach to reduce the SiO2 leaching in water. *Chem Mater* 2009; 21:4135-415.

[98] Pritesh A. Patel, Jessica Eckart, Maria C. Advincula, A. Jon Goldberg, Patrick T. Mather. Rapid synthesis of polymer-silica hybrid nanofibers by biomimetic mineralization. *Polymer* 2009,50: 1214-1222.

[99] Dai, Y.; Liu, W.; Formo, E.; Sun, Y.; Xia, Y. Ceramic nanofibers fabricated by electrospinning and their applications in catalysis, environmental science, and energy technology. *Polym. Adv. Technol.* 2011, 22: 326-338.

[100] Poologasundarampillai, G.; Ionescu, C.; Tsigkou, O.;Murugesan, M.; Hill, R. G.; Stevens, M. M.; Hanna, J. V.; Smith, M. E.; Jones, J. R. Synthesis of bioactive class II poly(γ-glutamic acid)/silica hybrids for boneregeneration. *J. Mater. Chem.* 2010, 20: 8952-8961.

[101] Larsen G, Velarde-Ortiz R, Minchow K, Barrero A, Loscertales IG. A Method for Making Inorganic and Hybrid (Organic/Inorganic) Fibers and Vesicles with Diameters in the Submicrometer and Micrometer Range *via* Sol–Gel Chemistry and Electrically Forced Liquid Jets. *J. Am. Chem. Soc.* 2003;125:1154-1155.

[102] Zhao, R. Su. B. Self-assembly of phosphorylated poly(ethyleneimine) for use as biomimetic templates in the formation of hybrid hollow silica spheres. *Mater. Lett.* 2012,74: 163-166.

[103] Kjeld JC, Bommel V, Jong HJ, Shinkai S. Poly(L-lysine) Aggregates as Templates for the Formation of Hollow Silica Spheres. *Adv Mater* 2001; 13:1472-1476.

[104] Kröger N, Loren S, Brunner E, Sumper M. Self-assembly of highly phosphorylated silaffins and their function in biosilica morphogenesis. *Science* 2002; 298:584-586.

[105] Sumper M, Lorenz S, Brunner E. Biomimetic control of size in the polyamine-directed formation of silica nanospheres. *Angew Chem Int Ed* 2003; 42:5192-5195.

[106] Tomczak MM, Glawe DD, Drummy LF, Lawrence CG, Stone MO, Perry CC, Pochan DJ, Deming TJ, Naik RR. Polypeptide-Templated Synthesis of Hexagonal Silica Platelets. *J Am Chem Soc* 2005; 127:12577-12582.

[107] Cha JN, Shimizu K, Zhou Y, Christiansen SC, Chmelka BF, Stucky GD, Silicatein filaments and subunits from a marine sponge direct the polymerization of silica and silicones *in vitro*. *Proc. Natl. Acad. Sci. U. S. A*, 1999; 96(2):361-5.

[108] Knecht Marc R, Wright David W. Functional analysis of the biomimetic silica precipitating activity of the R5 peptide from Cylindrotheca fusiformis. *Chem Comm*, 2003; 24: 3038-3039.

[109] Pohnert G. Biomineralization in diatoms mediated through peptide- and polyamine-assisted condensation of silica. *Angew Chem Int Ed* 2002; 41:3167-3169.

[110] Lo´pez-Noriega, A. Arcos, D. Izquierdo-Barba, I. Sakamoto, Y. Terasaki, O. Vallet-Regi. M. Ordered Mesoporous Bioactive Glasses for Bone Tissue Regeneration. *Chem. Mater.* 2006, 18: 3137-3144.

INDEX

A

Acid, glycolic 6, 24, 32, 164, 222

Active pharmaceutical ingredients (API) 232, 233

Adhesion, focal 15, 18-20, 80, 81

Adipose progenitor cells (APCs) 23

A-hydroxy acids 6, 7, 9, 12

Air jet spinning (AJS) 40, 58

Aliphatic polyesters 133, 161, 162

Alizarin Red S (ARS) 261

Alkaline Phosphatase (ALP) 18, 38, 40, 58, 80, 81, 134, 144

Alumina 102, 120

Amorphous 289, 290

Amorphous calcium phosphate (ACP) 102, 103, 108, 120

Angiogenesis 45, 56, 199, 204, 205, 213

Antifouling surfaces 70, 86

Apoptosis 288, 292

Applications

   cardiovascular 91, 175, 176

   engineering 32, 34, 39, 82, 112, 134, 140, 155, 198, 312, 314

   nanomaterial 220

Architecture, nanofibrous 7, 16-18

Artificial implants 101, 116

Atrial natriuretic peptide (ANP) 56, 58

B

Bacterial cells 93, 114

Bioactive glass 103, 106, 109, 111, 112, 114, 119, 120, 148, 306

Bioactive glass (BG) 103, 105, 106, 109, 111-14, 119, 120, 135, 148, 306, 313, 314

Bioactive glasses (BGs) 105, 148, 306, 313, 314

Bioactivity 102, 103, 105, 109, 111, 113, 114, 119, 163, 205, 207, 226, 313

F

G

Gelatin molecules 13
Gelatin solution 13, 14, 202
Gelatin substrates 18, 19
Gelatin type 163, 201-3
Genipin 201-4, 206-9, 213
Glutaraldehyde 47, 48, 52, 53, 201, 203
GNPs 275, 278, 279, 281, 282, 284-87, 291-93, 296
    biodistribution of 292
    cytotoxicity of 285, 286
    rod-shaped 287
    spherical-shaped 287
Gold nanoparticles 227, 229, 274
Gold nanorods 285, 287
Grain boundaries 79, 107
Groups, silanol 280, 308, 311
Growth factor release 198
Growth factors 23, 32, 33, 52, 111, 113, 116, 129, 132, 136, 148, 198, 199, 202,
    204-6, 230, 242, 304, 305

H

Hank's balanced salt solution (HBSS) 207, 208, 214
Hard tissue repair applications 109, 119
HeLa cells 84, 90, 285-87
HMSCs 15, 16, 33, 207, 212-14
Human bone marrow osteoblast cells 83
Human dental pulp cells (HDPC) 134, 135
Human umbilical vein endothelial cells (HUVECs) 279, 282, 288-90
Hyaluronic acid 33, 53, 54, 136, 201, 226
Hybrid mats 245, 253, 254, 256-58
Hydrogel networks 9, 307
Hydrogels 9, 20, 22, 36, 50, 54, 144, 156, 226, 306, 307

L

M

T

U

www.ingramcontent.com/pod-product-compliance
Lightning Source LLC
Chambersburg PA
CBHW050805220326
41598CB00006B/123